Lecture Notes in Computer Science   8641

Commenced Publication in 1973
Founding and Former Series Editors:
Gerhard Goos, Juris Hartmanis, and Jan van Leeuwen

T0212690

Yongjie Jessica Zhang
João Manuel R.S. Tavares (Eds.)

Computational Modeling of Objects Presented in Images

Fundamentals, Methods, and Applications

4th International Conference, CompIMAGE 2014
Pittsburgh, PA, USA, September 3-5, 2014
Proceedings

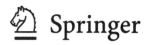 Springer

Volume Editors

Yongjie Jessica Zhang
Carnegie Mellon University
Department of Mechanical Engineering
5000 Forbes Avenue, Pittsburgh, PA 5213, USA
E-mail: jessicaz@andrew.cmu.edu

João Manuel R.S. Tavares
Universidade do Porto, Faculdade de Engenharia
Departamento de Engenharia Mecânica
Rua Dr. Roberto Frias, s/n, 4200-465 Porto, Portugal
E-mail: tavares@fe.up.pt

ISSN 0302-9743   e-ISSN 1611-3349
ISBN 978-3-319-09993-4   e-ISBN 978-3-319-09994-1
DOI 10.1007/978-3-319-09994-1
Springer Cham Heidelberg New York Dordrecht London

Library of Congress Control Number: 2014945253

LNCS Sublibrary: SL 6 – Image Processing, Computer Vision, Pattern Recognition, and Graphics

Typesetting: Camera-ready by author, data conversion by Scientific Publishing Services, Chennai, India

Printed on acid-free paper

Springer is part of Springer Science+Business Media (www.springer.com)

Preface

The 4th CompIMAGE conference (http://jessicaz.me.cmu.edu/CompImage 2014/) aimed to bring together researchers in the area of computational modeling of objects represented in images. Different approaches, such as level set methods, deformable models, optimization, geometric modeling, principal component analysis, stochastic methods, machine learning and fuzzy logic, among others, were discussed by experts to address problems from different applications, including medicine, biomechanics, biometrics, material science, robotics, surveillance, and defense. The CompImage 2014 conference was held in Pittsburgh, USA, during September 3–5, 2014. The previous CompIMAGE conferences were held in Rome, Italy (2012), Buffalo, USA (2010), and Coimbra, Portugal (2006).

There were 54 papers submitted to CompIMAGE 2014, and each paper was carefully reviewed by several Program Committee members and/or external reviewers. Papers were individually reviewed and subsequently opened for discussion by their reviewers to encourage debate and finding a consensus among reviewers. Eventually, 29 full papers were accepted. In addition, we solicited and accepted ten short or position papers. The proceedings are published by Springer in *Lecture Notes in Computer Science* and the authors of the best ranked papers were invited to submit extended versions to the journal *Computer Methods in Biomechanics and Biomedical Engineering: Imaging & Visualization*. The conference also featured six invited talks by Profs. Michael Sacks from The University of Texas at Austin, Jelena Kovačević from Carnegie Mellon University, Andrew D. McCulloch and Jiun-Shyan (JS) Chen from the University of California San Diego, Ross Whitaker from the University of Utah, and Marc Thiriet from the Université Pierre et Marie Curie.

We would like to thank the authors and participants at the conference, the international Program Committee members, and the external reviewers, all of whom made their best effort to ensure the high quality of the CompIMAGE 2014 technical program. We further thank Christine Lambrou, Keri Baker, and Mike Scampone from the Department of Mechanical Engineering, Carnegie Mellon University, for their very hard effort in organizing and handling all the events at CompIMAGE 2014.

July 2014

Yongjie Jessica Zhang
João Manuel R.S. Tavares

Organization

General Co-chairs

Jessica Zhang   Carnegie Mellon University, USA
Joao Manuel R.S. Tavares   Universidade do Porto, Portugal

Steering Committee

João Manuel R.S. Tavares   Universidade do Porto, Portugal
Renato M. Natal Jorge   Universidade do Porto, Portugal
Daniela Iacoviello   Università degli Studi di Roma "La Sapienza", Italy

Scientific Committee

Lyuba Alboul   Sheffield Hallam University, UK
Enrique Alegre   Universidad de Leon, Spain
Michel Audette   Old Dominion University, USA
Jorge M.G. Barbosa   Universidade do Porto, Portugal
Reneta Barneva   State University of New York, USA
George Bebis   University of Nevada, USA
Manuele Bicego   University of Verona, Italy
Elisabetta Binaghi   Università dell'Insubria Varese, Italy
Nguyen D. Binh   Hue University, Vietnam
John C. Brigham   University of Pittsburgh, USA
Valentin Brimkov   Buffalo State College, USA
Begoña Calvo Calzada   Universidad de Zaragoza, Spain
M. Emre Celebi   Louisiana State University in Shreveport, USA
Andrey Chernikov   Old Dominion University, USA
Gary Christensen   University of Iowa, USA
Michela Cigola   University of Cassino, Italy
Stefania Colonnese   Sapienza University of Rome, Italy
Miguel V. Correia   Universidade do Porto, Portugal
Alexandre Cunha   California Institute of Technology, Pasadena (CA), USA
Jorge Dias   Universidade de Coimbra, Portugal
Alexandre X. Falcão   Universidade Estadual de Campinas, Brazil
Yusheng Feng   The University of Texas at San Antonio, USA
José A.M. Ferreira   Universidade de Coimbra, Portugal
Ender Finol   The University of Texas at San Antonio, USA
Alejandro Frangi   The University of Sheffield, UK
Sidharta Gautama   Ghent University, Belgium

Supporting Organizations

Keynote Talks

On Development of an Anatomical, Structural, and Mechanical Integrated Model of the Mitral Valve

Michael Sacks

Professor of Biomedical Engineering
W.A. "Tex" Moncrief, Jr. Simulation-Based Engineering Science Chair I
Director of the ICES Center for Cardiovascular Simulation-based Engineering
Institute for Computational Engineering and Sciences
The University of Texas at Austin, USA

Abstract. The mitral valve (MV) is one of the four heart valves which locates in between the left atrium and left ventricle and regulates the unidirectional blood flow and normal functioning of the heart during cardiac cycles. Alternation of any component of the MV apparatus will typically lead to abnormal MV function. Currently 40,000 patients in the United States receive MV repair or replacement annually according to the American Heart Association. Clinically, this can be achieved iteratively by surgical repair that reinstate normal annular geometry (size and shape) and restore mobile leaflet tissue, resulting in reduced annular and chordae force distribution. High-fidelity computer simulations provide a means to connect the cellular function with the organ-level MV tissue mechanical responses, and to help the design of optimal MV repair strategy. As in many physiological systems, one can approach heart valve biomechanics from using multiscale modeling (MSM) methodologies, since mechanical stimuli occur and have biological impact at the organ, tissue, and cellular levels. Yet, MSM approaches of heart valves are scarce, largely due to the major difficulties in adapting conventional methods to the areas where we simply do not have requisite data. There also re-mains both theoretical and computational challenges to applying traditional MSM techniques to heart valves. Moreover, existing physiologically realistic computational models of heart valve function make many assumptions, such as a simplified micro-structural and anatomical representation of the MV apparatus, and thorough validations with in-vitro or in-vivo data are still limited. We present the details of the state-of-the-art of mitral valve modeling techniques, with an emphasis on what is known and investigated at various length scales.

Short Bio: Professor Michael Sacks is the W.A. "Tex" Moncrief, Jr. Simulation-Based Engineering Science Chair and a world authority on cardiovascular biomechanics. His research focuses on the quantification and modeling of the structure-mechanical properties of native and engineered cardiovascular soft tissues. He is a leading authority on the mechanical behavior and function of the native and engineered heart valves. He is also active in the biomechanics of engineered tissues, and in understanding the in-vitro and in-vivo remodeling processes from a functional biomechanical perspective.

His research includes multi-scale studies of cell/tissue/organ mechanical interactions in heart valves and is particularly interested in determining the local stress environment for heart valve interstitial cells. Recent research has included developing novel constitutive models of right ventricular myocardium that allow for the individual contributions of the myocyte and connective tissue networks.

Selected Recognitions:

Fellow, American Society of Mechanical Engineers

Fellow (Inaugural), Biomedical Engineering Society

Fellow, American Institute for Medical and Biological Engineering

Van C. Mow Medal, American Society for Mechanical Engineers Bioengineering Division

Chancellor's Distinguished Research Award, University of Pittsburgh

Ph.D., Biomedical Engineering, University of Texas Southwestern Medical Center at Dallas

M.S., Engineering Mechanics, Michigan State University

B.S. Engineering Mechanics, Michigan State University

Image Based Modeling of Biomaterials Based on Galerkin and Collocation Meshfree Method

Jiun-Shyan (JS) Chen

William Prager Chair Professor
Structure Engineering
University of California San Diego, USA

Abstract. This work introduces meshfree method for image based modeling of biomaterials. The proposed approach allows a direct construction of simulation model based on pixel data obtained the MRI images. The pixel points serve for dual purposes in the meshfree modeling: they are used to define the geometry of the subject and are employed as the discrete points to obtain approximate solution of the governing partial differential equations. The material properties and the fiber orientation information in the DTI data are stored at each pixel point, and the displacements, stresses and strains are solved at each pixel point as well. The meshfree approximation with smooth kernel allows a representation of material heterogeneity with smooth transition across the material interfaces. The point based reproducing kernel (RK) approximation also avoids the complexity in construction of the well shaped mesh in the conventional finite element method. Two types of meshfree method for image based modeling of biomaterials are introduced, one based on Gelerkin type weak formulation and the other based on a direct collocation of differential equations. In conjunction with the level set based image segmentation technique, we apply the proposed meshfree methods to multiscale modeling of bone materials as well as simulation of skeletal muscles under contraction.

Short Bio: Prof. Jiun-Shyan (JS) Chen is the William Prager Chair of Structural Engineering at UCSD. He earned his undergraduate degree from National Central University in Taiwan, and Master's and Ph.D. from Northwestern University. Before moving to UCSD in October 2013, he was the Chancellor's Professor of UCLA and has served as the Department Chair of Civil & Environmental Engineering Department (2007-2012). His research is in computational mechanics and multiscale materials modeling with specialization in development of meshfree methods. He is one of the original developers of the meshfree Reproducing Kernel Particle Method (RKPM). He has applied meshfree methods to large deformation and contact mechanics, geomechanics, shock waves, high strain rate fragment-impact problems, biomechanics, molecular mechanics, quantum mechanics, as well as multi-scale mechanics and materials.

He is the past President of US Association for Computational Mechanics (USACM) and is currently serving on the Executive Council of the International

Association for Computational Mechanics (IACM), the Executive Council of the USACM, the Executive Council of the International Chinese Association for Computational Mechanics (ICACM), and the Board of Governors of ASCE Engineering Mechanics Institute (EMI). He has received numerous awards, including GenCorp Technology Achievement Award; James Lightners Faculty Fellowship and The Faculty Scholar Award from The University of Iowa; Outstanding Alumnus of National Central University (Taiwan); Tongji Chair of Tongji University (China); the ICACM Award from International Chinese Association for Computational Mechanics; the Computational Mechanics Award from International Association for Computational Mechanics, among others. He is the Fellow of USACM, IACM, ASME, EMI, ICACM. He is serving as the Editor-in-Chief, Associate Editor, or Editorial Board member for nine international journals.

Problems in Biological Imaging: Opportunities for Signal Processing

Jelena Kovačević

Department Head of Electrical & Computer Engineering
Professor in Electrical & Computer Engineering and Biomedical Engineering
Director of Center for Bioimage Informatics
Carnegie Mellon University, Pittsburgh, PA, USA

Abstract. In recent years, the focus in biological sciences has shifted from understanding single parts of larger systems, sort of vertical approach, to understanding complex systems at the cellular and molecular levels, horizontal approach. Thus the revolution of "omics" projects, genomics and now proteomics. Understanding complexity of biological systems is a task that requires acquisition, analysis and sharing of huge databases, and in particular, high-dimensional databases. Processing such huge amount of bioimages visually by biologists is inefficient, time-consuming and error-prone. Therefore, we would like to move towards automated, efficient and robust processing of such bioimage data sets. Moreover, some information hidden in the images may not be readily visually available. Thus, we do not only help humans by using sophisticated algorithms for faster and more efficient processing but also because new knowledge is generated through use of such algorithms.

The ultimate dream is to have distributed yet integrated large bioimage databases which would allow researchers to upload their data, have it processed, share the data, download data as well as platform-optimized code, etc., and all this in a common format. To achieve this goal, we must draw upon a whole host of sophisticated tools from signal processing, machine learning and scientific computing. I will address some of these issues in this presentation, especially those where signal processing expertise can play a significant role.

Short Bio: Prof. Jelena Kovačević received a Ph.D. degree from Columbia University. She then joined Bell Labs, followed by Carnegie Mellon University in 2003, where she is currently Professor and Head of the Department of Electrical and Computer Engineering and a Professor in the Department of Biomedical Engineering. She received the Belgrade October Prize and the E.I. Jury Award at Columbia University. She is a coauthor on an SP Society award-winning paper and is a coauthor of the books "Wavelets and Subband Coding" and "Foundations of Signal Processing". Dr. Kovacevic is the Fellow of the IEEE and was the Editor-in-Chief of the IEEE Transactions on Image Processing. She was a keynote speaker at a number of meetings and has been involved in organizing numerous conferences. Her research interests include multiresolution techniques and biomedical applications.

Adaptivity and Conformity in Meshing: A Two Phase Strategy

Ross Whitaker

Professor in School of Computing
Scientific Computing and Imaging Institute
University of Utah, USA

Abstract. Despite a great deal of important research and many fundamental advances, the general problem of tetrahedral meshing remains unsolved and challenging. In particular, the contraints imposed by adaptive element size, good tetrahedral quality (shape measured by some local metric), and material boundaries are often in conflict, and attempts to satisfy these conditions simultaneously frustrate many conventional approaches, particularly those that rely on iterative local updates to the mesh. This talk presents results from a recent body of work where we decouple these problems of adaptivity and geometric conformity. The strategy is to construct an adaptive background mesh that ignores geometric boundaries, and then partition or cleave that mesh, so that the resulting mesh conforms to geometry and maintains certain gaurantees on important mesh properties. The resulting algorithm produces high-quality, adaptive meshes relatively quickly, but introduces several interesting and important technical challenges.

Short Bio: Ross Whitaker graduated Summa Cum Laude with B.S. degree in Electrical Engineering and Computer Science from Princeton University in 1986. From 1986 to 1988 he worked for the Boston Consulting Group, entering the University of North Carolina at Chapel Hill in 1989. At UNC he received the Alumni Scholarship Award, and completed his Ph.D. in Computer Science in 1994. From 1994–1996 he worked at the European Computer-Industry Research Centre in Munich Germany as a research scientist in the User Interaction and Visualization Group. From 1996–2000 he was an Assistant Professor in the Department of Electrical Engineering at the University of Tennessee and received an NSF Career Award. Since 2000 he has been at the University of Utah where he is faculty member of the Scientific Computing and Imaging Institute and a Professor and the Director of the School of Computing. He teaches discrete math, scientific visualization, and image processing. Professor Whitaker leads a graduate-level research group in image analysis, geometry processing, and scientific computing, with a variety of projects supported by both federal agencies and industrial contracts. He is an IEEE Fellow and a member of the Computing Community Consortium.

A Predictive Mathematical Model of Acupuncture Based on an Explanation Biological Model

Marc Thiriet

Laboratoire Jacques-Louis Lions (LJLL)
Université Pierre et Marie Curie - Paris 6 (UPMC)
France

Abstract. Acupuncture requires a long-term training to handle acupoints. Four techniques exist: (1) development of a local mechanical stress field by needle motions (lifting - thrusting cycle or rotation) at acupoints; (2) development of a local temperature field by directly applying a heating moxa (mugwort herb) stick on the skin or indirectly by applying this stick on the acupuncture needle (moxibustion) at acupoints; (3) development of a local electrical field by applying a small electric current between a pair of acupuncture needles (electroacupuncture, or percutaneous electrical nerve stimulation [PENS]) at acupoints; and (4) laser light excitation independently of heating and other physical means probably via proper G-protein-coupled receptors on the surface of mastocytes.

Acupoints are enriched of mastocytes, among other biological structures and cells. Mastocytes are activation by a mechanical stress field (mechanotransduction), heating (thermotransduction), or a electrical field (electrotransduction). Whatever the operation mode, calcium entry in the mastocyte triggers degranulation and release of chemoattractants, neural stimulants, and endocrine substances. The process is sustained by recruitment of mastocytes (chemotaxis).

Acupuncture effects result from a set of signals sent from activated mastocytes at given acupoints to local nerve endings and capillaries that are transmitted to the brain and heart for processing and augmenting the flow rate, especially in the vasodilated acupoint. Released substances targets their cognate receptors on nerves and lymph and blood vessels. These two types of conduits deliver fast cues (electrochemical waves) and delayed information (blood transport) to the central nervous system, where they are processed for a desired output.

The mathematical model is a system of 5 partial differential equations. Its simplest form describes the evolution of the density of mastocytes and the chemoattractant concentration. A mathematical analysis of a simplified version of the equation set leads to a theorem for blow-up condition (the expected solution) as well as an analytical solution useful for validation. Numerical simulations are also carried out using a finite element method with mesh adaptivity. The computational model based on the home-made FreeFEM++ software demonstrated the occurrence of a stress field that excite mastocytes. It also shows that only adequate pools of mastocyte, that is, acupoints, must be targeted to have marked effects.

Short Bio: Marc Thiriet was educated at Medicine Faculty of Lille and University Pierre and Marie Curie ([UPMC] MD), and then at Technology University of Compiègne (3rd cycle Doctorate in Biomechanics), and Physics College of University Denis Diderot (Accreditation to Supervise Research). He was assistant physician in the lung disease department of Pontoise hospital. He is currently a member of the INRIA-UPMC-CNRS team REO in Laboratory Jacques-Louis Lions (applied math.) of UPMC. He worked in flows in collapsible tubes applied to airways and veins, 3D unsteady developing laminar flows in bend and branchings, both experimentally and numerically, as well as in models derived from 3D reconstruction of human anatomy. He is now involved in mathematical modeling of biological processes.

Marc Thiriet is the author of Biology and Mechanics of Blood Flows (2∼Vols.) and the book series "Biomathematical and Biomechanical Modeling of the Circulatory and Ventilatory Systems" (9 Vols., 6 published books). He is associate editor for the medical encyclopedia "Pan Vascular II". He also wrote the chapter Biofluid Flow and Heat Transfer for the next edition of Handbook of Fluid Dynamics. He is President of the french committee for Intensive Computation in Biology and Medicine and was involved in European committees for HPC (HPC-Europa-2 and PRACE). He is an Internal Reviewer of several Evaluation Groups of the Canadian Granting Agency (NSERC, mainly Mech. Eng. and also Life Sciences, Chemistry, Material and Chem. Eng., Computer Sci., and Mathematics). He was a Member of the "Biology" Panel of the french National Strategy for Research and Innovation (SNRI). He won the Grand Prix de la Fondation scientifique Franco-Taiwanaise in 2011 from the french Academy of Sciences and Taiwainese Science Council with his colleague Tony WH Sheu for their contribution in high-intensity focused ultrasound (HIFU)-based treatment of liver cancer and the first modeling of acupuncture.

Multi-Scale Image-Based Modeling
of the Failing Heart: From Cell to Patient

Andrew D. McCulloch

Distinguished Professor of Bioengineering and Medicine
Jacobs School Distinguished Scholar
University of California San Diego
La Jolla, CA 92093-0412, USA

Abstract. Multi-scale models of the heart have been developed that integrate both functionally across biomechanical, electrophysiological and regulatory functions and structurally across physical scales of organization from molecule to organ system. Imaging is central to the development of multi-scale cardiac models at all scales of biological organization, especially in disease states such as heart failure where structural remodeling of cells, tissue and the whole heart are all key contributors to mechanical dysfunction and arrhythmia risk. Here, we illustrate the development and application of these imaged-derived computational models to improving understanding and treatment of heart disease using several examples including: Microanatomically detailed models of subcellular and cellular biophysics generated from 3D electron tomograms; multi-scale models of murine ventricular mechanics derived from mouse cardiac magnetic resonance imaging; and patient-specific computational models of human atrial fibrillation and dyssynchronous heart failure to improve diagnosis and treatment efficacy.

Short Bio: Prof. Andrew McCulloch is Distinguished Professor of Bioengineering and Medicine and Jacobs School Distinguished Scholar at the University of California San Diego, where he joined the faculty in 1987. He is member of the UCSD Institute for Engineering in Medicine, the Qualcomm Institute, a Senior Fellow of the San Diego Supercomputer Center, and a member of the UCSD Center for Research on Biological Systems. Dr. McCulloch is a Principal Investigator of the National Biomedical Computation Resource and the Cardiac Atlas project, and Co-Director of the Cardiac Biomedical Science and Engineering Center at UCSD. He served as Vice Chair of the Bioengineering Department from 2002 to 2005 and Chair from 2005 to 2008. Dr. McCulloch is Director of the HHMI-NIBIB Interfaces Graduate Training Program and the accompanying UCSD Interdisciplinary Ph.D. Specialization in Multi-Scale Biology.

Table of Contents

Medical Treatment, Imaging and Analysis

Image Registration, Denoising and Feature Identification

Image Segmentation

Shape Analysis, Meshing and Graphs

Medical Image Processing and Simulations

Image Recognition, Reconstruction and Predictive Modeling

Image-Based Modeling and Simulations

Computer Vision and Data-Driven Investigations

HIFU Treatment of Liver Cancer –
Reciprocal Effect of Blood Flow and US Studied
from a Patient-Specific Configuration

Marc Thiriet, Maxim Solovchuk[4,5], and Tony Wen-Hann Sheu[4,5]

[1] Sorbonne Universités, UPMC Univ Paris 06, UMR 7598,
Laboratoire Jacques-Louis Lions, 75005, Paris, France
[2] CNRS, UMR 7598, Laboratoire Jacques-Louis Lions, 75005, Paris, France
[3] INRIA-Paris-Rocquencourt, EPC ***, Domaine de Voluceau, BP105,
78153 Le Chesnay Cedex, France
[4] Department of Engineering Science and Ocean Engineering,
National Taiwan University, Taipei, Taiwan
[5] Center for Advanced Study in Theoretical Sciences (CASTS),
National Taiwan University, Taipei, Taiwan

Abstract. The present computational model is aimed at predicting the
temperature field in a region of the hepatic parenchyma with a cancer resulting from applied high-intensity focused ultrasounds (HIFU)
for thermal ablation of the tumor in a patient-specific geometry. The
three-dimensional (3D) acoustic–thermal–hydrodynamic coupling model
computes the pressure, temperature, and blood velocity fields expressed
by the nonlinear Westervelt equation with relaxation effects and bioheat equations in both the hepatic parenchyma and blood vessels (sink).
The classical nonlinear Navier–Stokes equations related to mass and momentum conservation in large hepatic blood vessels are employed both
for convective cooling and acoustic streaming. This 3D three-field coupling MODEL demonstrates that both convective cooling and acoustic
streaming change the temperature considerably near large blood vessels.
In addition, acoustic streaming cannot be neglected due to resulting velocity magnitude and blood redistribution in the local vascular circuit.

Keywords: 3D reconstruction, acoustic streaming, blood flow, hepatic
cancer, HIFU.

1   Introduction

Liver cancer is the second leading cause of death in Asia and pertains to the most
common malignancy worldwide. In addition to the open and minimally invasive surgery, cryotherapy, radio-frequency (RF) ablation, microwave coagulation
therapy, laser-induced thermotherapy, and catheter-based infusion chemotherapy followed by transarterial chemoembolizationinfusion chemotherapy (TACE),
high-intensity focused ultrasound (HIFU)-based treatment is noninvasive, non-
ionizing technique. Thermal ablation relies on the observation that a temperature

Y.J. Zhang and J.M.R.S. Tavares (Eds.): CompIMAGE 2014, LNCS 8641, pp. 1–11, 2014.
© Springer International Publishing Switzerland 2014

above 56°C applied during 1 second by a energy source (pressure or electromagnetic waves) causes irreversible tissue damage.

The HIFU beam should be properly focused to heat ($T > 56°C$) and subsequently necrose only a localized tumoral region. The propagation of sound in a dispersive medium is investigated by solving the Westervelt equation. The acoustic energy distributed over the transducer face is concentrated into a volume that roughly has the size of a rice grain. Acoustic energy propagates through dispersive biological tissues; hence, it is attenuated. The attenuation depends on frequency. The numerical model must tackle the frequency content of the acoustic signal. The heat deposition due to absorption of acoustic energy in the biological tissue is then determined.

The target tissue temperature should rise to lethal levels without affecting healthy surrounding tissue, especially blood vessels to avoid vascular damage, although some organs such as the liver has a strong self-renewal, which enables fast regeneration. On the other hand, blood flow cooling reduces the necrosed volume.

Blood supply by both the hepatic artery and portal vein and drainage by hepatic veins is particulalrly important, as the liver is the body's chemical processor. Destroying the microcirculatory network surrounding the tumor has little effect, as it contributes to cancer scavenging on the one hand and the liver is endowed with a strong renewal capacity on the other. Damaging segments of the macrocirculation can cause huge bleeding.

Creating a medicosurgical platform requires a proper HIFU equipment and a simulation device that incorporates multiple GPU processors for fast and efficient computations. Image processing tools are mandatory for optimized procedures. Simulations carried out on patient-specific geometries are aimed at training, predicting, and planning the treatment. Numerical investigation also enables to relatively easily test the effects of nonlinear wave propagation, blood flow cooling, and acoustic streaming on HIFU tumor ablation.

The three-dimensional (3D) acoustic–thermal–hydrodynamic coupling model computes the pressure, temperature, and blood velocity fields expressed by the nonlinear Westervelt equation with relaxation effects and bioheat equations in both the hepatic parenchyma and blood vessels. The classical nonlinear Navier–Stokes equations related to mass and momentum conservation in large hepatic blood vessels are employed both for convective cooling and acoustic streaming. The 3D problem is solved using the finite-volume method [5–8].

Intrahepatic blood flow and ultrasound-induced heat exert reciprocal influences. The flowing blood participates in heat transfer as a sink. On the other hand, ultrasounds disturb the local blood flow as well as its regional distribution.

2   Method

The Westervelt wave equation describes the nonlinear propagation of small-amplitude sound in a dispersive medium. The dispersive feature of a sonicated medium relies on the frequency-dependent attenuation. This equation is coupled

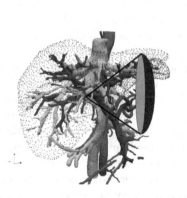
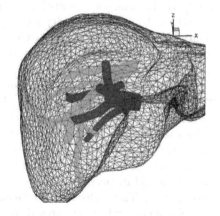

Fig. 1. Patient-specific 3D reconstruction of the liver and its vasculature

to Pennes bioheat and Navier–Stokes equations to numerically determine the resulting heat deposition.

2.1 Mathematical Model

The mathematical model relies on a coupling of: (1) nonlinear Westervelt equation; (2) heat equations in biological tissues; and (3) acoustic streaming hydrodynamic equations. The computational domain is meshed from a patient-specific 3D reconstruction that includes the hepatic and portal veins (Fig. 1). The total number of tetrahedral elements is 910,000. In the focal region, the grid is refined, thereby generating a cell length of 0.2 mm.

Three-dimensional ultrasound propagation creates an acoustic field that delivers energy especially in the focused beam area (heat source). The HIFU beam is spherically focused from an aperture of 12 cm and a focal length of 12 cm (frequency 1 MHz). The solid tumor is exposed to a 650-ms ultrasound. The peak positive and negative pressures equal 14.3 and -6.3 MPa. Acoustic intensity equals 2400 W/cm^2.

Resulting heat is transferred to the biological tissue that possesses sinks. These sinks are represented by the micro- and macrocirculation. In the region devoid of large vessels, heat transfer relies on Pennes bioheat equation [4]. In the neighboring region containing large vessels heat is convected by the local blood flow. Conversely, ultrasounds alter the local blood circulation by acoustic streaming.

A finite-amplitude wave propagation in a homogeneous medium obeys the Westervelt wave equation:

$$\nabla^2 p - \frac{1}{c^2}\partial_t^2 p + \left(\frac{\mathcal{D}}{c^4} + \frac{2}{c^3}\sum_k \frac{c_k \tau_k}{1 + \tau_k \partial_t}\right)\partial_t^3 p + \frac{\kappa}{\rho_0 c^4}\partial_t^2 p^2 = 0, \qquad (1)$$

where p is the acoustic pressure, c the characteristic medium sound speed, ρ_0 the medium density at rest, $\mathcal{D}$ the acoustic diffusivity ($2c^3\alpha/\omega^2$ in a thermoviscous fluid), α the acoustic absorption coefficient, ω the angular frequency, and $\kappa = 1 + B/2A$ ($B/2A$: nonlinearity parameter, an index of sound pressure vs. density relation). The third term (T_3) is a loss term that results from thermal conduction and viscous dissipation. The forth term (T_4) describes the nonlinear distorsion of the pressure wave.

The harmonic compression–expansion longitudinal sound wave oscillating in time with a given frequency (ω) applied along a given direction in a composite medium with a multiconstituent structure such as biological tissues undergoes a dispersion. Sound dispersion arises from the medium with its given physical properties as well as from possible boundaries (geometrical dispersion) and other dispersion sources independent of the propagation medium properties. In particular, sound dispersion is related to relaxation processes occuring during its propagation. The molecular displacement, especially vibrations, results from a transfer of energy from the sound wave with a certain delay, the relaxation time. A substantial frequency dispersion of the sound absorption coefficient can be observed in dispersive media, at least in the ultrasonic range.

Both the acoustic attenuation coefficient (α) and sound speed (c) depend on the ultrasound frequency (f). In a concentrated solution of polymer chains immersed in a solvent, the absorption coefficient α/f^2 scales as $f^{-1/2}$ when f ranges from 1 to 10 MHz [2]. The frequency dependence of the absorption coefficient becomes higher when the frequency increases.

The complex propagation factor $\gamma(\omega) = -\alpha(\omega) + \imath\beta(\omega)$ in the frequency domain (α: frequency-dependent attenuation; β: frequency-dependent dispersive component) is related to the relaxation time (τ) that characterizes the rate of the fluctuation relaxation and sound dispersion.

The Westerwelt equation is equivalent to the coupled system of partial differential equations:

$$\nabla^2 p - \frac{1}{c^2}\frac{\partial^2 p}{\partial t^2} + \frac{\mathcal{D}}{c^4}\frac{\partial^3 p}{\partial t^3} + \frac{\kappa}{\rho_0 c^4}\frac{\partial^2 p^2}{\partial t^2} + \sum_k P_k = 0,$$
$$\left(1 + \tau_k\frac{\partial}{\partial t}\right) P_k = \frac{2}{c^3}c_k\tau_k\frac{\partial^3 p}{\partial t^3},$$

where τ_i and c_i are the characteristic relaxation time and small sound speed component.

First-order non-reflecting boundary conditions are imposed:

$$\frac{\partial p}{\partial n} = \frac{1}{c}\frac{\partial p}{\partial t},$$

where $\mathbf{n}$ is the outward normal.

The heat equation incorporates a heat source, ultrasounds, and a sink, the local blood flow with a given velocity distribution ($\mathbf{v}$). The equation of energy field in the flowing blood domain is given by

$$\rho c_p\, D_t T = \nabla \cdot (\mathcal{G}_T \nabla T) + 2\mu \mathbf{D} : \mathbf{D} + S, \tag{2}$$

Table 1. Acoustic and thermal properties of the hepatic parenchyma and blood (c_p: specific heat capacity at constant pressure; $\mathcal{G}_T$: thermal conductivity)

	c (m/s)	ρ (kg/m^3)	c_p (J/[kg·K])	$\mathcal{G}_T$ (W/[m·K])
Liver	1550	1055	3600	0.51
Blood	1540	1060	3770	0.53
Tumor	1550	1000	3800	0.55

where $D_t = \partial_t + (\mathbf{v} \cdot \nabla)$ is the time derivative, $\mathbf{D} = (\nabla \mathbf{v} + (\nabla \mathbf{v})^T)/2$ the rate of deformation tensor for a Newtonian fluid, and S a source term (physical dimension $M/(LT^3)$). When the viscous dissipation is neglected, the heat transfer due to blood convection is given by:

$$\rho c_p \frac{DT}{Dt} = \mathcal{G}_T \nabla^2 T + S, \qquad (3)$$

The Pennes bioheat equation is

$$\rho_{\text{tis}} c_{\text{tis}} \partial_t T = \mathcal{G}_{\text{tis}} \nabla^2 T + q_b c_b (T - T_a) + q_{\text{met}} + q_s \qquad (4)$$

where c_{tis} is the specific heat of biological tissue (b: blood), ρ_{tis} the density of biological tissue, $\mathcal{G}_{\text{tis}}$ the thermal conductivity, q_b the perfusion rate (microcirculatory flow), T_a the arterial temperature, q_{met} the metabolic heat source (usually neglected), and q_s the heat source, that is, the ultrasound power deposition per unit volume. The physical quantities of the bioheat equation are given in Table 1.

In the linear case, the intensity is equal to $I_{lin} = p^2/2\rho c_0$, where c_0 is the speed of sound in the propagation medium. In the nonlinear case, the total intensity is

$$I = \sum_{n=1}^{\infty} I_n, \qquad (5)$$

where I_n are intensities for the respective harmonics $n f_0$. The ultrasound power deposition per unit volume is calculated as follows:

$$q_s = \sum_{n=1}^{\infty} 2\alpha(n f_0) I_n \qquad (6)$$

The acoustic streaming obeys the following equation, in the absence of body forces, the force vector exerted by an imposed ultrasound beam being assumed to act on blood along the acoustic axis ($\mathbf{n}$):

$$\rho D_t \mathbf{v} = -\nabla p + \nu \nabla^2 \mathbf{v} + \mathsf{F}, \qquad (7)$$

where F (physical dimension $M/(LT)^2$) is given by:

$$\mathsf{F} \cdot \mathbf{n} = \frac{q_s}{c_0}.$$

2.2 Relaxation Model for the Frequency-Dependent Attenuation Law in Tissue

The tissue absorption coefficient obeys the following power law (p=1):

$$\alpha = \alpha_0 \left(\frac{f}{f_0}\right)^p = \alpha_0 \left(\frac{\omega}{\omega_0}\right)^p. \tag{8}$$

The original Westervelt equation was derived for thermoviscous fluids. Dispersive biological tissues are characterized by a frequency-dependent phase velocity and attenuation. The acoustic attenuation depends linearly on frequency. Each relaxation process has its characteristic relaxation time (τ_i) and small sound speed increment (c_i).

The absorption coefficient at frequency $\omega_n = n\omega_0$ has the following form:

$$\alpha(\omega_n) = \frac{\delta\omega_n^2}{2c_0^3} + \frac{1}{c_0^2}\sum_{k=1}^{2}\frac{c_k\tau_k\omega_n}{1+(\tau_k\omega_n)^2}. \tag{9}$$

Five unknown parameters $\{\delta, \{c_k\}_1^2, \{\tau_k\}_1^2\}$ in the Westervelt equation are calculated by minimizing a mean square error between the experimental tissue attenuation (using Eq. 8 with $p = 1$) and the relaxation model (Eq. 9) in the frequency range from 0.5 to 20 MHz (Table 2).

Table 2. Values of quantities related to tissue attenuation in the Westervelt equation

Parameter	Value
δ	0.0022
c_1	5.3 m/s
c_2	4.3 m/s
τ_1	2.3×10^{-6} s
τ_2	2.4×10^{-7} s

2.3 Solving Procedure

The temporal terms are discretized using 2nd-order accuracy scheme and the nonlinear temporal term is linearized:

$$\frac{\partial^2 p^2}{\partial t^2} = 2\left(2\frac{\partial p}{\partial t}^n\frac{\partial p}{\partial t}^{n+1} + p^n\frac{\partial^2 p}{\partial t^2}^{n+1} + p^{n+1}\frac{\partial^2 p}{\partial t^2}^n - 2\left(\frac{\partial p}{\partial t}^n\right)^2 - 2p^n\frac{\partial^2 p}{\partial t^2}^n\right); \tag{10}$$

$$\frac{\partial p}{\partial t}^{n+1} = \frac{1}{2\Delta t}(3p^{n+1} - 4p^n + p^{n-1});$$

$$\frac{\partial^2 p}{\partial^2 t}^{n+1} = \frac{1}{(\Delta t)^2}(2p^{n+1} - 5p^n + 4p^{n-1} - p^{n-2});$$

$$\frac{\partial^3 p}{\partial t^3}^{n+1} = \frac{1}{2(\Delta t)^3}(6p^{n+1} - 23p^n + 34p^{n-1} - 24p^{n-2} + 8p^{n-3} - p^{n-4}).$$

The term P_k in the ultrasound wave equation is approximated by a scheme of second-order temporal accuracy

$$\frac{\partial}{\partial t}P_k^{n+1} = \frac{1}{\Delta t}(3P_k^{n+1} + 4P_k^n + P_k^{n-1})$$

The discretized formulas are then substituted into the Westervelt equation to get the Helmholtz equation. The Helmholz equation is then solved using the three-point sixth-order accurate scheme.

The numerical scheme used to solve the Westerwelt equation was validated by comparing the numerical pressure field with experimental results [7]. The Westerwelt equation is a more general form of the widely used Khokhlov–Zaboltskaya–Kuznetzov (KZK) equation. This equation was validated up to a peak acoustic pressure of 80 MPa [1]. In the present paper, the maximal acoustic pressure is lower than 25 MPa.

First, the acoustic pressure is calculated (once for a given set of transducer parameters). Afterward ultrasound power deposition and acoustic streaming force are determined and stored. Blood flow velocity is computed at every time step incorporating the acoustic streaming effect. Blood flow velocity is then updated in the bioheat equation. Using known blood flow velocities and power deposition, the temperature field is computed both in the hepatic parenchyma and blood vessels. The initial temperature is set to 37°C. On the wall, a constant temperature of 37°C is prescribed. A temperature continuity at the fluid–solid interface is imposed as that applied in a conjugate heat transfer problem. The interface boundary condition takes into account thermal conduction in liver and convection in blood vessel domain.

2.4 Validation

The mesh effect was explored. A temperature difference of 1% is observed for a cell number incrememt of 30%. Numerical results have been compared with experimental data obtained in a water tank (25°C). The pressure profiles in the focal plane are superimposed. Numerical results have also been compared with literature data (frequency 1.0 MHz; duration 5 s; flow velocity 0.67 cm/s) on organ phantom with blood vessel (bore 2.6 mm) [3]. The T_{max} vs. p curves were also superimposed.

Last, but not least, predicted and measured temperature elevations in a porcine muscle were compared. The porcine muscle was heated during 30 s by focused ultrasound transducer with an acoustic power ranging from 24 to 56 W using a home-made MR-guided HIFU system [9]. Excellent agreement was found

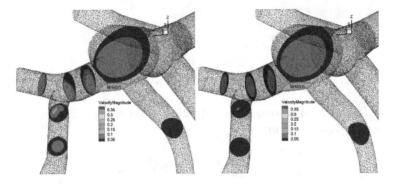

Fig. 2. Velocity distribution in various sections of the local portal venous circuit close to the tumor (light blue). (**Left**) With computed acoustic streaming (maximal velocity 40 cm/s). (**Right**) Without acoustic streaming effect (maximal velocity 7 cm/s).

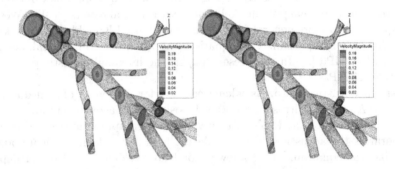

Fig. 3. Velocity distribution in various sections of the hepatic veinous drainage. (**Left**) With computed acoustic streaming. (**Right**) Without acoustic streaming effect.

using power of 80 and 140 W at the focal point for a 30-s sonication. For peak temperatures above 85 to 90°C (power of 160 and 200 W), cavitation appears and lesion distortion starts; small discrepancy can then be observed between measured and simulated temporal evolutions of the temperature.

2.5   Acoustic Streaming

Acoustic streaming is usually considered as a second order physical effect and consequently neglected. Acoustic streaming effect during a thermal ablation of hepatic cancer is thus explored. The blood velocity field is computed with and without acoustic streaming (Figs. 2 and 3 and Tables 3 and 4). Acoustic streaming velocity magnitude can be several times larger than the initial blood vessel velocity. Maximum velocity magnitudes in the portal vein with and without acoustic streaming equal 40 and 7 cm/s, respectively. Acoustic streaming thus increases the blood flow cooling.

Table 3. Blood mass flow (10^{-3} kg/s) distribution among branches (B) of the portal vein when acoustic streaming (AS) is incorporated or not. The closer the branch to the ultrasound focus, the larger the acoustic streaming effect.

	B1	B2	B3	B4	B5	B6	Inlet
Without AS	3.3	0.58	0.53	1.5	1.28	1.13	8.32
With AS	2.49	0.92	0.14	3.17	0.76	0.84	8.32
Difference (%)	−24	+60	−73	+112	−40	−26	

Table 4. Maximum acoustic streaming velocity U_{max} (m/s) at various distances between the focal point and blood vessel wall (columns 2–4) or axis (columns 5–6). The caliber of the blood vessel equals 3 mm and its axis is parallel to the acoustic axis. For low power (327 W), when the focal point localizes to the blood vessel centerline, the velocity field exhibits flow reversals at both sides of the centerline. When the focal point is outside the vessel axis, a single larger flow reversal appears in the opposite half-section of the vascular lumen and the velocity is higher near the focal point. For high power (2400 W), the velocity magnitude is nearly invariant whatever the focal point location, but is 3- to 40-times larger than usual blood flow velocity.

Intensity (W/cm^2)	U_{max} (cm/s)				
	gap				
	focus outside the vascular lumen			focus inside	
	1 mm	0.5 mm	0 mm	0.5 mm	0 mm
327	1.5	4.9	11	12.7	10
2470	10	30	60	69	70

The results (Table 4) show that

1. the higher the intensity, the greater the acoustic streaming;
2. the closer the vessel to focal point, the larger the acoustic streaming;
3. the lower the blood flow velocity, the greater the acoustic streaming attenuation of temperature elevation at both focal point and vessel wall.

The simulated temperature field is influenced by acoustic streaming (Fig. 5). A very sharp temperature difference appears near the venous wall. In addition, blood flow cooling causes a strong asymmetry in the temperature field inside the lesion. Simulations can thus optimize the procedure strategy by chosing an appropriate sonication time, ultrasound power, and focal point location.

Concluding Remarks

The proposed three-dimensional computational model of HIFU therapy is carried out on a mesh derived form 3D reconstruction of the liver and its major vessels.

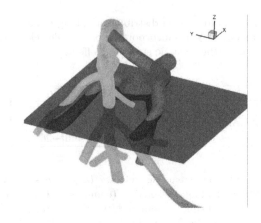

Fig. 4. Location of the visualization plane (Fig 5)

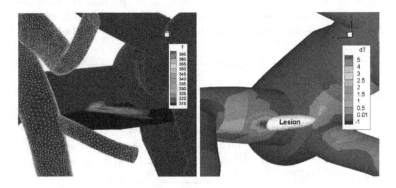

Fig. 5. Temperature contours in the tumor and portal vein in the plane $z = 0.16$ at time $t = 0.65$ s (end of sonication). (**Left**) Tumor. (**Right**) Portal vein branch. Temperature difference on the portal vein wall with and without acoustic streaming reaches a maximum of 7 K

A priori, the lower the flow velocity, the smaller the ablation zone volume should be due to the presence of a large blood vessel with respect to a target parenchyma free of large blood vessels. However, the treatment efficiency is markedly influenced not only by blood flow cooling, but also by acoustic streaming. At high intensities, cooling by acoustic streaming can prevail over the simple cooling by blood flow through large intrahepatic blood vessels. Acoustic streaming may thus enhance therapy safety.

References

1. Canney, M.S., Bailey, M.R., Crum, L.A., Khokhlova, V.A., Sapozhnikov, O.A.: Acoustic characterization of high intensity focused ultrasound fields: A combined measurement and modeling approach. Journal of the Acoustical Society of America 124, 2406–2420 (2008)
2. Gotlib, Y.Y., Salikhov, K.M.: Theory of ultrasonic absorption in concentrated polymer solutions. Akusticheskij Zhurnal 9, 301–308 (1963)
3. Huang, J., Holt, R.G., Cleveland, R.O., Roy, R.A.: Experimental validation of a tractable numerical model for focused ultrasound heating in flow-through tissue phantoms. J. Acoust. Soc. Am. 116, 2451–2458 (2004)
4. Pennes, H.H.: Analysis of tissue and arterial blood temperature in the resting human forearm. J. Appl. Physiol. 1, 93–122 (1948)
5. Sheu, T.W.H., Solovchuk, M.A., Chen, A.W.J., Thiriet, M.: On an acoustics–thermal–fluid coupling model for the prediction of temperature elevation in liver tumor. International Journal of Heat and Mass Transfer 54, 4117–4126 (2011)
6. Solovchuk, M.A., Sheu, T.W.H., Lin, W.L., Kuo, I., Thiriet, M.: Simulation study on acoustic streaming and convective cooling in blood vessels during a high-intensity focused ultrasound thermal ablation. International Journal of Heat and Mass Transfer 55, 1261–1270 (2012)
7. Solovchuk, M.A., Sheu, T.W.H., Thiriet, M.: Simulation of nonlinear Westervelt equation for the investigation of acoustic streaming and nonlinear propagation effects. J. Acoust. Soc. Am. 134, 3931–3942 (2013)
8. Solovchuk, M.A., Sheu, T.W.H., Thiriet, M., Lin, W.L.: On a computational study for investigating acoustic streaming and heating during focused ultrasound ablation of liver tumor. Applied Thermal Engineering 56, 62–76 (2013)
9. Solovchuk, M.A., Hwang, S.C., Chang, H., Thiriet, M., Sheu, T.W.: Temperature elevation by HIFU in ex vivo porcine muscle: MRI measurement and simulation study. Medical Physics 41, 052903 (2014)

An Inter-Projection Interpolation (IPI) Approach with Geometric Model Restriction to Reduce Image Dose in Cone Beam CT (CBCT)

Hong Zhang[1], Fengchong Kong[1], Lei Ren[2], and Jian-Yue Jin[1,3]

[1] Department of Radiation Oncology, Georgia Regents University, USA
[2] Department of Radiation Oncology, Duke University, USA
[3] Department of Radiology, Georgia Regents University, USA
{honzhang,fekong,jjin}@gru.edu, lei.ren@duke.edu

Abstract. Cone beam computed tomography (CBCT) imaging is a key step in image guided radiation therapy (IGRT) to improve tumor targeting. The quality and imaging dose of CBCT are two important factors. However, X-ray scatter in the large cone beam field usually induces image artifacts and degrades the image quality for CBCT. A synchronized moving grid (SMOG) approach has recently been proposed to resolve this issue and shows great promise. However, the SMOG technique requires two projections in the same gantry angle to obtain full information due to signal blockage by the grid. This study aims to develop an inter-projection interpolation (IPI) method to estimate the blocked image information. This approach will require only one projection in each gantry angle, thus reducing the scan time and patient dose. IPI is also potentially suitable for sparse-view CBCT reconstruction to reduce the imaging dose. To be compared with other state-of-the-art spatial interpolation (called inpainting) methods in terms of signal-to-noise ratio (SNR) on a Catphan and head phantoms, IPI increases SNR from 15.3dB and 12.7dB to 29.0dB and 28.1dB, respectively. The SNR of IPI on sparse-view CBCT reconstruction can achieve from 28dB to 17dB for undersample projection sets with gantry angle interval varying from 1 to 3 degrees for both phantoms.

Keywords: Scatter correction, Dose reduction, CBCT, SMOG, Moving grids, Interpolation, Geometric model.

1 Introduction

In recent years, on board cone beam computed tomography (CBCT) has been developed as an important imaging modality in image guided radiation therapy (IGRT) [1]. In IGRT, CBCT is performed before radiation delivery with a patient holding a treatment position similar to the position when the simulation/planning computed tomography (CT) was taken [2]. The CBCT image is then registered with the simulation CT, and the patient's treatment position is adjusted and aligned according to the registration to ensure a precise radiation dose delivery [3]. The image quality of CBCT is critical, especially for

Y.J. Zhang and J.M.R.S. Tavares (Eds.): CompIMAGE 2014, LNCS 8641, pp. 12–23, 2014.
© Springer International Publishing Switzerland 2014

cancer treatments requiring high accurate dose delivery. Also, the imaging dose is another important factor due to the frequent CBCT scans because radiation therapy usually requires 30-40 fractions of treatments.

Unfortunately, CBCT image quality is largely degraded by scatter artifacts because a large volume of the imaging object is irradiated for each projection [4]. Many approaches have been proposed to reduce the scatter artifacts and improve the CBCT image quality. Among them, the synchronized moving grid (SMOG) [5,6] is one of the most promising techniques. The SMOG approach utilizes a grid to divide the large cone beam field into multiple small narrow strips, and thus reduce the amount of scatter. In addition, the remaining scatter can be measured and thus be corrected by the shadow regions blocked by the grid. However, the imaging information in these shadow regions is also blocked by the grid (Fig.1(b) and Fig.2(b)). The SMOG approach resolves this issue by acquiring two complementary projections at each gantry angle (a linear accelerator is mounted on the gantry and the gantry angle is the rotation angle of the gantry) to obtain full information by shifting the grid a proper distance before taking the second projection. The SMOG approach may also potentially reduce the image lag-induced artifacts [5]. However, the SMOG approach is technically challenging since it requires a fast moving grid, especially for fast gantry rotation. More importantly, the CBCT control system needs to be redesigned completely with a capacity of taking at least two projections at the same gantry angle. This may increase the scan time and dose due to the limitation of the frame rate of the flat panel imager.

This study aims to derive the blocked information without taking an additional projection; thus, it may also reduce the imaging dose by half. Approaches based on total variance (TV) [7] have been proposed, but usually these TV-based methods are time-consuming due to iteratively repeated projection calculations. An efficient method would be interpolation. The interpolation process is called image inpainting which is used in the field of computer vision for old picture repairing. The inpainting technique could be roughly classified into several groups: 1) texture synthesis-based [8], 2) partial differential equation (PDE)-based [9], 3) exemplar-based [10] and 4) hybrid [11]. Texture synthesis-based inpainting uses similar unblocked neighbourhoods of the blocked pixels to synthesize the missing texture in blocked regions. PDE-based inpainting iteratively perfuses and propagates the information of unblocked pixels at the border of blocked regions in the direction of minimal change using 'isophote lines'. Exemplar-based inpainting selects the most similar patches from unblocked regions and pastes them back to blocked regions. Hybrid-based inpainting is a combination of the above methods. Although the inpainting starts to be used in fan-beam CT reconstruction [12], most of the above methods lack CBCT imaging geometric model restrictions. Thus, these inpainting results are very hard to validate and some artifacts are generated, as shown in the Results section. Generally, it is impossible to recover complete information in the blocked regions with inpainting.

In this study, we propose an inter-projection interpolation (IPI) method, which utilizes two adjacent projections as references and extracts groups of paired corresponding pixels on the two projections based on the CBCT geometric model. The method uses a similar SMOG approach. Instead of moving the grid and taking two projections at each gantry angle, the new approach takes only one projection at each gantry angle and moves the grid at the same distance for the next gantry angle. Thus, the blocked regions in each projection correspond to open regions in the two adjacent projections. The missing pixels are finally estimated from the paired pixels with the highest similarity. We compared the reconstruction result of IPI and exemplar-based inpainting method in terms of signal-to-noise ratio (SNR) on two phantoms (Catphan phantom and head phantom). The proposed method increased SNR significantly. In addition, we applied IPI on sparse view CBCT reconstruction and found that SNR was kept in a reasonable range with increase of the interval.

The paper is organized as follows. The IPI framework, including the geometric model, cost function and optimization method, is described in Section 2. The results are presented and discussed in Section 3. Finally, the conclusion is given in Section 4.

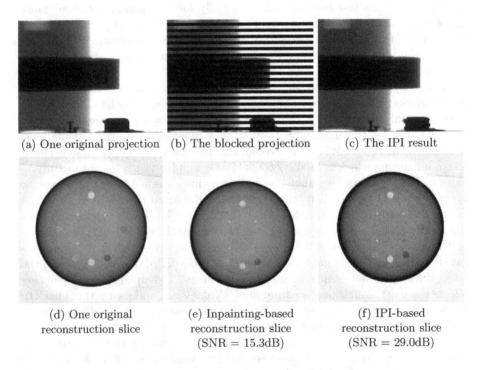

(a) One original projection   (b) The blocked projection   (c) The IPI result

(d) One original
reconstruction slice

(e) Inpainting-based
reconstruction slice
(SNR = 15.3dB)

(f) IPI-based
reconstruction slice
(SNR = 29.0dB)

Fig. 1. Comparison between inpainting and IPI of Catphan phantom

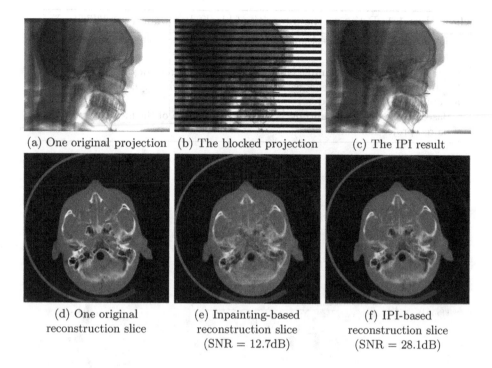

(a) One original projection   (b) The blocked projection   (c) The IPI result

(d) One original
reconstruction slice

(e) Inpainting-based
reconstruction slice
(SNR = 12.7dB)

(f) IPI-based
reconstruction slice
(SNR = 28.1dB)

Fig. 2. Comparison between inpainting and IPI of head phantom

2   Materials and Methods

2.1   Inter-projection Interpolation

The value of each pixel on each projection could be viewed as the line integral of
attenuation of all points along the ray connecting the source and the pixel. Due
to the continuity of a patient's anatomy, if the gantry angle interval between two
consecutive projections is sufficiently small, the values of the corresponding pixel
in three consecutive projections are usually similar, unless there is an 'abrupt'
point, such as an edge of a bone, along the ray corresponding to the pixel. A
geometric model was developed to approximately determine the location as well
as the density change of this 'abrupt' point from two sets of corresponding pixels
in the two nearest neighboring projections. Along the artificial ray, we sampled
some equidistant points, and the paired projection pixels of each point onto the
two nearest neighboring projections were identified via the geometric model. In
this way, a group of paired projection pixels were detected and the two pixels
corresponding to the 'abrupt' point are expected to have the smallest similarity
cost. Thus, the location and corresponding pixel value of this 'abrupt' point was
identified by picking up a pair of the 'closest' pixels. The pipeline of the process
is shown in pseudocode:

Algorithm 1.1. Estimate the intensity of blocked scanline $PS_g^{scanline}(v_g)$

1. Locate the paired projection pixels on two unblocked neighboring projections based on geometric model
2. Along $\overrightarrow{S_g E_{g,j}(u_g, v_g)}$, sample equidistantly with different depths
3. After minimizing the energy along the scanline with dynamic programming, 'abrupt' points are searched
4. Based on the depths of 'abrupt' points, the estimation of the intensity is the mean of paired projection pixels

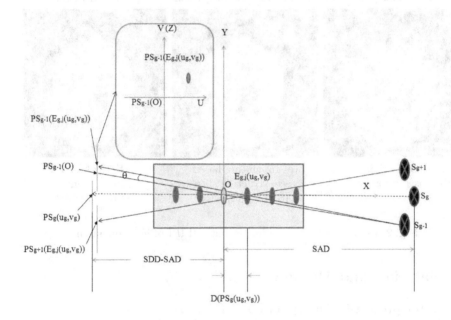

Fig. 3. The geometric model

Nomenclature for Fig. 3

S_{g-1}, S_g, S_{g+1}: the locations of source in continued gantry angle.

SAD: source-to-axis distance.

SDD: source-to-detector distance.

O: origin of global coordinate.

$PS_g(u_g, v_g)$: a blocked pixel on the detector projection plane of source S_g with local coordinate of (u_g, v_g).

$E_{g,j}(u_g, v_g)$: a sampling point on the ray between S_g and $PS_g(u_g, v_g)$.

$D(PS_g(u_g, v_g))$: the depth of 'abrupt' point of $PS_g(u_g, v_g)$.

$PS_{g-1}(E_{g,j}(u_g, v_g)), PS_{g+1}(E_{g,j}(u_g, v_g))$: the unblocked projection pixel of $E_{g,j}(u_g, v_g)$ under source S_{g-1} and S_{g+1} on the detector, respectively.

$PS_{g-1}(O)$: the projection global coordinate origin under source S_{g-1} on the detector.

U,V(Z): local coordinate of the detector projection plane and the global axis; Z is the same as axis V.

X,Y,Z: global coordinate.

2.2 Paired Projection Pixels Localization

The proposed geometric model is shown in Fig. 3 and the nomenclature is listed. Based on the geometric model, we first need to calculate the local coordinate of $PS_{g-1}(E_{g,j}(u_g, v_g))$ and $PS_{g+1}(E_{g,j}(u_g, v_g))$. Since the rotation orbit is perpendicular to the Z axis, $PS_g(u_g, v_g)$, $PS_{g-1}(E_{g,j}(u_g, v_g))$ and $PS_{g+1}(E_{g,j}(u_g, v_g))$ have the same known Z coordinate v_g (i.e., local V coordinate), and we just need to calculate the local U coordinate. Taking $PS_{g-1}(E_{g,j}(u_g, v_g))$ as an example, the U coordinate can be derived from θ between $\overrightarrow{S_{g-1}O}$ and $\overrightarrow{S_{g-1}E_{g,j}(u_g, v_g)}$. The θ is calculated as:

$$\theta = \arccos(\frac{\overrightarrow{S_{g-1}E_{g,j}(u_g, v_g)}}{\|\overrightarrow{S_{g-1}E_{g,j}(u_g, v_g)}\|} \cdot \frac{\overrightarrow{S_{g-1}O}}{\|\overrightarrow{S_{g-1}O}\|}) \tag{1}$$

and the distance between $PS_{g-1}(E_{g,j}(u_g, v_g))$ and $PS_{g-1}(O)$ is derived as:

$$\|\overrightarrow{PS_{g-1}(E_{g,j}(u_g, v_g))PS_{g-1}(O)}\| = SDD * \tan(\theta). \tag{2}$$

Finally, the local U coordinate is

$$|PS_{g-1}(E_{g,j}(u_g, v_g))_U| = \sqrt{(SDD * \tan(\theta))^2 - v_g^2} \tag{3}$$

where $PS_{g-1}(E_{g,j}(u_g, v_g))_U$ is the local U coordinate. The sign of the U coordinate is the same as the Z coordinate of $\overrightarrow{S_{g-1}E_{g,j}(u_g, v_g)} \times \overrightarrow{S_{g-1}O}$. In the same way, the local coordinate of $PS_{g+1}(E_{g,j}(u_g, v_g))$ can be calculated.

Therefore, a pair of projection pixels, $PS_{g-1}(E_{g,j}(u_g, v_g))$ and $PS_{g+1}(E_{g,j}(u_g, v_g))$, can be localized analytically for any sample point $E_{g,j}(u_g, v_g)$ under the geometric restriction.

2.3 'Abrupt' Point Searching

After locating the paired projection pixels, we can sample along the ray $\overrightarrow{S_g E_{g,j}(u_g, v_g)}$ equidistantly and find the 'abrupt' point defined as the depth of blocked pixel $PS_g(u_g, v_g)$ (i.e., $D(PS_g(u_g, v_g))$) based on the similarity of the corresponding paired projection unblocked pixels. The problem is called the 'stereo matching' [13] problem in computer vision and roughly can be divided into two steps: cost calculation and optimization. For the first step, a lot of similarity cost measurements have been proposed, including the sum of absolute difference, the sum of squared difference, and the normalized cross correlation [14,15]. Some of them target at the occlusion and non-rigid transformation problems, which can be omitted in our case [16]. Thus, we used the sum of squared difference to balance the speed and accuracy. For the second step, a large number of optimization methods are also developed, including Markov Random Field [17], graph-cut [18] and dynamic programming [19]. Among them, scanline-based dynamic programming is the fastest and most suitable for our case, since the paired projection pixels of the same scanline parallel to the U axis on projections share the same Z axis as we mentioned before.

Similarity Cost. After rewriting the paired pixels of a sample point $E_{g,j}(u_g, v_g)$ in local coordinate format as $(PS_{g-1}(u_{g-1}, v_{g-1}), PS_{g+1}(u_{g+1}, v_{g+1}))$ to simplify the formula, we sampled a 2D window with width w (5 is used in our case) centered at each pixel. The similarity cost is defined as:

$$
Cost(E_{g,j}(u_g, v_g)) = Similarity(PS_{g-1}(u_{g-1}, v_{g-1}), S_{g+1}(u_{g+1}, v_{g+1}))
$$
$$
= \sum_{i=-(w-1)/2}^{i=(w-1)/2} (S_{g-1}(u_{g-1}+i, v_{g-1}) - S_{g+1}(u_{g+1}+i, v_{g+1}))^2.
$$
$$(4)$$

Optimization. If we simply used the cost for each sample point of a missing pixel $PS_g(u_g, v_g)$ to search the 'abrupt' pixel individually as below:

$$
D(PS_g(u_g, v_g)) = \underset{j}{\arg\min}\, Cost(E_{g,j}(u_g, v_g)),
\tag{5}
$$

the smoothness along the scanline (i.e., $PS_g^{scanline}(v_g) = PS_g(1...width, v_g)$ where $width$ is the width of the detector in pixels) can not be guaranteed. Thus, we built up an energy function:

$$
E(PS_g^{scanline}(v_g)) = E_{data} + \lambda E_{smooth}
$$
$$
= \sum_{i=1}^{i=width} Cost(E_{g,j}(i, v_g)) + \lambda \sum_{i=1}^{i=width-1} |D(PS_g(i, v_g))
$$
$$
- D(PS_g(i+1, v_g))|
$$
$$(6)$$

where E_{data} is the sum of the data cost from the whole scanline and E_{smooth} is the sum of the difference of depths between two adjacent pixels in the scanline while λ adjusts the weight between the data and smooth terms. This energy can be minimized by rewriting the energy in recursive format and applying dynamic programming [20]:

$$
E(PS_g^{scanline}(v_g)) = E(PS_g(1...width, v_g))
$$
$$
= \underset{j}{\min}(Cost(E_{g,j}(1, v_g)) + \lambda|D(PS_g(1, v_g))
\tag{7}
$$
$$
- D(PS_g(2, v_g))| + E(PS_g(2...width, v_g))).
$$

In this way, the sum of energy along the scanline is split into three parts: the first part is the cost of the first pixel defined in formula 4; the second part is the difference of depths between the first and second pixel; the third part is the sum of energy along the scanline expected for the first pixel. Iteratively, the sum of the energy could be split into a group of the first part and a group of the second part. Starting from the last pixel, we could trace back the depths of all pixels along the scanline with minimized energy. After finding the corresponding pair based on the optimized depths, the missing pixel intensity is estimated as the mean of the intensity of the corresponding paired projection pixels.

2.4   SMOG Simulation and Evaluation of the IPI Technique

A Catphan phantom and a head phantom were scanned using the onboard CBCT system on a Varian® Trilogy™machine using a half fan mode, with the X-ray tube voltage of 120 kVp. In each scan, approximately 650 projections were acquired and each projection's dimensions were 1024×768 with resolutions of $0.388\text{mm} \times 0.388\text{mm}$. The reconstruction images contain $384 \times 384 \times 64$ voxels with resolutions of $0.651\text{mm} \times 0.651\text{mm} \times 2.5\text{mm}$.

The SMOG was simulated by erasing the information (filling with '0') of the areas in each projection corresponding to the grid, which is designed as 1:1 space ratio and 21 pixels width. The artificial grid moves back and forth on each projection at the step of the grid width. In this way, a blocked projection pixel in one gantry angle is guaranteed to be 'seen' in the two adjacent gantry angles. The blocked image information was derived from the information in the two neighboring projections immediately before and after the projection using the IPI algorithm. A complete projection was derived, and the CBCT image was reconstructed using the FDK [21] reconstruction algorithm. SNR was calculated by comparing the CBCT images with the original unblocked CBCT image. The IPI method was also compared with an examplar-based inpainting interpolation method in terms of the SNR [22].

The gantry angle step effect was also studied in the IPI technique. For the original 650 projections with an gantry angle step of ≈0.5 degree, we undersampled the projections by deleting 1/2, 2/3, 3/4, 4/5 and 5/6 of the projections evenly so that the gantry angle step was around 1, 1.5, 2, 2.5 and 3 degrees, respectively. The IPI technique was then used to recover the deleted projections, and CBCT images were reconstructed after that. The image quality of the IPI-recovered CBCT images with various gantry angle steps was evaluated by comparing with the original CBCT images and calculating the SNR.

3   Results and Discussion

3.1   IPI Technique to Recover Blocked Information for the SMOG-Based CBCT

Fig. 1 shows the result for the Catphan phantom. We noted that the CBCT image from the IPI-recovered projection had a SNR of 29dB in comparison to a SNR of 15.3dB for the inpainting-based interpolation.

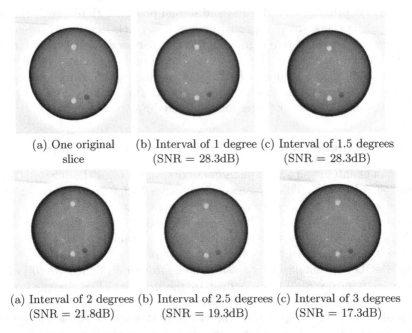

(a) One original
slice

(b) Interval of 1 degree
(SNR = 28.3dB)

(c) Interval of 1.5 degrees
(SNR = 28.3dB)

(a) Interval of 2 degrees
(SNR = 21.8dB)

(b) Interval of 2.5 degrees
(SNR = 19.3dB)

(c) Interval of 3 degrees
(SNR = 17.3dB)

Fig. 4. Undersampled reconstruction after IPI results at different intervals of Catphan phantom

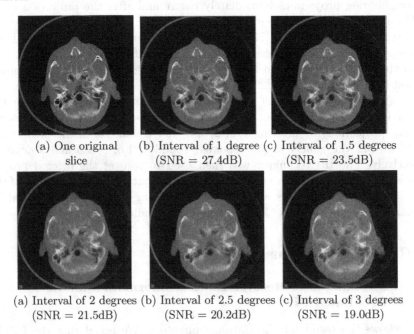

(a) One original
slice

(b) Interval of 1 degree
(SNR = 27.4dB)

(c) Interval of 1.5 degrees
(SNR = 23.5dB)

(a) Interval of 2 degrees
(SNR = 21.5dB)

(b) Interval of 2.5 degrees
(SNR = 20.2dB)

(c) Interval of 3 degrees
(SNR = 19.0dB)

Fig. 5. Undersampled reconstruction after IPI results at different intervals of head phantom

Similarly, Fig. 2 shows the result for the head phantom. We noted that the CBCT image from the IPI-recovered projection had a SNR of 28.1dB in comparison to a SNR of 12.7dB for the inpainting-based interpolation.

These results demonstrate that the IPI technique can provide superior results to the inpainting-based interpolation. The SNR values of 29.0dB and 28.1dB are quite high, suggesting that the IPI technique is reliable. The IPI technique may allow us to directly add the SMOG system in the current clinical on-board CBCT system without significantly modifying the CBCT control system.

3.2   Gantry Angle Interval Effect in IPI Technique

The undersampled projection sets with various gantry angle intervals (1, 1.5, 2, 2.5 and 3 degrees) were used to study the gantry angle interval effect for the IPI technique. Fig. 4 shows the comparison of an axial cut of the CBCT images of the Catphan phantom with the missing projections recovered by the IPI technique for these undersampled projections. We noted that the SNRs were 28.3, 28.3, 21.8, 19.3 and 17.3dB for the gantry angle intervals of 1, 1.5, 2, 2.5, and 3 degrees, respectively.

Similarly, Fig. 5 shows the comparison of an axial cut of the CBCT images of the head phantom with the missing projections recovered by the IPI technique for the undersampled projections. We noted that the SNRs were 27.4, 23.5, 21.5, 20.2 and 19.0dB for the gantry angle intervals of 1, 1.5, 2, 2.5, and 3 degrees, respectively.

The SNR was reduced with the increasing gantry angle interval. The Catphan tended to have a better SNR than the head phantom when the gantry angle interval was very small (less than 2 degrees). The head phantom tended to have a better SNR for relatively large gantry angle intervals.

The IPI may also be used on sparse-view CBCT reconstruction to reduce the imaging dose (*i.e.*, reconstruction based on partial projections in sparse gantry view). When the gantry angle interval is less than 2 degrees, the SNR is still larger than 20dB and thus the image deviation due to the IPI estimation may still be acceptable.

4   Conclusion

The IPI technique is a new interpolation method utilizing neighboring projections to estimate the blocked projection following a geometric model. It shows a much higher accuracy level than the inpainting algorithm to recover the blocked information. The technique may allow us to directly add a SMOG system in the current clinical on-board CBCT system without significantly modifying the CBCT control program. In combination with SMOG, it may reduce the scatter artifacts and reduce the image dose. It may also be used for sparse-view CBCT reconstruction to further reduce the imaging dose.

Acknowledgments. This study was supported by Award Number 1R01CA166948-01 from the National Cancer Institute. The content is solely the responsibility of the authors and does not necessarily represent the official views of the National Cancer Institute or the National Institutes of Health.

References

1. Xing, L., Thorndyke, B., Schreibmann, E., Yang, Y., Li, T.F., Kim, G.Y., Luxton, G., Koong, A.: Overview of image-guided radiation therapy. Medical Dosimetry 31(2), 91–112 (2006)
2. Schaly, B., Kempe, J., Bauman, G., Battista, J., Van Dyk, J.: Tracking the dose distribution in radiation therapy by accounting for variable anatomy. Physics in Medicine and Biology 49(5), 791 (2004)
3. Dawson, L.A., Sharpe, M.B.: Image-guided radiotherapy: rationale, benefits, and limitations. The Lancet Oncology 7(10), 848–858 (2006)
4. Zhu, L., Xie, Y., Wang, J., Xing, L.: Scatter correction for cone-beam ct in radiation therapy. Medical Physics 36(6), 2258–2268 (2009)
5. Jin, J.Y., Ren, L., Liu, Q., Kim, J., Wen, N., Guan, H., Movsas, B., Chetty, I.J.: Combining scatter reduction and correction to improve image quality in cone-beam computed tomography (cbct). Medical Physics 37(11), 5634–5644 (2010)
6. Ren, L., Yin, F.F., Chetty, I.J., Jaffray, D.A., Jin, J.Y.: Feasibility study of a synchronized-moving-grid (smog) system to improve image quality in cone-beam computed tomography (cbct). Medical Physics 39(8), 5099–5110 (2012)
7. Ouyang, L., Song, K., Wang, J.: A moving blocker system for cone-beam computed tomography scatter correction. Medical Physics 40(7), 071903 (2013)
8. Heeger, D.J., Bergen, J.R.: Pyramid-based texture analysis/synthesis. In: Proceedings of the 22nd Annual Conference on Computer Graphics and Interactive Techniques, pp. 229–238 (1995)
9. Bertalmio, M., Sapiro, G., Caselles, V., Ballester, C.: Image inpainting. In: Proceedings of the 27th Annual Conference on Computer Graphics and Interactive Techniques, pp. 417–424 (2000)
10. Yang, J., Hua, K., Wang, Y., Wang, W., Wang, H., Shen, J.: Automatic objects removal for scene completion. In: IEEE INFOCOM Workshop on Security and Privacy in Big Data (2014)
11. Wu, J., Ruan, Q.: A novel hybrid image inpainting model. In: International Conference on Audio, Language and Image Processing, pp. 138–142 (2008)
12. Li, Y., Chen, Y., Hu, Y., Oukili, A., Luo, L., Chen, W., Toumoulin, C.: Strategy of computed tomography sinogram inpainting based on sinusoid-like curve decomposition and eigenvector-guided interpolation. Journal of the Optical Society of America A 29(1), 153–163 (2012)
13. Scharstein, D., Szeliski, R.: A taxonomy and evaluation of dense two-frame stereo correspondence algorithms. International Journal of Computer Vision 47(1-3), 7–42 (2002)
14. Kanade, T., Okutomi, M.: A stereo matching algorithm with an adaptive window: Theory and experiment. IEEE Transactions on Pattern Analysis and Machine Intelligence 16(9), 920–932 (1994)
15. Simoncelli, E.P., Adelson, E.H., Heeger, D.J.: Probability distributions of optical flow. In: IEEE Computer Society Conference on Computer Vision and Pattern Recognition, pp. 310–315 (1991)

16. Kolmogorov, V., Zabih, R.: Computing visual correspondence with occlusions using graph cuts. In: IEEE International Conference on Computer Vision, vol. 2, pp. 508–515 (2001)
17. Black, M.J., Rangarajan, A.: On the unification of line processes, outlier rejection, and robust statistics with applications in early vision. International Journal of Computer Vision 19(1), 57–91 (1996)
18. Boykov, Y., Veksler, O., Zabih, R.: Fast approximate energy minimization via graph cuts. IEEE Transactions on Pattern Analysis and Machine Intelligence 23(11), 1222–1239 (2001)
19. Ohta, Y., Kanade, T.: Stereo by intra-and inter-scanline search using dynamic programming. IEEE Transactions on Pattern Analysis and Machine Intelligence (2), 139–154 (1985)
20. Veksler, O.: Stereo correspondence by dynamic programming on a tree. In: IEEE Computer Society Conference on Computer Vision and Pattern Recognition, vol. 2, pp. 384–390 (2005)
21. Feldkamp, L., Davis, L., Kress, J.: Practical cone-beam algorithm. Journal of the Optical Society of America A 1(6), 612–619 (1984)
22. Jia, J., Tang, C.K.: Image repairing: Robust image synthesis by adaptive nd tensor voting. In: IEEE Computer Society Conference on Computer Vision and Pattern Recognition, vol. 1, pp. I–643 (2003)

Adaptive Sampling and Non Linear Reconstruction for Cardiac Magnetic Resonance Imaging

Giuseppe Placidi[1], Danilo Avola[1], Luigi Cinque[2],
Guido Macchiarelli[1], Andrea Petracca[1], and Matteo Spezialetti[1]

[1] Department of Life, Health and Environmental Sciences, University of L'Aquila
Via Vetoio Coppito 2, 67100, L'Aquila, Italy
{giuseppe.placidi,danilo.avola,andrea.petracca,
matteo.spezzialetti}@univaq.it, guido.macchiarelli@cc.univaq.it
[2] Department of Computer Science, Sapienza University
Via Salaria 113, 00198, Rome, Italy
cinque@di.uniroma1.it

Abstract. We show how an adaptive acquisition sequence and a non linear reconstruction can be efficiently used to reconstruct undersampled cardiac MRI data. We demonstrate that, by using the adaptive method and L_0-homotopic minimization, we can reconstruct an image with a number of samples which is very close to the sparsity coefficient of the image without knowing a-priori the sparsity of the image. We highlight two important aspects: 1) how the shape and the cardinality of the starting dataset influence the acquisition/reconstruction process; 2) how well the termination criteria allows to fit the optimal number of coefficients. The method is tested on MRI cardiac images and it is also compared to the weighted Compressed Sensing. All the experiments and results are reported and discussed.

Keywords: adaptive sampling, compressed sensing, non linear reconstruction, MRI, cardiac imaging, image reconstruction, imaging.

1 Introduction

Magnetic Resonance Imaging (MRI) has become a major non-invasive imaging modality due to its ability to provide structural details of human body and additional functional information. Cardiac imaging, in particular, represents one of the challenging applications where MRI can be effectively used. Being cardiac imaging a dynamic application, particular triggering techniques have to be used to avoid motion artifacts. However, acquisition time is usually long if a complete set of k-space trajectories has to be collected [1]. In order to decrease acquisition time, a reduced number of trajectories could be accepted through undersampling.

Undersampling is the violation of the Nyquist's criterion where images are reconstructed by using a number of samples lower than what is theoretically required to obtain a fully sampled image. Some methods [2], [3], [4] presented

Y.J. Zhang and J.M.R.S. Tavares (Eds.): CompIMAGE 2014, LNCS 8641, pp. 24–35, 2014.

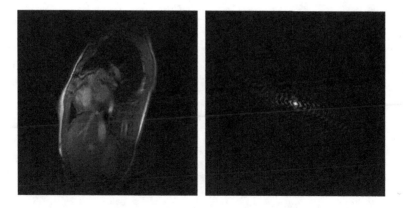

Fig. 1. Original cardiac image (a) and its Fourier coefficients (b) choosen as k-space samples

adaptive acquisition techniques for MRI from projections. One of these [4] defined the entropy function on the power spectrum of the collected projections to evaluate their information content, thus driving the acquisition where data variability is maximum. The choice of the projections was made during the acquisition process; this allowed the reduction of acquisition time, by reducing the scanned directions. A modified Fourier reconstruction algorithm, including an interpolation method [5], was used to reconstruct the image from the sparse set of projections. Other authors [6], [7], [8], [9], [10] presented the theory of Compressed Sensing (CS) and the details of its implementation for rapid MRI and demonstrated that if an image is sparse in some domain, then it can be recovered from randomly undersampled raw data, having supposed that a non linear reconstruction algorithm is used. A well-performant non linear reconstruction algorithm has been proposed in [11] and [12] and it is based on homotopic approximation of the L_0-norm. Non linear reconstruction can also be improved by increasing samples in the central region of the k-space where low frequency terms contain most of the energy of the image, as demonstrated in weighed CS [13], [14].

In the present paper we show how an adaptive acquisition sequence and non linear reconstruction [15], [16] can be efficiently used to reconstruct undersampled cardiac MRI data. Moreover, it is discussed how the adaptive method is effective in collecting the near optimal number of data to reconstruct the unknown image (at least two times lower than the number fixed by CS) and how the termination strategy is capable to stop the acquisition just to the correct number, adapted to the image shape. Numerical simulations are reported and compared with weighted CS to show its performances.

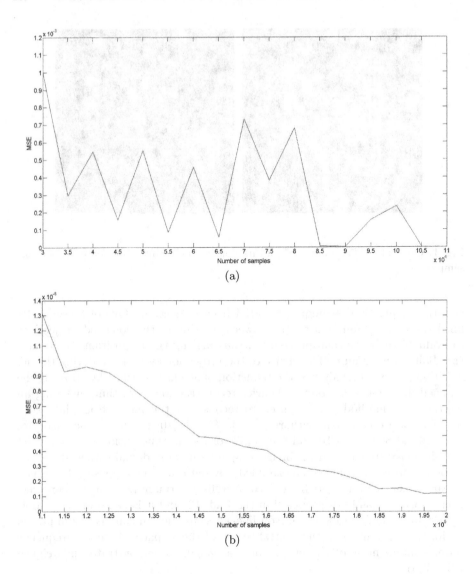

Fig. 2. MSE values calculated on the CS images reconstructed by using increasing datasets from 30000 to 200000 samples (by steps of 5000). The plot is divided in two to appreciate MSE amplitude variations.

2   The Acquisition/Reconstruction Method

The used adaptive acquisition method, described in [15], consists of two phases. Consider the k-space image support as a M × M matrix. In a first phase, the acquisition process collects a set of random Cartesian trajectories, having a Gaussian distribution in a central region of the k-space whose width is a portion p

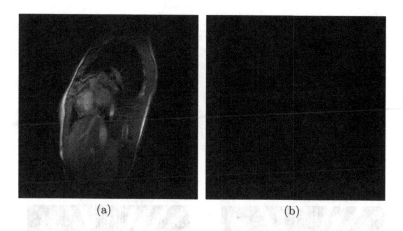

(a)   (b)

Fig. 3. CS reconstruction with 115000 samples (a) and difference between the theoretical image (Figure 1(a)) and CS reconstruction (b)

of the k-space, both along the rows and along the columns. Each trajectory is completely sampled but the number of total trajectories is lower than p. Lines are collected by randomizing the phase-encoding gradient and the columns are collected by reversing the phase-encoding gradient with the frequency-encoding gradient (also in this case, the randomization process involves phase-encoding). The square central region W, whose size is p × p, provides the foundation for the proposed adaptive sampling where an equispaced set of 20 radial projections is calculated and whose entropy is calculated as:

$$E = \frac{1}{q_j} \sum_{i=1}^{q_j} v_i \log v_i \quad \forall j = 1, \cdots, 20 \tag{1}$$

The parameter q_j is the number of measured coefficients in W falling on the j-th radial projection and v_i is the power of the i-th coefficient allowing to the j-th projection. Once calculated the entropy of each projection, the average value is chosen as a threshold value T. A *blade* composed by 9 parallel lines of k-space coefficients is collected around the projections whose entropy is above T (a sort of PROPELLER [17], [18]). Since the adaptive dataset follows the most informative directions, its shape is usually irregular. For this reason, the image is reconstructed by using a non linear reconstruction method. The dataset is suitable for non linear L_0-norm reconstruction [12], [15], in line with the theory of CS [13], [4]. Standard compressed sensing requires that, given an S-sparse image in some domain (in this case the Fourier domain), the number of measured k-space samples, Φf, must be $\Phi f > 2S$ and, experimentally, $3S \leq \Phi f \leq 5S$ is usually chosen (having supposed that 5S is lower than M × M). On the other hand, the reconstruction method described in [11], [12] addresses directly the ideal L_0-norm minimization problem. This method minimizes iteratively continuous

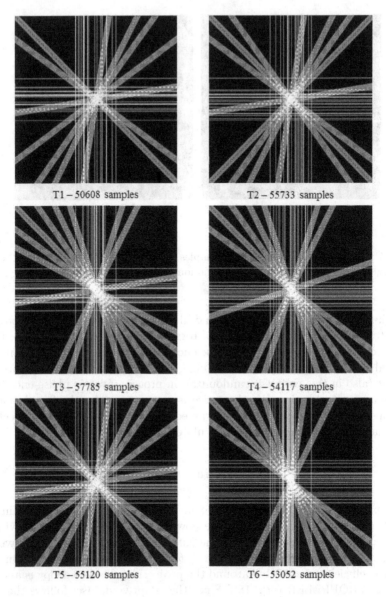

T1 – 50608 samples

T2 – 55733 samples

T3 – 57785 samples

T4 – 54117 samples

T5 – 55120 samples

T6 – 53052 samples

Fig. 4. Adaptive masks for T1:T6 obtained with $\sigma = 0.25$, p = M/4 and 20572 starting samples

approximations of the L_0-norm. Although the achieving of the global minimum is not ensured, the L_0-homotopic minimization method typically allows accurate image reconstruction by using a number of samples which is arbitrarily close to the theoretical minimum number for CS associated with direct L_0 minimization (2S measurements).

3   Numerical Experiments

Our aim is to demonstrate experimentally on cardiac MRI images that, by using the adaptive method and L_0-homotopic minimization, we can reconstruct an image with a number of samples very close to the sparsity coefficient, S, of the image without knowing a-priori the sparsity of the image (the value of S). In order to do that, we show how the weighted CS converges to the theoretical reconstruction, by using the L_0-homotopic minimization strategy, as the number of collected samples increases. Moreover, we show how important are, in the adaptive strategy, shape and cardinality of the starting dataset and how well the termination criterion allows to calculate the optimal number of coefficients. In order to do that, simulations have been performed on cardiac MRI completely sampled 512×512 images. To simulate the MRI acquisition, Fast Fourier Transform (FFT) of each image was performed and the obtained coefficients were treated as the k-space experimentally collected data, assuming that the image and the whole k-space dataset were not known a-priori (we found this procedure useful to compare the undersampled reconstructed images with the complete, theoretical, image). One of these images is reported on Figure 1(a). Figure 1(b) shows its Fourier coefficients (simulating k-space samples). Of the reported image, we also calculated the number of non-zero coefficients with respect to the total number: it was 51993 of a total of 262144 (S = 51993). The treated 25 images of the same subject, corresponding to 25 different phases of the cardiac cycle. Being the treated images very similar each other (the variations consisted in the movements of the heart), and very similar were also their S values (S = 52750 $\pm$ 2745) and the acquisition/reconstruction results, we show and discuss just the results referred to the image reported in Figure 1.

For the reported image, at least 104000 samples would be necessary for CS to obtain a good reconstruction with L_0-homotopic minimization. To show this, we extracted a series of datasets, of different cardinality, for CS reconstruction. The datasets used for weighted CS were extracted by using a Gaussian weight extraction, both along the rows and the columns, in equal parts, in order to allow a more dense sampling in the central region of the k-space with respect to the peripheral zones. The Gaussian distribution function had zero mean and $\sigma = 1$. The number of samples in the extracted series of Gaussian weighted CS subsets gone from 30000 samples to 200000 samples (in step of 5000). These tests served to show how CS converged to the optimal reconstruction and to verify the correctness of the previously estimated sparsity value S, to allow a very good reconstruction, in a mean squared error (MSE) sense, with respect to the completely sampled image. The MSE values, calculated on the CS images reconstructed by using increasing datasets variations, are reported in Figure 2. Figure 2 (splitted in two to better visualize MSE variations) shows a strong non-monotonic behaviour between 30000 and 100000 samples, and a quite regular descendent behaviour above 105000 with reduced improvements above 150000. This demonstrates a sort of saturation, an arrival point, at about 150000 (about 3S). Moreover, at 115000, the MSE function showed a consistent decreasing: this number was very close to the optimal for CS (about 2S) for the given image. However CS, having no information about the image

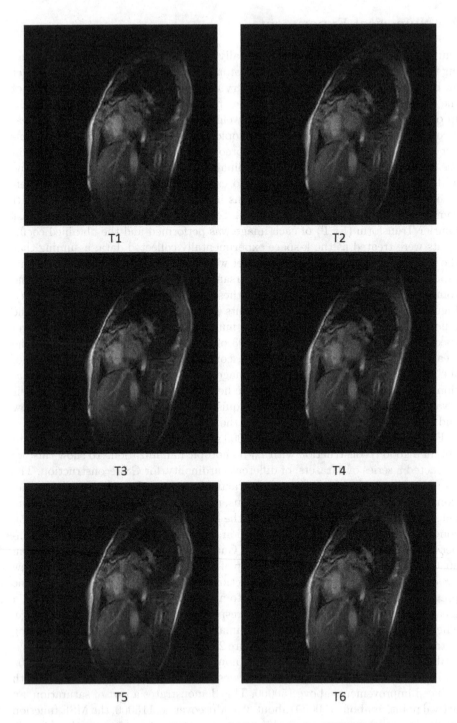

Fig. 5. Images reconstructed with the masks of Figure 4

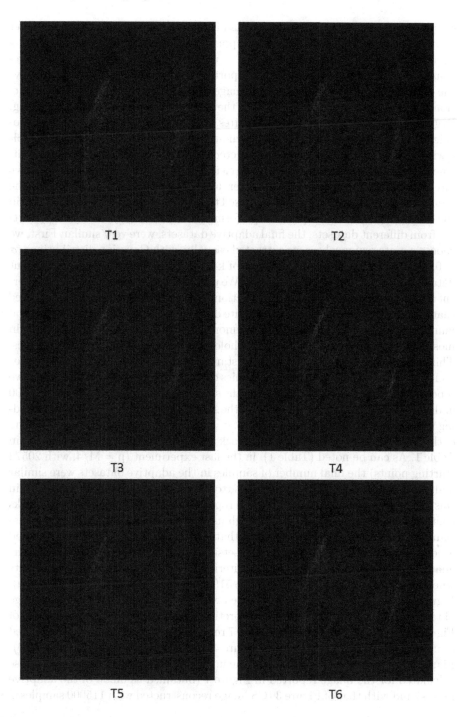

Fig. 6. Images obtained as difference between the theoretical image of Figure 1(a) and the images in Figure 5

shape and, hence, about this number, had no choice than to increase the number of collected coefficients above 2S. It is important to note that, for datasets between 50000 and 70000, besides noise, residual structured aliasing is present. The CS reconstruction with 115000 samples is reported in Figure 3(a). Figure 3(b) shows the difference between the theoretical image (Figure 1(a)) and the CS reconstruction (Figure 3(a)). Figure 3(b) confirms the good reconstruction without aliasing. Regarding the adaptive method, it requires that an initial, cross shaped, set of coefficients has to be used for entropy calculation to drive the acquisition of the following blades [15], [16], adaptively collected in base of their information content. The initial dataset has been proven to be crucial to include all the most informative directions of the image and two parameters are important: its extension (p) and the number of its coefficients. Having supposed that the center of the cross is located in the central region of the k-space, we performed different trials to verify that, starting from different datasets, the final adaptive datasets, were very similar. First, we choose a cross region where we extracted casually, with Gaussian distributions (σ = 0.06, p = M/16), rows and columns of k-space samples to generate 6 different datasets of about 10000 (10640) points. We used these datasets to perform 6 different adaptive acquisitions and reconstructions. From this first experiment, we noted that the final adaptive datasets were quite different both in shape and in the total number of the collected samples, thus demonstrating that the adaptive method, in most cases, was unable to collect the whole set of the most informative samples. This was mainly due to the fact that the starting datasets were too poor of samples and too narrow to capture all the dynamics of the whole image. For this reason, we repeated the experiments by increasing the starting number of coefficients to 20000 and by gradually increasing the width of the starting datasets (σ = 0.06 corresponding to p = M/16, σ = 0.12 and p = M/8, σ = 0.25 and p = M/4). For each setting of the parameters, 6 different starting mask were collected. Results are reported in Table 1. As can be noted (Table 1), in the last experiment (p = M/4, with 20572 starting points) the final number of samples in the adaptive datasets were similar and, more important, they were very close to the calculated value of S. Moreover, in this last example, whose final masks are reported in Figure 4, the obtained masks contained very similar directions, though using different casually collected Gaussian starting masks. This demonstrates that 20572 and p = M/4 can be considered acceptable parameters for the starting sets and that, with such starting sets, the adaptive method and its termination criterion allow to obtain a set of coefficients whose cardinality, 54400, is very close to 51993 (the sparsity value for this image). Figure 5 reports the images reconstructed with the masks of Figure 4. The image obtained as difference between the theoretical image of Figure 1(a) and those of Figure 5 are reported in Figure 6. Figure 7 reports the mask (Figure 7(a)) obtained as union of the 6 adaptive masks of Figure 4 and its reconstruction (Figure 7(b)). Figure 8 indicates the MSE values for the images of Figure 5 as compared to those calculated for the image reported in Figure 7 (obtained as union of the adaptive masks) and with that of Figure 3 (CS image reconstructed with 115000 samples).

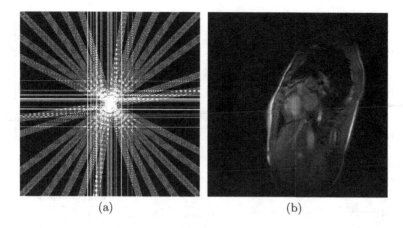

(a)   (b)

Fig. 7. (a) Union mask (79066 samples) obtained as union of the masks T_1:T_6 of Figure 4, (b) image reconstructed by the using mask (a)

Table 1. Number of samples collected for the 6 trials (T_i) performed for each setting of the parameters

σ	p	Starting Points	T1	T2	T3	T4	T5	T6
0.06	M/16	20572	48092	54442	55082	55216	51282	54789
0.12	M/8	20572	54166	54149	56008	50968	58896	58340
0.25	M/4	20572	50608	55733	57785	54117	55120	53052

The adaptive method obtained good reconstructions (as confirmed by MSE values) without residual structured aliasing (as confirmed by analysing the reconstructed images), though it used very small datasets for reconstruction (their cardinality was very close to S). In particular, the obtained results were very similar to those obtained by the union of the adaptive masks or to the CS image obtained with 115000 samples. This demonstrates that the adaptive method allows to reduce the acquisition time of at least a factor of 2 with respect to the CS strategy. Moreover, the adaptive strategy demonstrates that also starting with different sets of samples, the method and the termination criterion allowed to converge to similar datasets, though with some difference. However, the differences included image similarities because all these final adaptive sets included the necessary information to recover good images (the union of the adaptive mask did not improve appreciably the reconstructed image).

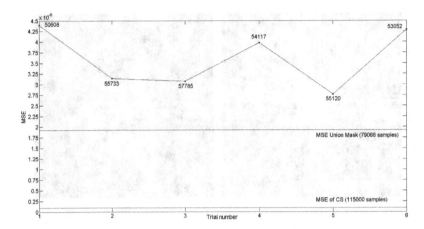

Fig. 8. MSE values for the 6 images of Figure 5, compared to the MSE error for the image in Figure 7 (obtained as the union of the adaptive masks, and composed by 79066 samples) and with the image in Figure 3 (CS image reconstructed with 115000 samples). MSE values for the union mask and CS were constant because each of them was referred to a single dataset.

4 Conclusions and Future Developments

An adaptive acquisition method for MRI has been applied to cardiac MRI images. The results of the proposed method were equivalent to weighted CS, through it used about half of the samples necessary for CS (CS results, for the same number of samples as the adaptive method, had worse MSE and produced residual structured aliasing). Through the performed experiments we demonstrated that with a starting mask obtained with $\sigma = 0.25$ and p = M/4 we obtained acceptable numbers and width for the starting sets. We also demonstrated that, with such starting sets the adaptive method and its termination criterion allowed to obtain a set of coefficients whose average number of coefficients was very close to the sparsity value and the reconstructed images were very similar to the original, completely sampled, image. Besides, it furnished a criterion to estimate the near optimal number of coefficients to obtain a good reconstruction for the given image: this was impossible for CS that, being it a blind method, required that the number of collected data had to be fixed in advance, independently of the image shape. For this reason, the adaptive method allowed to reduce the acquisition time of at least a factor of 2 with respect to the CS strategy: this is very important for cardiac imaging. In the future we plan to apply the proposed method on volumetric MRI datasets and to use spatial/temporal similarities and information to reduce further the number of collected samples.

References

1. O'sullivan, J.: A fast sinc function gridding algorithm for fourier inversion in computer tomography. IEEE Transactions on Medical Imaging 4(4), 200–207 (1985)
2. Placidi, G., Alecci, M., Sotgiu, A.: ω-space adaptive acquisition technique for magnetic resonance imaging from projections. Journal of Magnetic Resonance 143(1), 197–207 (2000)
3. Placidi, G., Alecci, M., Sotgiu, A.: Theory of adaptive acquisition method for image reconstruction from projections and application to epr imaging. Journal of Magnetic Resonance, Series A 108(1), 50–57 (1995)
4. Placidi, G.: MRI: essentials for innovative technologies. CRC Press (2012)
5. Placidi, G., Alecci, M., Colacicchi, S., Sotgiu, A.: Fourier reconstruction as a valid alternative to filtered back projection in iterative applications: implementation of fourier spectral spatial epr imaging. Journal of Magnetic Resonance 134(2), 280–286 (1998)
6. Candès, E.J., Romberg, J., Tao, T.: Robust uncertainty principles: Exact signal reconstruction from highly incomplete frequency information. IEEE Transactions on Information Theory 52(2), 489–509 (2006)
7. Donoho, D.L.: Compressed sensing. IEEE Transactions on Information Theory 52(4), 1289–1306 (2006)
8. Lustig, M., Donoho, D., Pauly, J.M.: Sparse mri: The application of compressed sensing for rapid mr imaging. Magnetic Resonance in Medicine 58(6), 1182–1195 (2007)
9. Elad, M.: Sparse and redundant representations: from theory to applications in signal and image processing. Springer (2010)
10. Usman, M., Prieto, C., Schaeffter, T., Batchelor, P.: k-t group sparse: A method for accelerating dynamic mri. Magnetic Resonance in Medicine 66(4), 1163–1176 (2011)
11. Trzasko, J.D., Manduca, A.: A fixed point method for homotopic l0-minimization with application to mr image recovery. In: Medical Imaging, International Society for Optics and Photonics, pp. 69130F–69130F (2008)
12. Trzasko, J., Manduca, A.: Highly undersampled magnetic resonance image reconstruction via homotopic-minimization. IEEE Transactions on Medical imaging 28(1), 106–121 (2009)
13. Lustig, M.: Sparse MRI. ProQuest (2008)
14. Wang, Z., Arce, G.R.: Variable density compressed image sampling. IEEE Transactions on Image Processing 19(1), 264–270 (2010)
15. Ciancarella, L., Avola, D., Placidi, G.: Adaptive sampling and reconstruction for sparse magnetic resonance imaging. In: Computational Modeling of Objects Presented in Images, pp. 115–130. Springer (2014)
16. Ciancarella, L., Avola, D., Marcucci, E., Placidi, G.: A hybrid sampling strategy for sparse magnetic resonance imaging. Computational Modelling of Objects Represented in Images III: Fundamentals, Methods and Applications, 285 (2012)
17. Pipe, J.G., et al.: Motion correction with propeller mri: application to head motion and free-breathing cardiac imaging. Magnetic Resonance in Medicine 42(5), 963–969 (1999)
18. Arfanakis, K., Tamhane, A.A., Pipe, J.G., Anastasio, M.A.: k-space undersampling in propeller imaging. Magnetic Resonance in Medicine 53(3), 675–683 (2005)

A Feasibility Study on Kinematic Feature Extraction from the Human Interventricular Septum toward Hypertension Classification

Jing Xu[1], Jia Wu[2], Bahram Notghi[1], Marc Simon[3,4], and John C. Brigham[1,4]

[1] Department of Civil and Environmental Engineering,
University of Pittsburgh, USA
[2] Department of Radiology, University of Pennsylvania, USA
[3] Cardiovascular Institute, School of Medicine, University of Pittsburgh, USA
[4] Department of Bioengineering, University of Pittsburgh, USA
brigham@pitt.edu

Abstract. The current work is intended to present the first steps in examining the feasibility of improving the diagnosis and understanding of cardiovascular diseases, particularly pulmonary hypertension (PH), by analyzing the shape of the right side of the interventricular septum. Although there clearly exists a connection between the septum shape and PH, there is still no quantitative and clear understanding of how this shape change relates to the disease state. Therefore, there exists a great need for techniques that are capable of quantitatively analyzing variations in septum shape and to perform a study that analyzes these shape changes relating to various states of PH. Such advancements could directly improve the diagnostic process for this deadly disease, including early detection overcoming the early nonspecific symptoms of PH and better understanding the progression of the disease by identifying behaviors that relate to either beneficial or deleterious cardiac adaptation. The details of a potential shape analysis approach for the interventricular septum is presented, including a surface parameterization approach and direct application of proper orthogonal decomposition for feature extraction. To show the feasibility of implementing this approach, the decomposition of a single patient's interventricular septum at several phases in a single cardiac cycle is shown. The results show the capability to obtain distinct features of the septal wall shape in a generally applicable way, and provide a path for future large-scale analyses of groups of patients.

1 Introduction

Pulmonary hypertension (PH) is a critical cardio-pulmonary illness, which has often been observed to induce substantial deleterious changes to the human cardiac (especially the left and right ventricle) shape and function [1,2,3]. One particular observation about cardiac function changes due to PH is increasingly abnormal interventricular septal motion as the pressure in right ventricle (RV) increases and the the disease progresses. Furthermore, several previous studies

Y.J. Zhang and J.M.R.S. Tavares (Eds.): CompIMAGE 2014, LNCS 8641, pp. 36–47, 2014.

have noted certain specific aspects of the changes in the interventricular septum due to pressure changes [4,5,6,7]. Beyar, et al. [8] showed that the increasing left ventricle (LV) end-diastolic pressure does not lead to any noticeable changes in the shape of septum, however, when the RV has a similarly high end-diastolic pressure level, the septum moved to the left side and there were clear changes to the curvature. Mori, et al. [9] investigated the clinical and hemodynamic implication of the interventricular septal motion in patients with PH through echocardiography. It was shown that there were two specific motions of the interventricular septum detected by M-mode echocardiography: early systolic anterior motion (Type A) and early diastolic posterior motion (Type B). The results further showed that the type A motion was more morbid clinically than motion (B). Maffessanti, et al. [10] went even further in the analysis by reconstructing dynamic three-dimensional (3D) left ventricular endocardial surfaces based on cardiac magnetic resonance (CMR) imaging and analyzed the septal wall curvature throughout the cardiac cycle and considered the relationship of this metric to PH.

Although work exists (such as the above-referenced literature) analyzing the relationship between the interventricular septum and hypertension, no specific feature has been identified yet that precisely discerns the state of the heart function as relates to PH. However, developments continue to be made in medical imaging techniques and computer-aided diagnosis (CAD) to aid physicians in both observing the nature of disease-related shape changes in biological structures and identifying diagnostic relationships between a shape change and a particular pathology. One such shape analysis framework has already been proposed by the authors to detect and better understand the onset and progression of PH by analyzing the kinematic features of the right ventricle endocardial surface [11,12]. Such an approach allows for data-driven automatic extraction of the most relevant (in a certain sense) features of a digitized geometry, and could potentially expose features that are significant in better understanding the relationship between the septum shape and PH.

The present study is intended to display the feasibility of a generally applicable approach to use 3D statistical shape analysis to analyze the shape of the human interventricular septum from cardiac imaging data and to show how this approach could be applied to analyze the right side of a human interventricular septum endocardial surface. In particular, the present study is an extension of the previous work by the authors [11,12], which examined the entire right ventricle endocardial surface, to explore the necessary changes in the methods and potential results that can be extracted by exclusively examining the septal wall portion of the right ventricle. The approach is anatomically consistent, allows direct comparison across populations of individuals, and can potentially provide new metrics to improve the diagnosis and understanding of PH (unique to what could be extracted by analyzing the right ventricle as a whole). Section 2 presents the statistical shape analysis methods proposed and the imaging dataset obtained from cardiac computed tomography (CT) used to display the details of the process. Section 3 shows the results of the analysis of this example single human right ventricle at several phases in a cardiac cycle. Lastly, Section 4 discusses the conclusions and potential future directions for this research effort.

2   Data and Analysis Methods

The following describes the workflow of the statistical shape analysis methods applied in the present work to obtain kinematic features of the interventricular septum endocardial surface (see [11,12] for additional details of these shape analysis methods):

1. Segment the image stacks to obtain 3D surfaces (i.e., point clouds) of the RV at multiple phases in the cardiac cycle and/or for multiple patients.
2. Smooth the surfaces of the RV with a standard Gaussian filter and convert the surfaces into 3D meshes suitable for numerical analysis (e.g., finite element meshes).
3. Topologically map (i.e., parameterize) every septum portion of each 3D mesh to a unit hemisphere through a harmonic mapping approach.
4. Apply the proper orthogonal decomposition method to the complete set of septum shape functions (i.e., topologically mapped septa) to determine and rank a set of kinematic features (i.e., modes and corresponding transient coefficients from decomposition).

2.1   Imaging Data

In order to display the details of each step in the analysis process, the details will be discussed within the context of one example imaging dataset. This work utilized a clinically obtained set of ECG-gated multislice cardiac CT images, which are from a research study about regional RV structural and functional adaptation to PH as reported in [13]. Scan parameters were as follows: kV 120; mA approximately 400 without ECG-dose modulation; rotation time 350 ms; pitch dependent on heart rate; 1.25 mm slice thickness (for 16 detector scanner); kV 120, mA approximately 500 with ECG-dose modulation adjusted to peak at 6580% RR interval; rotation time 350 ms; pitch dependent on heart rate; 0.625 mm slice thickness (for 64 detector scanner). To examine the capabilities of the proposed approach, a single patient with normal hemodynamics (i.e., pulmonary arterial pressure less than 25 $mmHg$) was selected from the study for analysis. The imaging set for the patient included nine time frames (i.e., snapshots) over one entire cardiac cycle, distributed approximately uniformly from end diastole to end diastole during a single breath hold, all of which were analyzed through the following approach.

2.2   Segmentation and Mesh Generation

Since there were nine unique time frames in the image set, there were nine unique 3D surface descriptions of the RV shape that needed to be segmented for analysis. This was by far the most laborious portion of the described workflow, in that the RV endocardial surface (RVES) needed to be manually segmented from each image in the CT image stacks and for each of the nine phases, then the slices could be interpolated to create a set of nine 3D shapes. Segmentation was done manually to ensure that the most anatomically consistent representation of the RV shape could be obtained at each phase. After initial segmentation and interpolation each RVES shape was smoothed using a standard recursive and discrete Gaussian filter within the commercial medical image processing software Simpleware [1]. After this processing each of the 3D surfaces could be viewed as a continuous, linearly-interpolated, mesh-based representation.

2.3   Surface Parameterization

To parameterize each RV interventricular septum so that they could each be consistently quantitatively compared to each other, a variation of a harmonic topological mapping approach was applied to each RVES shape. A harmonic mapping should be capable of being applied to any 3D non-overlapping surface and can be simply thought of as a parameterization method that satisfies Laplace's equation for each new parameter [14,15,16]. Previous work showed that the 3D closed RVES shape could be consistently mapped using a harmonic mapping to the surface of a unit sphere (i.e., each point on the RVES was mapped to a unique value of latitude and longitude) [11,12]. Similarly, for the present work, since the interventricular septum is only a portion of the RVES (and an open surface), it was assumed that each point on the septum could be mapped to a unique value of latitude (θ) and longitude (ϕ) on a hemisphere (rather than a complete sphere), which could be determined through the harmonic mapping with

$$\nabla^2 \theta(\boldsymbol{x}) = 0, \ \forall \boldsymbol{x} \in \Omega_k, \qquad \nabla^2 \phi(\boldsymbol{x}) = 0, \ \forall \boldsymbol{x} \in \Omega_k, \qquad (1)$$

where $\Omega_k \subset \Re^3$ is the kth 3D continuous non-overlapping surface domain of the RVES.

Then, it is only necessary to provide sufficient boundary conditions for the latitude and longitude on the RVES domain when solving (1) to ensure that the septum (alone) can be extracted in a anatomically consistent and comparable format. Two "poles" (two points) are required to uniquely define the latitude and two "datelines" were used to uniquely define the longitude for each septum, such that

$$\theta = 0, \ \forall \boldsymbol{x} \in P_n, \quad \theta = \pi, \ \forall \boldsymbol{x} \in P_s, \quad \phi = 0, \ \forall \boldsymbol{x} \in \Gamma_d, \quad \phi = \pi, \ \forall \boldsymbol{x} \in \Gamma_e, \qquad (2)$$

where P_n is the point on the RVES designated as the north pole, P_s is the point on the RVES designated as the south pole, Γ_d is the line on the RVES designated as the dateline, and Γ_e is the line on the RVES designated as the east dateline. In addition, to ensure anatomical consistency these boundary conditions should correspond to unique and consistently identifiable anatomical features on the

---

[1] www.simpleware.com

RVES. As shown in Fig. 1 for an example RVES mesh, for the present study the dateline was selected as the anterior border between the free wall and septum with endpoints at the intersection with the pulmonary valve and apex, with these intersections also serving as the north and south poles, respectively, and the east dateline was selected as the posterior border between the free wall and septum. The standard finite element method was applied for the present study to solve

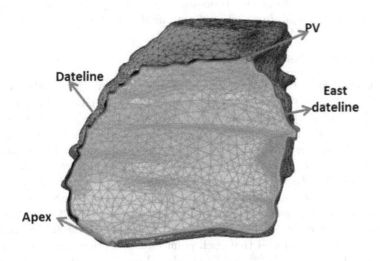

Fig. 1. Representative example of an RVES with each of the harmonic mapping boundary condition features labeled

(1) given these anatomical features as boundary conditions for each RVES in the dataset. Fig. 2 shows an example of the latitude and longitude mapping results for an RVES from the set. In addition, Fig. 3 shows the original shape of the interventricular septum extracted from the RVES and the location of each of the nodes and elements of that septum mesh mapped to the θ-ϕ parameterization domain. Each of the nine shapes in the dataset were similarly mapped to obtain a unique description of each interventricular septum shape (i.e., each coordinate on the septum surface) in terms of $\theta \in [0, \pi]$ and $\phi \in [0, \pi]$.

2.4   Statistical Decomposition

Lastly, the shapes were decomposed by applying the Proper Orthogonal Decomposition (POD) method [17,18] to derive the fundamental shape features from the set of parameterized 3D surfaces, where the set of surfaces can be represented as 3D functional representations of shape after topological mapping, $\{\boldsymbol{x}_k(\theta, \phi)\}_{k=1}^{9}$. Simply put, the main objective of the standard POD approach used for this work is to obtain the m fundamental features, $\{\boldsymbol{v}_i(\theta, \phi)\}_{i=1}^{m}$, that

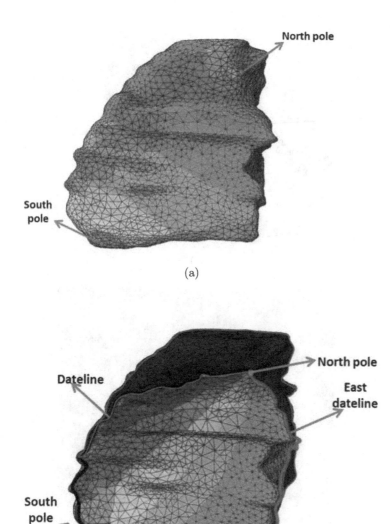

Fig. 2. Example topological mapping results for the (a) latitude and (b) longitude values for a RVES

can optimally (in some sense) describe the set of shapes, such that any shape (i.e., the kth septum shape) in the set could be described as

$$\boldsymbol{x}_k(\theta, \phi) \approx \sum_{i=1}^{m} a_{ki}\boldsymbol{v}_i(\theta, \phi), \tag{3}$$

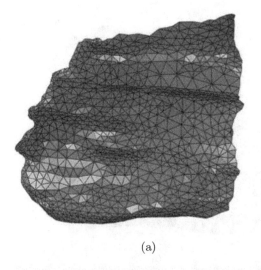

(a)

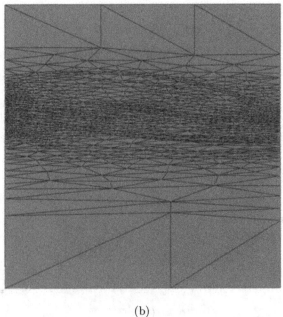

(b)

Fig. 3. Example of (a) the 3D mesh for the original segmented RV interventricular septum and (b) the corresponding mesh topologically mapped to the θ-ϕ domain

where the coefficient a_{ki} is defined as the modal coefficient that represents the contribution of the ith POD mode to the kth interventricular shape. Then, the optimal set of modes (i.e., POD basis) can be obtained by solving the minimization problem

$$\underset{\{v_i(\theta,\phi)\}_{i=1}^{m}}{\text{Minimize}} \left\langle \|x_k(\theta,\phi) - x_k^*(\theta,\phi)\|_{L_2}^2 \right\rangle \tag{4}$$

where $x_k^*(\theta, \phi)$ is the best approximation to the kth shape for the basis (i.e., the projection), $\langle . \rangle$ is the averaging operator, and $\|.\|_{L_2}$ is the standard L_2-norm. Therefore, the POD basis is that which best approximates the original set of shapes in an optimal average L_2 sense.

Applying the method of snapshots [17] the optimal set of modes can be calculated deterministically through the following eigenvalue problem

$$\frac{1}{n} \sum_{k=1}^{n} A_{jk} C_k^{(i)} = \lambda^{(i)} C_j^{(i)},$$ (5)

where

$$A_{jk} = \int_0^\pi \int_0^\pi x_j \cdot x_k \sin(\theta) d\theta d\phi,$$ (6)

and

$$C_k^{(i)} = \int_0^\pi \int_0^\pi x_k \cdot v_i \sin(\theta) d\theta d\phi.$$ (7)

Finally, after solving the eigenvalue problem, the optimal basis can be calculated with

$$v_i(\theta, \phi) = \frac{1}{\lambda^{(i)} n} \sum_{k=1}^{n} x_k(\theta, \phi) C_k^{(i)}.$$ (8)

Applying this method the optimal modes can be obtained, and these modes can be ranked in terms of importance (i.e., relative contribution to the set of shapes) by the relative eigenvalue. In other words, the modes corresponding to higher eigenvalues are more important to the representation of the shape set. As an added benefit, the modes corresponding to the lowest eigenvalues are typically associated with noise, which can then be removed. In practice, the modes themselves could provide a physical understanding of the fundamental aspects of shape and kinematics of the biological structure being analyzed. For classification purposes, the highest energy modes are chosen, with a typical heuristic being to choose the highest energy modes that contain just over 99% of the total eigenvalue sum of the set, and the coefficients of these modes for each surface in the set are used to define and classify the population.

3   Decomposition Results for the Interventricular Septum Shape Set

After applying the topological mapping and the POD approach to the set of nine interventricular septa, the shape of the septum could then be analyzed in terms of the POD modal shapes themselves (i.e., the fundamental features of this particular shape) and the modal coefficients over the cardiac cycle (i.e., how each mode contributes to the shape of the septum over the cardiac cycle). To show how the modes contribute to the shape of the septum Fig. 4 shows the contributions of the POD modes to the reconstruction of the septum shape at end diastole and end systole. Clearly, the first mode (i.e., the most significant

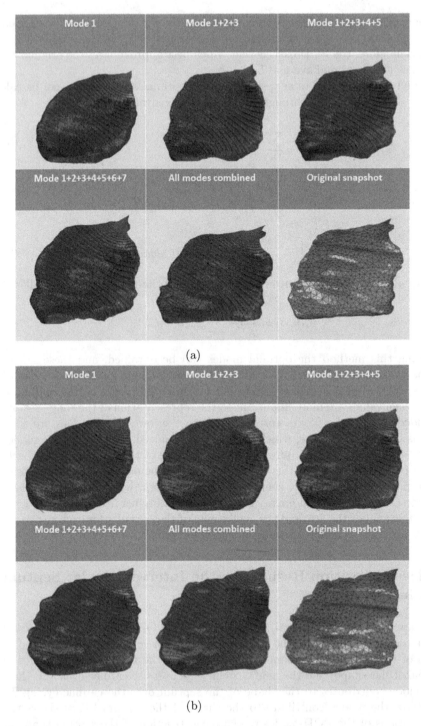

(a)

(b)

Fig. 4. Modal reconstruction of the septum at (a) end diastole and (b) end systole

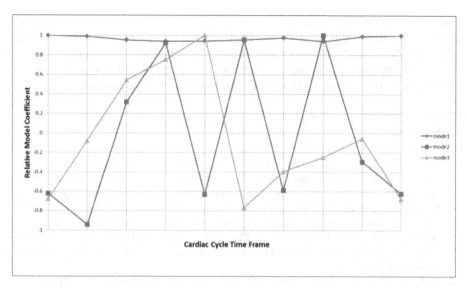

Fig. 5. Relative modal coefficient values for first three POD modes of the interventricular septum over the cardiac cycle, from end diastole to end diastole

mode to the reconstruction) represents the smoothed-out average shape of the septum over the cardiac cycle. Then the latter modes (the second mode and higher) represent the more subtle shape variations that occur throughout the cardiac cycle, with the very high modes likely representative of noise in the shape dataset. These observations are further reinforced when considering the relative amplitude of the modal coefficients over the cardiac cycle. Fig. 5 shows the relative modal coefficient value for the first three highest energy modes of the septum over the cardiac cycle (from end diastole to end diastole). It can be seen that the first mode stays nearly constant over the cardiac cycle, in some sense representing the base shape of the septum, while the second and third modes vary significantly throughout the cardiac cycle and appear to capture the finer-scale variations as the heart beats.

4   Conclusions and Future Directions

An approach was presented to obtain the fundamental shape features of the human interventricular septum from untagged medical images throughout the cardiac cycle that is generally applicable, in particular being applicable to a multi-patient set. The stages of the approach were presented, including a topological mapping technique and a direct application of the POD method. The feasibility of this approach was confirmed with the application to decompose the septum of one patient, with images acquired for that patient at nine phases over a cardiac cycle. The decomposition results show the capability to obtain distinct and meaningful features of the septal wall shape in a generally applicable way, and provide a path for future large-scale analyses of groups of patients. In future work a patient set will be decomposed following the format described herein, and then the modal coefficients will be used to define new and unique patient clusterings and potentially build classifiers to understand and better predict the adaptation of the human right ventricle to pulmonary hypertension.

References

1. Simonneau, G., Robbins, I.M., Beghetti, M., Channick, R.N., Delcroix, M., Denton, C.P., Elliott, C.G., Gaine, S.P., Gladwin, M.T., Jing, Z.C., Krowka, M.J., Langleben, D., Nakanishi, N., Souza, R.: Updated clinical classification of pulmonary hypertension. Journal of the American College of Cardiology 54(suppl.1), 43–54 (2009); Proceedings of the 4th World Symposium on Pulmonary Hypertension.
2. Hyduk, A., Croft, J.B., Ayala, C., Zheng, K., Zheng, Z.J., Mensah, G.A.: Pulmonary hypertension surveillance— united states, 1980–2002. MMWR Surveill. Summ. 54, 1–28 (2005)
3. Rich, S., Dantzker, D.R., Ayres, S.M., Bergofsky, E.H., Brundage, B.H., Detre, K.M., Fishman, A.P., Goldring, R.M., Groves, B.M., Koerner, S.K.: Primary pulmonary hypertension—a national prospective study. Ann. Intern. Med. 107, 216–223 (1987)
4. King, M., Braun, H., Goldblatt, A., Liberthson, R., Weyman, A.: Interventricular septal configuration as a predictor of right ventricular systolic hypertension in children: a cross-sectional echocardiographic study. Circulation 68(1), 68–75 (1983)
5. López-Candales, A., Rajagopalan, N., Kochar, M., Gulyasy, B., Edelman, K.: Systolic eccentricity index identifies right ventricular dysfunction in pulmonary hypertension. International Journal of Cardiology 129(3), 424–426 (2008)
6. Nelson, G.S., Sayed-Ahmed, E.Y., Kroeker, C.A.G., Sun, Y.H., Keurs, H.E.D.J.T., Shrive, N.G., Tyberg, J.V.: Compression of interventricular septum during right ventricular pressure loading. American Journal of Physiology - Heart and Circulatory Physiology 280, H2639–H2648 (2001)
7. Roeleveld, R.J., Marcus, J.T., Faes, T.J., Gan, T.J., Boonstra, A., Postmus, P.E., Vonk-Noordegraaf, A.: Interventricular septal configuration at mr imaging and pulmonary arterial pressure in pulmonary hypertension. Radiology, 710–717 (2005)
8. Beyar, R., Dong, S.J., Smith, E.R., Belenkie, I., Tyberg, J.V.: Ventricular interaction and septal deformation: a model compared with experimental data. The American Journal of Physiology (1993)
9. Mori, S., Nakatani, S., Kanzaki, H., Yamagata, K., Take, Y., Matsuura, Y., Kyotani, S., Nakanishi, N., Kitakaze, M.: Patterns of the interventricular septal motion can predict conditions of patients with pulmonary hypertension. Journal of the American Society of Echocardiography 21(4), 386–393 (2008)
10. Maffessanti, F., Sciancalepore, M.A., Patel, A.R., Gomberg-Maitland, M., Chandra, S., Caiani, E., Freed, B., Lang, R., Mor-Avi, V.: Three-dimensional analysis of septal curvature from cardiac magnetic resonance images for the evaluation of severity of pulmonary hypertension. In: Computing in Cardiology, pp. 801–804 (September 2010)
11. Wu, J., Wang, Y., Simon, M.A., Brigham, J.C.: A new approach to kinematic feature extraction from the human right ventricle for classification of hypertension: a feasibility study. Physics in Medicine and Biology 57(23), 7905–7922 (2012)

12. Wu, J., Wang, Y., Simon, M.A., Sacks, M.A., Brigham, J.C.: A new computational framework for anatomically consistent 3d statistical shape analysis with clinical imaging applications. Computer Methods in Biomechanics and Biomedical Engineering: Imaging and Visualization 1(1), 13–27 (2013)
13. Simon, M.A., Deible, C., Mathier, M.A., Lacomis, J., Goitein, O., Shroff, S.G., Pinsky, M.R.: Phenotyping the right ventricle in patients with pulmonary hypertension. Clinical and Translational Science 2(4), 294–299 (2009)
14. Floater, M.S., Hormann, K.: Surface parameterization: a tutorial and survey. In: Advances in Multiresolution for Geometric Modelling, pp. 157–186. Springer (2005)
15. Hormann, K., Lévy, B., Sheffer, A.: Mesh parameterization: Theory and practice video files associated with this course are available from the citation page. In: ACM SIGGRAPH 2007 Courses, SIGGRAPH 2007. ACM, New York (2007)
16. Sheffer, A., Praun, E., Rose, K.: Mesh parameterization methods and their applications. Found. Trends. Comput. Graph. Vis. 2(2), 105–171 (2006)
17. Aquino, W.: An object-oriented framework for reduced-order models using proper orthogonal decomposition (pod). Computer Methods in Applied Mechanics and Engineering 196(41-44), 4375–4390 (2007)
18. Brigham, J.C., Aquino, W.: Inverse viscoelastic material characterization using pod reduced-order modeling in acoustic–structure interaction. Computer Methods in Applied Mechanics and Engineering 198(9-12), 893–903 (2009)

Analysis of Cardiac MRI Based Regional Timing of Left Ventricular Mechanical Contraction as a Biomarker for Electrical Dyssynchrony in Heart-Failure Patients

Prahlad G. Menon[1,2,3,*], Srilakshmi M. Adhyapak[4], and V. Rao Parachuri[5]

[1] Sun Yat-sen University - Carnegie Mellon University (SYSU-CMU)
Joint Institute of Engineering, Sun Yat-sen University, Guangdong, China
[2] SYSU-CMU, Shunde International Joint Research Institute, Guangdong, China
[3] QuantMD, LLC, Pittsburgh, PA, USA
[4] St. John's Medical College Hospital, Bangalore, India
[5] Narayana Hrudayalaya Institute of Medical Sciences, Bangalore, India
pgmenon@andrew.cmu.edu

Abstract. Cardiac resynchronization therapy (CRT) is relatively new treatment for symptoms associated with congestive heart failure (HF) which is achieved by simultaneously pacing both the left and right ventricles of the heart. Current clinical guidelines support the use of CRT in moderate or severe HF patients with a left ventricular (LV) ejection fraction of ≤35% and a prolonged QRS interval (≥120 ms), characteristic of electrical dyssynchrony. Several clinical studies have reported high non-response rates to CRT and have questioned the accuracy of currently practiced patient-selection criteria for this therapy. In this study we demonstrate the translational application of medical imaging biomarkers of phase of ventricular contraction quantified from cardiac magnetic resonance (CMR) imaging, in defining correlations between mechanical dyssynchrony (MD) and electrical dyssynchrony, in an effort to identify a means to relate the best-practices for positioning an LV pacing lead (viz. localized to the latest mechanically activating, non-scarred regions) with the clinical guidelines for electrical dyssynchrony in a cohort of heart failure (HF). We retrospectively examine two cohorts of HF patients with different electrical conduction characteristics: a) Left bundle branch block (LBBB) and wide QRS interval – defining the Class I indication for CRT – characteristic of electrical dyssynchrony as evidenced from electrocardiograms; and b) HF with large antero-apical aneurysms and scarring but narrow QRS interval. Indices of mean and standard deviation in phase of regional contraction were examined across the entire LV of each patient, including scarred territories. Additionally, contraction timing delay between the septal and lateral cardiac walls were also examined in the basal LV territories which were free from adverse remodelling and scar. The results from this pilot study show that MD assessment using CMR imaging based biomarkers of phase of LV contraction is highly accurate in predicting electrical dyssynchrony defined by QRS duration ≥150 ms, with receiver operator characteristics evidencing close to perfect accuracy when MD was analyzed in LV territories which excluded scar.

Keywords: Cardiac Resynchronization Therapy, Cardiac Magnetic Resonance Imaging, Heart Failure, Fourier Analysis, Left Ventricular Contraction.

---

* Corresponding author.

Y.J. Zhang and J.M.R.S. Tavares (Eds.): CompIMAGE 2014, LNCS 8641, pp. 48–56, 2014.
© Springer International Publishing Switzerland 2014

1   Introduction

Cardiac resynchronization therapy (CRT) is a cutting-edge new treatment for symptoms associated with congestive heart failure (HF) with discoordinated contraction due to intra-ventricular conduction delay which is achieved by simultaneously pacing both the left and right ventricles of the heart. CRT has been shown to improve the rate of survival, quality of life, exercise capacity, and functional status in patients with electrical dyssynchrony as evidenced by a prolonged QRS interval in electrocardiograms (ECG) [1, 2]. CRT is thought to improve the left ventricular (LV) ejection fraction and functional status by minimizing regional LV conduction delay, reducing mitral regurgitation and LV reverse remodeling, benefiting moderate-to-severe heart failure that are resistant to optimal medical therapy. Current guidelines support the use of CRT in patients with an ejection fraction $\leq 35\%$ having   moderate or severe heart failure i.e. New York Heart Association (NYHA) Class III or IV, and a prolonged QRS interval ($\geq$120 ms) [3], but not patients with narrow QRS intervals [4]. Despite encouraging results, cumulative evidence shows that only a fraction of patients exhibit a favourable clinical or echocardiographic response to CRT [5] with more than 30% of the patients in large clinical trials like MIRACLE (Multicenter InSync Randomized Clinical Evaluation) and the MIRACLE-ICD (Multicenter In-Sync Implantable Cardioverter Defibrillator) [6] having fulfilled the aforementioned clinical inclusion criteria has encouraged the research of novel indices and strategies that can reliably predict response to CRT.

LV conduction delay is manifested by a prolonged QRS complex duration and is common among patients with systolic dysfunction and HF. It is associated with an increased prevalence of mechanical dyssynchrony (MD). However, MD may also be caused by scar-related adverse remodeling of the LV which occurs as a result of myocardial infarction (MI). Such LV remodeling usually begins within the first few hours after an MI and may progress over time with abnormal myocardial wall thinning (termed infarct expansion) and dilatation of the necrotic zone. It has been shown that scar burden is linked to CRT response and ideally, patients with an LV scar burden < 15% show optimal response to CRT [7], however, MD caused by remodeling or scarring may not be concordant with electrical dyssynchrony in terms of QRS duration on the 12 lead ECG. The distinction between MD resulting from scarred and remodelled LV territories as opposed to MD resulting from inherent conduction dyssynchrony is important to study in order to better identify likely responders to CRT. Scar-induced mechanical discoordination in contraction could potentially confound statistics in regard to the efficacy of MD in the prediction of CRT response. In fact, recent reports from the multi-center PROSPECT (Predictors of Response to CRT) trial indicate that no single LV MD parameter could accurately predict response to CRT [8]. Moreover, a significant percentage of the patients showing an improvement in clinical status did not exhibit improvements in LV systolic function or reverse LV remodelling (i.e reduction in LV volumes).

Therefore, the purpose of this study is to examine the potential role of MD based on a comprehensive MD analysis made by regional quantification of LV contraction timing, starting with cardiac magnetic resonance (CMR) imaging of endocardial motion, in identifying the relationship between mechanical and electrical dyssynchrony in these two distinct groups viz.: a) HF patients with left bundle branch block (LBBB) and wide QRS intervals – characteristic of electrical dyssynchrony as evidenced from ECG data; and b) HF patients with large antero-apical aneurysms and scarring but having narrow QRS interval. The overarching goal of this study is to help in identifying a bridge between the established best-practices for intra-operative positioning an LV pacing lead localized to regions of non-scarred regions of latest mechanical activation [9-12] and the clinical guidelines for patient-selection based on electrical dyssynchrony.

The methods followed in this study have been organized into sections which begin with a detailed delineation our strategy for quantifying MD using fundamental frequency component analysis of time-varying endocardial motion data across the entire LV of each patient extracted from CMR imaging. This is followed up with methods for rendering results in cardiologist-friendly formats as well as statistical analysis for binary classification of patients in our study cohort by QRS interval using our quantified metrics of MD. Finally, we compare the classification efficacy of our MD indices computed across the entire LV (including scarred territories) against a metric for contraction timing delay between septal and lateral myocardial walls in only unscarred LV regions and comment upon the clinical implications of this study in terms the effect of scar on analysis of MD.

2   Methods

2.1   Imaging Data

Our study cohort included 15 HF patient imaging datasets which were retrospectively acquired after local IRB approval and patient consent. ECG-gated, short-axis, steady state free precession (SSFP) cine CMR image sequences (8mm thick slices, 20 phases) of: a) 3 patients that presented with HF and left bundle branch block (LBBB) having wide QRS intervals (QRS> 150 ms), defining the Class I indication for CRT; as well as b) 12 patients that presented with congestive HF following transmural myocardial infarctions and had extensive scarring as well as adverse antero-apical remodeling but narrow QRS intervals (mean QRS duration 124±23 ms), were analyzed for regional mechanical contraction. Further, the extent of myocardial scarring in these patients was quantified using late gadolinium enhancement (LGE) CMR data, which made it possible to objectively demarcate scar in short axis cardiac slices.

2.2   Assessment of Intra-ventricular Dyssynchrony

ECG-gated short-axis steady state free precession (SSFP) cine cardiac MR (CMR) image sequences (8mm thick slices, 20 phases) were obtained after local IRB approval and patient consent, as DICOM image stacks. 3D surface contours of the inner blood-contacting wall and outer wall of the LV endocardium were semi-automatically segmented, in MedViso Segment (Medviso AB, Lund, Sweden) [13] at each cardiac phase. An in-house Matlab code (The Mathworks Inc., Natick, MA) was developed to track endocardial motion as identified from these segmented contours and report regional endocardial displacement between consecutive cardiac phases. Endocardial displacement was approximated as the difference between regional endocardial radius and the maximum regional radius achieved over the cardiac cycle. This radial endocardial displacement was studied in each slice level with respect to a fixed centroid located inside of the LV, pre-computed based on the three-dimensional segmentation of the LV at end-diastole. The endocardial displacement results were averaged within circumferentially divided segmental regions of the endocardium, in each short-axis slice level, represented cumulatively as a polar plot, similar to the American Heart Association (AHA) polar plot of the LV. The standard AHA polar plot defines how the myocardium can be divided into 17 segments for the regional analysis of left ventricular function. However, to prepare the polar plot representations in this study, the LV was first divided into equally thick slices perpendicular to the long axis of the heart, equal in number to the number of short-axis CMR images available from base to apex of the LV, resulting in a series of circular sections of the LV, spanning from the basal, mid-cavity and apical regions. Each section was further divided circumferentially into six segments with an angular interval of 60° each. The segment nomenclature along the circumference is: anterior, anteroseptal, inferoseptal, inferior, inferolateral, and anterolateral, in a clockwise fashion from the attachment of the right ventricular wall to the LV (i.e. identifying the septum), as seen in the short-axis CMR images. This has been illustrated alongside Fig 1A. The averaged endocardial displacement in each of these segmental regions, for each slice level, was provided as input for the next phase of the analysis pipeline.

Next, the radial displacement characteristics per segment were further analyzed for phase of the fundamental frequency component of time-varying endocardial displacement, using a method of Fourier decomposition. As illustrated in Equation (1), given knowledge of the time-period of the cardiac cycle, T, for each segment, i, the Fourier decomposition of endocardial displacement was computed as:

$$f_i(t) = a_0 + \sum_{n=1}^{\infty}\left(a_n \cos\left(\frac{2nt\pi}{T}\right) + b_n \sin\left(\frac{2nt\pi}{T}\right)\right) \tag{1}$$

The phase, ϕ_i, of the fundamental frequency component of endocardial displacement in each segment, i, was computed using Equation (2) as:

$$\phi_i = \tan^{-1}\left(\frac{b_1}{a_1}\right) \tag{2}$$

The phase, ϕ, evidences the cardiac phase of peak regional contraction. ϕ was also plotted in the polar plot representation for visual analysis of regional variation of contraction timing across the LV, for each patient. Phase of contraction polar plots were plotted using a color-scale of 0 to 360 degrees representative of the time duration of one cardiac cycle, T.

The timing of contraction was also possible to estimate in milli-seconds (ms) based on information in the DICOM image headers. The mean and standard deviation in phase (i.e. time instant relative to the time-period of the cardiac cycle) of peak contraction across was LV endocardium was recorded for each patient in the study cohort and then investigated in their potential for being used as biomarkers for automatic retrospective binary classification of the patients (in a blinded fashion) into the categories of patients viz. narrow and wide QRS.

The extent of scarred regions from LGE images was characterized as a percentage scar extent for each patient, using the Otsu's method of thresholding, available in Medviso Segment. The basal slices of the LV were observed in all patients in the study cohort were found to have limited scarring and therefore, in order to identify the possible role of scar on affecting our aforementioned Fourier analysis of phase of contraction, we additionally reported the mean septal to lateral contraction timing delay (in milli-seconds, ms) in the basal slices of each patient. This metric of septal to lateral delay in the unscarred basal regions was additionally evaluated for accuracy in automatically classifying narrow and wide QRS patients in a blinded fashion.

3   Results and Discussion

The mean EDV in the 12 patients with narrow QRS was 186.95±75.2 ml, with mean LVEF being 19.4±7.14 %. The mean LV end-diastolic volume (EDV) in patients with LBBB was 334.65±40.77 ml, with the mean LV ejection fraction (EF) being 19.66±1.0 %. The LV-EDV of the patients with LBBB was significantly greater than the patients with narrow QRS (p=0.0005). The LV-EF of two groups was not significantly different (p=0.8). The amount of scar in the post myocardial infarction patients was 39.88±8.84%, which in itself is an exclusion criterion for CRT.

Polar plots of phase of peak contraction, ϕ, resulted in objective color-mapped renderings of MD (see Fig 1). All patients in the LBBB group had a septal to lateral wall delay, while all patients in the narrow QRS group had a lateral wall to septal delay due to presence of large amounts of scar in the septum (see representative radial endocardial displacement plots in Fig 2). In the narrow QRS cohort, the late-contracting LV territories (black in Fig 1) were mostly localized to the left-anterior descending coronary arterial perfusion territories in the anterior wall, in mid-level and apical LV slices, which were congruent with the spatial location of scar in these patients. The mean phase to peak contraction and phase standard deviation were significantly greater in these patients than the patients with LBBB (p=0.002), evidencing higher global extent of mechanical discoordination in contraction. This is congruent with expectations of MD based on large extents of myocardial scarring.

When timing of contraction was re-analyzed in the basal LV slices which had minimum scarring, a significantly greater mean and standard deviation in phase of peak contraction was found in the narrow QRS group i.e. mean phase of 173.07±25.4 degrees in narrow QRS group, versus 134.5±26.4 degrees in wide QRS group (p=0.03), and phase standard deviation of 67.6±13.6 degrees in the narrow QRS group versus 43.2±3.0 degrees in the wide QRS group (p=0.01). Comparison of the basal-regional septal to lateral wall delay (after exclusion of the mid-ventricular and apical slices containing scar) in the two groups revealed that the narrow QRS group had significantly lesser dyssynchrony in the basal regions excluding scar (-11.7±52.5 ms versus 55.16±12 ms in wide QRS group, p=0.04).

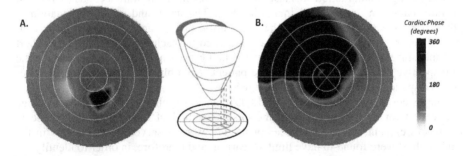

Fig. 1. Polar plots of phase of peak regional contraction in discrete segments of the LV (segmental demarcations shown and illustrated on top-right), resulting from Fourier analysis of phase of contraction, starting from time-varying regional endocardial motion in: A) a representative wide-QRS LBBB patient; and B) a narrow QRS HF patient with extensive scarring.

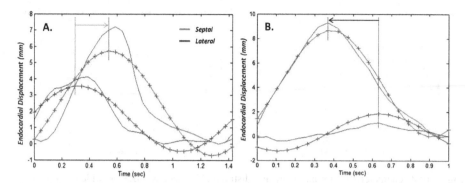

Fig. 2. Septal to Lateral delay in endocardial contraction, visualized as a line plot of time-varying mean septal (blue) and lateral (red) endocardial displacement, in a representative patient from: A) the wide-QRS LBBB cohort, which exhibited septal to lateral delay charactersitics; and B) the narrow-QRS HF cohort, which exhibited lateral to septal delay characterstics. The corresponding smooth first-order Fourier curve fits used to compute septal-to-lateral delay time are also superimposed upon each plotted endocardial displacement curve. Note that in these plots the first time-instant (0 ms) represents the displacement from the first to second cardiac phase of the cine CMR imaging data.

Further, LV-EDV was found to have a significant positive correlation with the mean and standard deviation phase indices in patients with wide QRS intervals (r^2=1.0, p<0.001), and LV-EF had a significant negative correlation with both mean and standard deviation in phase in these patients (r^2= -1.0, p<0.001). The septal to lateral wall delay also had a significant positive correlation with the LV-EDV (r^2=1.0, p<0.001) and negative correlation with the LV-EF (r^2=-1.0, p<0.001). However, neither LV-EDV and LV-EF correlated with any of these three indices of contracting timing in patients with narrow QRS intervals (r^2=0.089, p=0.37 and r^2=0.05, p=0.49 and r^2=0.04, p=0.52, for mean phase of contraction, standard deviation in phase of contraction and septal-to-lateral delay, respectively), although the narrow QRS patients demonstrated greater MD as per both indices of mean and standard deviation of phase of peak contraction (see Table 1). However, the amount of scar correlated positively with the mean phase (r^2=0.3, p=0.07) and with the phase standard deviation (r^2=0.23, p=0.08) in the narrow QRS group.

Table 1. Comparison of left ventricular dyssynchrony indices of mean phase to peak regional contraction, phase standard deviation and septal to lateral wall delay (after exclusion of the mid-ventricular and apical slices containing scar) in the two sub-groups of the study cohort viz. narrow & wide QRS interval. Legend: LV EDV- Left ventricular End Diastolic volume, LVEF - Left ventricular ejection fraction, LBBB - Left bundle branch block, SD - Standard Deviation.

QRS	LV EDV (ml)	LVEF (%)	Phase of Contraction, ϕ		Septal to Lateral delay (ms)
			Mean (deg)	Std Dev (deg)	
>150ms	334.65±40.8	19.66±1.0	134.5±26.4	43.2±3.0	55.16±12
<150ms	186.95±75.2	19.4±7.14	173.07±25.4	67.6±13.6	-11.7±52.5

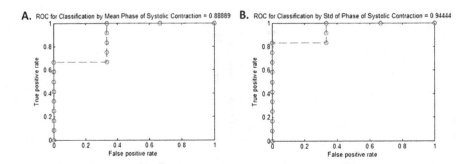

Fig. 3. ROC characteristics for automatically distinguishing narrow QRS vs. wide QRS patients using the presented metrics of MD viz. mean and standard deviation in phase of endocardial contraction as classifier parameters.

Receiver operator characteristics (ROC) were studied for each of the indices in Table 1 in order to gauge the efficacy of automatic classification wide and narrow QRS patients blindly using only the new biomarkers extracted from Fourier analysis of phase of regional contraction (see Fig 3). Mean phase of regional contraction across the LV was able to automatically identify wide QRS patients with an area under the curve (AUC) of 89% as per the ROC analysis. Phase standard deviation was accurate in classifying wide QRS patients with an AUC of 94% (see Fig 4, left).

When used in combination, using a cut-off for mean phase of contraction ≥126.37 degrees and a cut-off ≥43.2 degrees for phase standard deviation, an improved classification was possible, as per the classification tree shown in Fig 4A. In contrast with the two phase metrics computed across the entire LV (which included scarred regions), septal to lateral wall delay in non-scarred basal-LV regions was the most successful metric in classifying patients. Using a cut-off of delay ≥ 21.568 ms in the basal slices (i.e excluding the scarred of mid-ventricular and apical slices) an AUC of 100% was achieved (see Fig 4B).

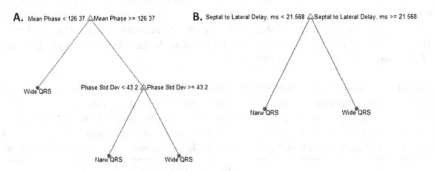

Fig. 4. LEFT: Classification tree defining rules to optimally identify narrow QRS vs. wide QRS (i.e. LBBB) patients using both mean and standard deviation in phase to peak endocardial contraction (in degrees, 0 to 360), together, as input features. RIGHT: The same classification exercise was noted to have an accuracy of 100% by using septal to lateral delay in the instant of peak contraction (in ms) as a metric in only unscarred basal LV regions.

4   Conclusion

We present a method of applying Fourier analysis to the phase of LV mechanical contraction to derive metrics of MD. We apply these metrics to the problem of automatically classifying patients into two groups based on their inherent electrical dyssynchrony i.e wide and narrow QRS. The results of this pilot study show that the described technique of MD assessment from CMR images is highly specific in defining parameters which can predict electrical dyssynchrony defined by a QRS duration ≥ 150 ms. The septal to lateral wall delay for the basal LV regions (which excluded scarred territories in our study cohort), was highly specific in predicting QRS duration with an AUC of 100%, and individually performed better than metrics of both mean or standard deviation in phase of contraction which led less than perfect AUC values for the same classification exercise (viz. 89% and 94%, respectively). This leads us to the conclusion that that scarring in the LV is a potential confounding factor in terms of MD assessment using phase of contraction as a metric of identifying Class I indication CRT candidates (wide QRS group); therefore, scar must be excluded during regional analysis LV contraction timing.

Best practices for LV pacing lead placement during CRT suggest optimal benefit is derived when the LV lead is localized to the latest-activating, non-scarred region [9-12]. However, today LV lead implantation is performed with limited consideration of the LV scar or mechanical activation but rather with greater focus on metrics electrical dyssynchrony evidenced from ECG data, which have application at the patient-selection stage. The phase of regional contraction computed in this study objectively identifies these late mechanically activating regions and therefore may have additional application in CRT LV lead placement guidance. The establishment of objective LV lead placement sites using pre-operative CMR imaging is a subject of our ongoing endeavors.

References

1. Abraham, W.T., Fisher, W.G., Smith, A.L., et al.: Cardiac resynchronization in chronic heart failure. N. Engl. J. Med. 346(24), 1845–1853 (1845)
2. Cazeau, S., Leclercq, C., Lavergne, T., et al.: Effects of multisite biventricular pacing in patients with heart failure and intraventricular conduction delay. N. Engl. J. Med. 344(12), 873–880 (2001)
3. Strickberger, S.A., Conti, J., Daoud, E.G., et al.: Patient selection for cardiac resynchronization therapy: from the Council on Clinical Cardiology Subcommittee on Electrocardiography and Arrhythmias and the Quality of Care and Outcomes Research Interdisciplinary Working Group, in collaboration with the Heart Rhythm Society. Circulation 111, 2146–2150 (2005)
4. Beshai, J.F., Grimm, R.A., Nagueh, S.F., et al.: Cardiac-resynchronization therapy in heart failure with narrow QRS complexes. N. Engl. J. Med. 357(24), 2461–2471 (2007)
5. Bax, J.J., Gorcsan, J.: 3rd, Echocardiography and noninvasive imaging in cardiac resynchronization therapy: results of the PROSPECT (Predictors of Response to Cardiac Resynchronization Therapy) study in perspective. J. Am. Coll. Cardiol. 53(21), 1933–1943 (2009)

6. Young, J.B., Abraham, W.T., Smith, A.L., et al.: Combined cardiac resynchronization and implantable cardioversion defibrillation in advanced chronic heart failure: the MIRACLE ICD Trial. Jama 289(20), 2685–2694 (2003)
7. Leclercq, C., Kass, D.A.: Retiming the failing heart: principles and current clinical status of cardiac resynchronization. J. Am. Coll. Cardiol. 39(2), 194–201 (2002)
8. Chung, E.S., Leon, A.R., Tavazzi, L., et al.: Results of the Predictors of Response to CRT (PROSPECT) trial. Circulation, 2008 117(20), 2608–2616 (2008)
9. Boogers, M.J., Chen, J., van Bommel, R.J., et al.: Optimal left ventricular lead position assessed with phase analysis on gated myocardial perfusion SPECT. Eur. J. Nucl. Med. Mol Imaging 38(2), 230–238 (2011)
10. Delgado, V., van Bommel, R.J., Bertini, M., et al.: Relative merits of left ventricular dyssynchrony, left ventricular lead position, and myocardial scar to predict long-term survival of ischemic heart failure patients undergoing cardiac resynchronization therapy. Circulation 123(1), 70–78 (2011)
11. Ypenburg, C., van Bommel, R.J., Delgado, V., et al.: Optimal Left Ventricular Lead Position Predicts Reverse Remodeling and Survival After Cardiac Resynchronization Therapy. J. Am. Coll. Cardiol. 52(17), 1402–1409 (2008)
12. Khan, F.Z., Virdee, M.S., Palmer, C.R., et al.: Targeted Left Ventricular Lead Placement to Guide Cardiac Resynchronization Therapy: The TARGET Study: A Randomized, Controlled Trial. J. Am. Coll. Cardiol. 12, j.jacc.2011.12.030 (2011)
13. Heiberg, E., Sjogren, J., Ugander, M., et al.: Design and validation of Segment–freely available software for cardiovascular image analysis. BMC Med. Imaging 10(1), 1 (2010)

A Parallel Adaptive Physics-Based Non-rigid Registration Framework for Brain Tumor Resection

Fotis Drakopoulos and Nikos P. Chrisochoides

Department of Computer Science, Old Dominion University, Norfolk, VA, USA

Abstract. We present a Parallel Adaptive Physics-Based Non-Rigid Registration (PAPBNRR) framework for warping pre-operative to intra-operative brain Magnetic Resonance Images (MRI) of patients who have undergone a tumor resection. This method extends our previous APB-NRR framework based on ITK and contributes three new parallel modules: A Finite Element Method (FEM) Solver for assembling the system matrices of a heterogeneous biomechanical model, rejecting the feature outliers and estimating the model deformations; two correction modules, the first for the warped pre-operative segmented MRI and the second for the produced image deformation field, which take into account the tissue removal depicted in the iMRI. As a result, PAPBNRR not only accurately captures the large intra-operative deformations associated with the resection, but also further reduces the overheads due to the inherited -from APBNRR- adaptivity and brings the end-to-end execution within the time constraints imposed by the neurosurgical procedure. Our evaluation is based on 6 clinical volume MRI cases including: (i) partial and complete tumor resections, (ii) isotropic and anisotropic image spacings. In all the case studies, the PAPBNRR framework shows promising results. In a Linux Dell workstation with 12 Intel Xeon 3.47 GHz CPU cores and 96GB of RAM, it reduces the registration time from about 10 minutes to less than 140 seconds for the anisotropic data and from 2 minutes to less than 45 seconds for the isotropic data.

Keywords: non-rigid registration, ITK, biomechanical model, threads, FEM.

1 Introduction

Image registration in general is concerned with spatial alignment of corresponding features between two or more images. During registration, a spatial transformation is applied to one image, which is called moving, such that it is brought into alignment with the other image, which is called fixed. In the context of Image-Guided Neurosurgery (IGNS), the moving image corresponds to a brain pre-operative MRI, which is aligned with the position of the patient before the surgery using translations and rotations (rigid transformations), and the fixed image corresponds to an intra-operative MRI (iMRI) acquired during the

Y.J. Zhang and J.M.R.S. Tavares (Eds.): CompIMAGE 2014, LNCS 8641, pp. 57–68, 2014.
© Springer International Publishing Switzerland 2014

surgery. After the opening of the skull and dura, the brain changes its shape because of the cerebrospinal fluid leakage, the effect of gravity and the administration of osmotic diuretics, introducing discrepancies in relation to the preoperative configuration. The Non-Rigid Registration (NRR) usually can compensate for the brain shifts caused by all these factors. In the case of a tumor resection, however, NRR becomes a difficult ill-posed problem because: first, not all points in the pre-operative image have a correspondence in the intra-operative image; second, the discrepancies are larger; and third, NRR requires significant computing resources and time.

Our previous work [1] demonstrated a NRR framework for brain deformations induced by a tumor resection. Its accuracy was evaluated on 14 clinical cases provided by the Surgical Planning Laboratory at Brigham and Women's Hospital and the Department of Neurosurgery at Shanghai Huashan Hospital. In this work, we focus on the NRR performance, and we propose a framework that facilitates image-guidance during neurosurgery under the real-time constraints (about 1-2 minutes) required by the neurosurgical workflow.

In [2] a method for the biomechanical simulation of volumetric brain deformations was presented, achieving reasonably accurate image alignments within the IGNS time constraints and evaluated on two neurosurgery cases. A prospective study on NRR of pre-operative data (T1,fMRI, DTI) with intra-operative data (T1) was reported in [3]. The clinical cases obtained from 11 patients enrolled over 12 months. The computationally intensive components of this method were parallelized in [4] with a cluster of 300 workstations, and the image alignments were calculated in near real-time. Nevertheless, these methods and others [5,6] compensate only for small brain deformations (shifts). The complex neurosurgical procedure of the tumor resection, which invalidates the biomechanical model defined on the pre-operative MRI and compromises the fidelity of the IGNS is not addressed.

In [7] a robust Expectation-Maximization (EM) framework for the simultaneous segmentation and registration of volume MRIs with partial or missing data was presented. A Matlab implementation of this method required about 30 minutes to register a pair of $64 \times 64 \times 64$ volume MRIs on a 2.8GHz Linux machine. In this paper, we evaluate the performance of our method on larger images with sizes about $512 \times 448 \times 176$ voxels. On a Linux Dell workstation with 12 Intel Xeon 3.47 GHz CPU cores, our scheme registers the images in about 2 min or less.

In summary, this paper presents a Parallel Adaptive Physics-Based NRR (PAPBNRR) framework to compensate for the brain deformations induced by a tumor resection. The presented framework augments the APBNRR method [1] with the contribution of three new parallel modules. The first is a FEM Solver (PFEMS) that estimates the deformations of a multi-tissue biomechanical model and rejects the feature outliers. The second (PWSC) and third (PDFC) modules correct a warped segmented pre-operative MRI and the produced image deformation field, respectively, to take into consideration the resected tissue in the iMRI.

Our evaluation on 6 patients with anisotropic and isotropic volume MRI data indicates that the proposed scheme satisfies the real-time constraints of IGNS. We will show that compared to its predecessor method, the PAPBNRR reduces about 44% and 30.7% the end-to-end execution time for the anisotropic and isotropic data, respectively. Next we will briefly describe the PAPBNRR framework and outline the new contributions in more detail.

2   Method

The PAPBNRR framework is built on the ITK open-source system[1]. Figure 1 illustrates the new and the existing modules of our method. All modules are parallel implemented with the POSIX thread library since ITK has a cross-platform API infrastructure for the creation of multi-threaded templated filters.

The PAPBNRR iteratively estimates a dense deformation field that defines a transformation for every point in the intra-operative image to the pre-operative image. The estimation of the dense field is facilitated by a linear heterogeneous (brain parenchyma, tumor) biomechanical model of high quality tetrahedral elements. During the execution, the model deforms and adapts to the changes in the brain morphology caused by the tissue resection, the gravity and other factors. After each deformation, the quality of the elements deteriorates, so the model is globaly remeshed (to avoid the flipped or distorted tetrahedra) from a warped segmented pre-operative image. We should point out that an additive (total) image deformation field is used to warp the input pre-operative and segmented pre-operative images (Figure 1). In that way, independently of the number of PAPBNRR iterations, these input images are interpolated only once. The model deformation and consequently the image warping stops when $i = N_{iter}$ where N_{iter} is the desired number of adaptive iterations (Figure 1).

The next subsections give more details about the new modules. A complete description of all the existing modules can be found in [1].

2.1   Parallel FEM Solver (PFEMS)

The sequential FEM Solver (FEMS) was originally presented in [5]. It estimates the mesh deformations from an approximation to an interpolation-based formulation while it rejecting the feature outliers (blocks with a large error between the computed mesh deformations and the block matching displacements). In [8] we parallelized this method by employing ParMETIS[2] to implement a balanced parallel partitioning of the tetrahedral mesh among the processing cores, and PETSc [9] to assembled-solved the linear system of equations. Later, we integrated FEMS within ITK [6].

In this paper, we develope a new parallel implementation of FEMS within ITK (PFEMS). We avoid using ParMetis or PETSc because their integration

---

[1] http://www.itk.org/

[2] http://glaros.dtc.umn.edu/gkhome/metis/parmetis/overview

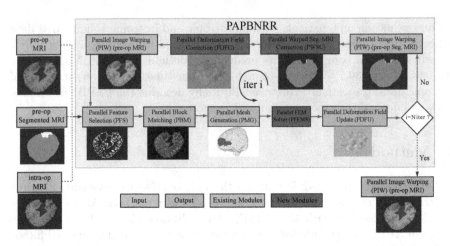

Fig. 1. The PAPBNRR framework. All the modules are implemented with the POSIX thread library for shared memory multiprocessor architectures. The red boxes represent the contributions compared to our previous work [1].

into the ITK is very cumbersome, and they present maintenance and portability issues.

Figure 2(a) depicts PFEMS. It takes as an input a mesh, the N_b selected blocks from the PFS module, the BM displacements from the PBM module and the corresponding parameters listed in Table 2. PFEMS estimates the deformations U on the mesh nodes in the following four steps: a) Parallel Initializations, b) Parallel Assembly, c) Parallel Outlier Rejection, and d) Parallel Interpolation.

Parallel Initializations. The first component of this step computes an image interpolation grid (Figure 2(a)). The image grid links the elements of the mesh to its own voxels. An element is linked to a voxel if the geometric center of the voxel is inside the element. Considering k threads and N_e elements, we assign $\lfloor N_e/k \rfloor$ elements to the first $k-1$ threads and $N_e - (k-1) \cdot \lfloor N_e/k \rfloor$ elements to the last thread. Then each thread links its assigned elements to the grid voxels. The voxels that lie outside the mesh do not have a linked element.

The second component computes a 3×3 stiffness tensor for each selected block. The tensor provides a three-dimensional measure of the block stiffness [5] regarding the linked element. All blocks have a linked element because the center of a block is always the center of a voxel in the interpolation grid. The parallelization of this component is implemented similar to the interpolation grid, but instead of elements, we assign feature blocks to each thread. Then the 3×3 tensors are computed in parallel.

Parallel Assembly. This step assembles the stiffness matrices K_b, K_m, K_g of the heterogeneous biomechanical model and the block displacements vector F.

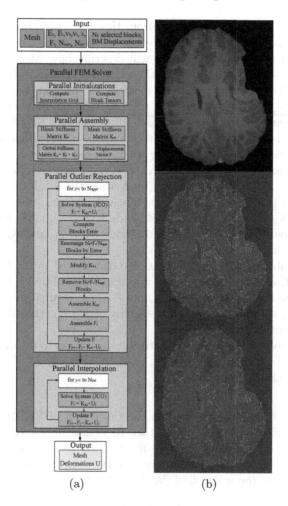

(a)   (b)

Fig. 2. (a): The Parallel FEM Solver (PFEMS). The green boxes represent the input, the gray the PFEMS steps, the cyan the components of each step, and the yellow the output. (b): The feature blocks before and after the Parallel Outlier Rejection for the clinical case 3 of Table 1. From top to bottom: warped pre-op MRI, feature blocks before the rejection superimposed on the warped pre-op MRI ($N_b = 287003$), feature blocks after the rejection superimposed on the warped pre-op MRI ($N_b \cdot (1 - F_r) = 215253$). N_b is the number of feature blocks, $F_r = 25\%$ is the rejection percentage.

K_b and K_m are $N \times N$ stiffness matrices of the feature blocks and the mesh, respectively; F is $N \times 1$; $N = 3 \cdot N_n$ where N_n is the number of mesh nodes. K_g is the $N \times N$ total stiffness matrix of the biomechanical model:

$$K_g = K_b + K_m \tag{1}$$

More details about the formulation of K_b, K_m, K_g and F are given in [5,6]. In this paper, we use ITPACK's [10] compressed storage matrix representation scheme because it is part of the ITK's distribution. However, all ITPACK subroutines are currently sequential. The parallel assembly of the compressed storage matrix structures is not supported. Next, we will describe how we implemented the parallel assembly of K_b and K_m using the existing ITPACK subroutines.

In the case of K_b, we assign $\lfloor N_b/k \rfloor$ blocks to the first $k - 1$ threads and $N_b - (k - 1) \cdot \lfloor N_b/k \rfloor$ blocks to the kth thread. N_b is the number of the feature blocks. Each thread $i = 1, 2, \ldots, k$ builds a stiffness matrix K_{b_i} from the assigned blocks. Then we recursively add K_{b_i} with maximum $\lfloor k/2 \rfloor$ threads. Specifically, in the first recursion $\lfloor k/2 \rfloor$ threads are used; thread 1 adds K_{b_1} and K_{b_2} and stores the result to $K_{b_{12}}$; thread 2 adds K_{b_3} and K_{b_4} and stores the result to $K_{b_{34}}$; finally, thread $\lfloor k/2 \rfloor$ adds $K_{b_{k-1}}$ and K_{b_k} and stores the result to $K_{b_{(k-1)k}}$. In the second recursion $\lfloor k/4 \rfloor$ threads are used; thread 1 adds $K_{b_{12}}$ and $K_{b_{34}}$; thread 2 adds $K_{b_{56}}$ and $K_{b_{78}}$; finally, thread $\lfloor k/4 \rfloor$ adds $K_{b_{(k-3)(k-2)}}$ and $K_{b_{(k-1)k}}$. In the last recursion one thread is used; thread 1 adds $K_{b_{12 \ldots k/2}}$ and $K_{b_{(k/2+1)(k/2+2) \ldots k}}$ and stores the result to K_b.

For the assembly of K_m, the elements are distributed to the threads similar to the computation of the interpolation grid. Each thread builds a mesh stiffness matrix K_{m_i} from the assigned elements, and K_{m_i} are recursively added with the procedure explained above. After the assembly of K_b, K_m the addition in (1) is performed sequentially.

For the assembly of vector F, we distribute N_b blocks to k threads similar to the case of K_b. Each thread $i = 1, 2, \ldots, k$ builds a vector F_i of size $N \times 1$ and F_i are added to the global vector F.

Parallel Outlier Rejection. This is the third step of PFEMS. It is shown in Figure 2(a) with grey. Parallel Outlier Rejection iteratively estimates the deformations U on the mesh nodes while it rejects the blocks (outliers) with large error between the estimated deformations and the block matching displacements. U is estimated after the solution of the linear system:

$$F = K_g \cdot U \tag{2}$$

In each iteration $j = 1, 2, \ldots, N_{appr}$ of the rejection loop, $N_b \cdot F_r/N_{appr}$ blocks with the highest error are rejected. F_r, N_{appr} are listed in Table 2 and N_b is the number of the selected blocks from PFS. Figure 2(b) shows an example of the feature blocks before and after the Parallel Outlier Rejection step for the adaptive iteration $i = 2$ of the clinical case 3 in Table 1.

In a rejection iteration j, first, we solve system (2) for U_j (Figure 2(a)). In this paper, we develope a new parallel implementation of the sequential Jacobi Conjugate Gradient (JCG) method [11] to solve system (2). In our JCG implementation, all vector-vector and matrix-vector multiplications are performed in parallel using the native ITPACK storage structures.

In order to parallelize the block error computation [5], we distribute $N_b - j \cdot (N_b \cdot F_r/N_{appr})$ blocks to k threads similar to the Parallel Assembly step. For the parallel rearrangement of the outliers based on their error, we employ the $nth\_element$ function of the GNU libstdc++ library.

Because outlier blocks are rejected in every iteration j (Figure 2(a)), their contribution should be also removed from matrix K_b. The modification of K_b is performed in parallel by distributing $N_b \cdot F_r/N_{appr}$ outliers to k threads. Each thread $i = 1, 2 \ldots k$ builds a block outlier matrix K'_{b_i}, and later K'_{b_i} and K_b are recursively subtracted (in the assembly of K_b we recursively added K_{b_i}). The result matrix is stored at $K_{b,j}$. Then $K_{g,j}$ is re-computed from (1). Likewise, the vector F_j is re-assembled from $N_b - j \cdot (N_b \cdot F_r/N_{appr})$ blocks with the procedure described in the Parallel Assembly step. Finally F_{j+1} is computed by adding the mesh internal forces $K_m \cdot U_j$ to F_j.

Parallel Interpolation. The interpolation step solves (2) N_{int} times for the mesh displacements U and updates the vector F. During the interpolation loop, the number of feature blocks is constant: $N_b - N_{appr} \cdot (N_b \cdot F_r/N_{appr})$.

2.2   Parallel Warped Segmented Pre-op MRI Correction (PWSC)

This module overlaps two images. The first is a warped pre-operative segmented MRI, and the second is a brain mask of the intra-op MRI. Then it removes from the first image the region of the tumor that falls into the background of the second image [1]. We call the modified region of the first image as corrected region. For the parallel implementation of the module, we partition the first image into k pieces where k is the number of threads. The overlap is performed concurrently between the piece of the thread $i = 1, 2, \ldots k$ and the second image.

2.3   Parallel Deformation Field Correction (PDFC)

This module detects voxels in the image deformation field that correspond to the corrected region (subsection 2.2) and sets their values equal to zero. The detection of the voxels is facilitated by a map image [1], which relates the warped pre-operative segmented MRI with the image deformation field. The computation of the map image and the correction of the deformation field is performed in parallel after their partition into k thread pieces like in subsection 2.2.

3   Results

We evaluate the performance of the proposed framework on 6 clinical MRI cases provided by the Department of Neurosurgery at Shanghai Huashan Hospital [12]. We compare PAPBNRR with the predecessor method APBNRR to show the impact of the new contributions on the registration performance. We conduct all the experiments in a Dell Linux workstation with 2 sockets of 6 Intel Xeon X5690@3.47 GHz CPU cores each, totaling 12 cores and 96 GB of RAM. In this paper, we do not evaluate the accuracy of the framework because the two methods share the same functionality, and the APBNRR was extensively evaluated (qualitatively and quantitatively) in our previous work [1].

Table 1 lists the MRI data of this study. From a total of 6 cases, 2 are Partial Tumor Resections (PTR), and 4 are Complete Tumor Resections (CTR). We resample cases 4-6 to an isotropic image spacing in order to investigate the influence of the image size on the registration performance. The original image sizes and spacings before the resampling are: $448 \times 512 \times 176$ and $0.488 \times 0.488 \times 1.00$ for case 4; $512 \times 448 \times 176$ and $0.488 \times 0.488 \times 1.00$ for case 5; $448 \times 448 \times 58$ and $0.496 \times 0.496 \times 1.622$ for case 6. For all the conducted experiments, we use linear displacement FE biomechanical models with 4-node tetrahedral elements, and we model the tissues (brain parenchyma, tumor) as elastic isotropic materials. Table 2 lists the parameters for the experiments. Because the input window size is given in voxels and the image spacing for the anisotropic and isotropic cases is different, we adjust W_s accordingly (Table 2). More details about the input parameters can be found in [1].

Table 1. The clinical MRI data of this study. Cases 1-3 and 4-6 have anisotropic and isotropic image spacing, respectively. PTR : Partial Tumor Resection, CTR : Complete Tumor Resection, x : axial, y : coronal, z : sagittal.

Voxel Type	Case	Genre	Type	Tumor Location	Image Size (voxels)	Image Spacing $s_x \times s_y \times s_z$ (mm)
Anisotropic	1	M	PTR	L parietal	$512 \times 448 \times 176$	$0.488 \times 0.488 \times 1.000$
	2	F	PTR	L frontal	$384 \times 512 \times 176$	$0.488 \times 0.488 \times 1.000$
	3	F	CTR	L frontal	$448 \times 512 \times 176$	$0.488 \times 0.488 \times 1.000$
Isotropic	4	F	CTR	L parietal	$219 \times 250 \times 176$	$1.000 \times 1.000 \times 1.000$
	5	M	CTR	L temporal	$250 \times 219 \times 176$	$1.000 \times 1.000 \times 1.000$
	6	F	CTR	L temporal	$240 \times 240 \times 134$	$1.000 \times 1.000 \times 1.000$

Table 2. The input parameters for the 6 clinical cases. PFS : Parallel Feature Selection, PBS : Parallel Block Matching, PMG : Parallel Mesh Generation, FEMS : FEM Solver, PFEMS : Parallel FEM Solver, x : axial, y : coronal, z : sagittal.

Parameter	Units	Value	Description	Module
$B_{s,x} \times B_{s,y} \times B_{s,z}$	voxels	$3 \times 3 \times 3$	Block size	PFS-PBM
$W_{s,x} \times W_{s,y} \times W_{s,z}$	voxels	$13 \times 13 \times 5$ (Case 1-3)	Window size	PBM
		$7 \times 7 \times 5$ (Case 4-6)		
F_s	-	5%	% of selected feature blocks	PFS
δ	-	5	Mesh size	PMG
E_b	Pa	$2.1 \cdot 10^3$	Brain Young's modulus	FEMS-PFEMS
E_t	Pa	$2.1 \cdot 10^4$	Tumor Young's modulus	FEMS-PFEMS
ν_b	-	0.45	Brain Poisson's ratio	FEMS-PFEMS
ν_t	-	0.45	Tumor Poisson's ratio	FEMS-PFEMS
λ	-	1	Trade off parameter	FEMS-PFEMS
F_r	-	25%	% of rejected outlier blocks	FEMS-PFEMS
N_{appr}	-	10	Number of outlier rej. steps	FEMS-PFEMS
N_{int}	-	5	Number of interpolation steps	FEMS-PFEMS
N_{iter}	-	5	Number of adaptive iterations	-

Figure 3 presents the PAPBNRR results for the anisotropic data. Qualitative results for isotropic data were presented in [1]. We show the same representative

MRI slice for all the images belonging to the same row. A visual inspection of the subtracted images (first column from the right) demonstrates the accuracy of the non-rigid alignments, particularly near the tumor resection margins.

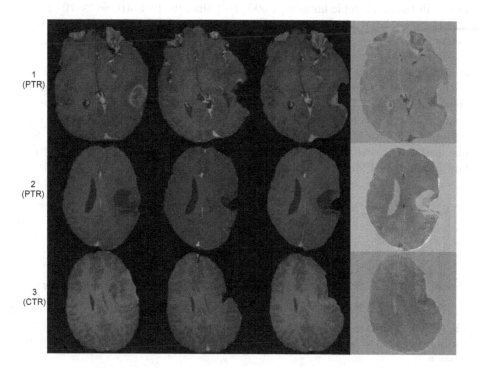

Fig. 3. The PAPBNRR results for the anisotropic cases 1-3. Each row represents a single case. The left margin indicates the number and the resection type for each case. From left to right column: pre-op MRI, intra-op MRI, warped pre-op MRI, warped pre-op MRI subtracted from intra-op MRI.

Figure 4 shows the total execution time for the 6 clinical cases using the two methods with 1, 2, 4, and 12 hardware cores. Both methods take about the same time to register the images with 1 thread; on average, 10 and 2 minutes for the anisotropic and isotropic cases, respectively. However, the PAPBNRR incorporates additional parallel modules, so the difference in the performance becomes significant depending on the number of the cores. With 12 cores, it requires less than 140 seconds for the anisotropic cases and less than 45 seconds for the isotropic cases, when the APBNRR needs less than 250 and 65 seconds, respectively. In other words, the PAPBNRR reduces the end-to-end execution time by 44% (1.78 times faster) for cases 1-3 and by 30.7% (1.44 times faster) for cases 4-6, compared to the APBNRR. This improvement is crucial considering the hard real-time constraints of IGNS.

We should point out that the total running time for the anisotropic images is considerably larger (about 10 min) than the isotropic (about 2 min) for both methods. The reason is that the former images are larger ($\approx 40 \cdot 10^6$ voxels) than the latter ($\approx 10 \cdot 10^6$ voxels). Consequently, the PFS module selects more feature blocks in the anisotropic images ($\approx 300 \cdot 10^3$) than in the isotropic ($\approx 70 \cdot 10^3$), and the associated block computations in modules PFS, PBM, PFEMS take longer.

Figure 5(a) illustrates how much faster the parallel implementation is with 12 cores, than the sequential, for both methods. For example, in case 1, the PAPB-NRR achieves a speedup of about 4.8 (orange bar) while APBNRR's speedup (blue bar) is only 2.71 (43.5% smaller). According to Figure 5(a), the proposed framework exhibits more parallelism than the APBNRR method, in all the experiments. Figure 5(b) illustrates the speedup of each PAPBNRR module for one anisotropic case. PBM [6] shows an excellent scaling. The speedup for the new modules PFEMS, PWSC, and PDFC is 2.89, 4.21, and 2.28, respectively.

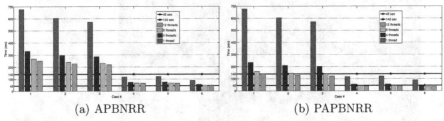

(a) APBNRR   (b) PAPBNRR

Fig. 4. The end-to-end execution time for the 6 clinical cases using 1, 4, 8, and 12 hardware cores. The black solid horizontal lines illustrate two thresholds; 45 and 140 seconds.

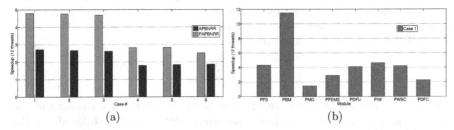

(a)   (b)

Fig. 5. (a): The end-to-end speedup with 12 cores for the 6 clinical cases. (b): The speedup with 12 cores of each PAPBNRR module for case 1.

Table 3 shows the performance of all the PFEMS components. Considering the fact that PFEMS is not only the most complex module of the framework but also -together with PBM- the most time consuming [1], the achieved speedup of 2.89 has proven beneficial for the overall performance of our method (Figures 4(b), 5(a)). In the future, we will focus on the improvement of those PFEMS components (Assemble F, Modify K_b, Initialize Interpolation Grid, and Assemble K_g)

Table 3. The performance of the new PAPBNRR modules for case 1. The PFEMS components are sorted according to the speedup. The speedup is not available (n/a) for the sequential components.

Module	Component	Time (sec)		% Total Time		Speedup
		1 thread	12 threads	1 thread	12 threads	
PFEMS	Compute Block Tensors	7.58	0.79	5.2	1.6	9.59
	Compute Blocks Error	22.67	3.22	15.5	6.4	7.04
	Assemble K_b	28.05	4.55	19.2	9.0	6.16
	Initialize Interpolation Grid	24.70	6.31	16.9	12.5	3.91
	Rearrange Blocks by Error	13.12	3.98	9.0	7.9	3.29
	Assemble F	23.61	9.10	16.1	18.0	2.59
	Assemble K_m	1.64	0.85	1.1	1.7	1.92
	Solve system (JCG)	6.56	4.52	4.5	8.9	1.45
	Modify K_b	10.14	9.04	6.9	17.8	1.12
	Assemble K_g	5.89	5.76	4.0	11.4	n/a
	Initialize Blocks	1.57	1.58	1.1	3.1	n/a
	Remove Blocks	0.84	0.86	0.6	1.7	n/a
	Update F	0.10	0.10	0.1	0.2	n/a
	Total	146.47	50.66	100	100	2.89
PDFC		10.47	4.59	100	100	2.28
PWSC		8.48	2.01	100	100	4.21

that consume more than 10% of its total time with 12 cores (Table 3). Therefore, we anticipate to register the anisotropic MRIs in less than 1 minute and the isotropic in less than 30 seconds.

4 Conclusion

We presented a Parallel Adaptive Non-Rigid Registration framework for warping pre-operative to intra-operative brain MRI of patients who have undergone a tumor resection.

We believe that the proposed framework is an important step toward a clinically applicable, real-time non-rigid registration technology for neurosurgical resection, for two reasons. First, PAPBNRR inherits the adaptive biomechanical model of its predecessor method. As a result, accurately compensates for the large deformations imposed by the resection, independently of the portion (partial or complete) of the resected tumor depicted in the intra-operative MRI. Second and most important for this study, our scheme shows potential to satisfy the hard real-time constraints required by the IGNS. In our clinical evaluation based on 6 patients, the PAPBNRR reduces the end-to-end execution time from about 10 minutes to 140 seconds for anisotropic volume MRI data and from 2 minutes to 45 seconds for isotropic data. Compared to our previous APBNRR framework, the new contributions reduce the execution time by 44% and 30.7% for the anisotropic and isotropic cases, respectively.

In the future, we will try to exploit more parallelism from our method by improving the performance of the computationally intensive PFEMS components. Our goal is to provide non-rigid alignments of anisotropic volume MRI of adult patients who have undergone a tumor resection, in less than 60 seconds. Additionally, we will incorporate more tissues into the adaptive heterogeneous biomechanical model like the the falx cerebri and the ventricles, for more accurate results.

Acknowledgements. This work is supported in part by NSF grants: CCF-1139864, CCF-1136538, CSI-1136536, by the CRCF grant No. MF14-F-007-LS, John Simon Guggenheim Foundation, the Modeling and Simulation fellowship, and the Richard T.Cheng Endowment.

References

1. Drakopoulos, F., Liu, Y., Foteinos, P., Chrisochoides, N.P.: Towards a real time multi-tissue adaptive physics based non-rigid registration framework for brain tumor resection. Frontiers in Neuroinformatics 8(11) (2014)
2. Warfield, S.K., Ferrant, M., Gallez, X., Nabavi, A., Jolesz, F.A.: Real-time biomechanical simulation of volumetric brain deformation for image guided neurosurgery. In: Proceedings of the 2000 ACM/IEEE Conference on Supercomputing, Supercomputing 2000. IEEE Computer Society, Washington, DC (2000)
3. Archip, N., Clatz, O., Fedorov, A., Kot, A., Whalen, S., Kacher, D., Chrisochoides, N., Jolesz, F., Golby, A., Black, P., Warfield, S.K.: Non-rigid alignment of preoperative mri, fmri, dt-mri, with intra-operative mri for enchanced visualization and navigation in image-guided neurosurgery. Neuroimage (2007)
4. Chrisochoides, N., Fedorov, A., Kot, A., Archip, N., Black, P., Clatz, O., Golby, A., Kikinis, R., Warfield, S.: Toward real-time image guided neurosurgery using distributed and grid computing (October 2006)
5. Clatz, O., Delingette, H., Talos, I.F., Golby, A., Kikinis, R., Jolesz, F., Ayache, N., Warfield, S.: Robust non-rigid registration to capture brain shift from intraoperative mri. IEEE Trans. Med. Imag. (2005)
6. Liu, Y., Kot, A., Drakopoulos, F., Yao, C., Fedorov, A., Enquobahrie, A., Clatz, O., Chrisochoides, N.P.: An itk implementation of a physics-based non-rigid registration method for brain deformation in image-guided neurosurgery. Frontiers in Neuroinformatics 8(33) (2014)
7. Periaswamy, S., Farid, H.: Medical image registration with partial data. Medical Image Analysis 10(3) (2006)
8. Liu, Y., Fedorov, A., Kikinis, R., Chrisochoides, N.: Real-time non-rigid registration of medical images on a cooperative parallel architecture. In: IEEE Intern. Conf. on Bioinformatics and Biomedicine (2009)
9. Balay, S., Gropp, W.D., McInnes, L.C., Smith, B.F.: Petsc 2.0 users manual. Tech. Rep. ANL-95/11 - Revision 2.0.28, Argonne National Laboratory (2000)
10. Kincaid, D.R., Respess, J.R., Young, D.M., Grimes, R.R.: Algorithm 586: Itpack 2c: A fortran package for solving large sparse linear systems by adaptive accelerated iterative methods. ACM Trans. Math. Softw. 8(3), 302–322 (1982)
11. Grimes, R., Kincaid, D., Macgregor, W., Young, D.: Itpack report: Adaptive iterative algorithms using symmetric sparse storage. CNA-139, Center for Numerical Analysis, University of Texas, Austin, Texas, 78712 (1978)
12. Chen, W., Ying, M., Jian-Hong, Z., Liang-Fu, Z.: The department of neurosurgery at shangai huashan hospital. Neurosurgery 62(4), 947–953 (2008)

Curvature-Based Registration for Slice Interpolation of Medical Images

Ahmadreza Baghaie[1] and Zeyun Yu[2]

[1] Department of Electrical Engineering, University of Wisconsin-Milwaukee, WI, USA
abaghaie@uwm.edu
[2] Department of Computer Science, University of Wisconsin-Milwaukee, WI, USA
yuz@uwm.edu

Abstract. Slice interpolation is a fast growing field in medical image processing. Intensity-based interpolation and object-based interpolation are two major groups of methods in the literature. In this paper an object based method for slice interpolation using a modified version of curvature registration is proposed. Due to non-linear nature of image registration the results of forward and backward registration can be different. Therefore assuming a linear displacement between corresponding pixels of reference and moving image, a functional is minimized and the displacement fields for both reference and moving images with respect to the missing in-between slice are computed and used for reconstruction of the missing slice. The proposed approach is evaluated quantitatively by using the Mean Squared Difference (MSD) as metric. The produced results show significant visual improvement in preserving sharp edges in images.

Keywords: Image Registration, Slice Interpolation, Optimization, Medical Images, Mean Squared Difference.

1 Introduction

Image interpolation is a well-known research topic in image processing and there have been many studies in this area especially in bio-medical applications. With modern image modalities (CT, MRI, light/electron microscopy, etc.), a sequence of 2D images can be provided and used in building 3D models. However, the resolutions of the images are often not identical in all three directions. Usually the resolution in the Z direction is significantly lower than the resolutions in the X and Y directions. For example, in a generic CT, resolution in X and Y direction, or in more accurate term the spacing, is between 0.5-2mm while the spacing in Z direction is in the range of 1-15mm. This asymmetry in the resolution causes problems such as step-shaped iso-surfaces and discontinuity in structures in 3D reconstructed models. Therefore utilizing a slice interpolation algorithm to augment the 3D data into a symmetric one is of high demand.

In general, slice interpolation methods can be divided into two groups: intensity-based interpolation, and object-based interpolation. In the first category, the final

Y.J. Zhang and J.M.R.S. Tavares (Eds.): CompIMAGE 2014, LNCS 8641, pp. 69–80, 2014.

result of interpolation is directly computed from the intensity values of input images. Linear and cubic spline interpolation methods are two examples of this group. The major advantages of these methods are their simplicity and low computational complexity, which lead to their wide uses in practice. As the final result is basically a weighted average of input images, however, these methods suffer from blurring effects on object boundaries, yielding unrealistic and visually unpleasing results.

In object-based methods, on the other hand, the extracted information from objects contained in input images is used in order to guide the interpolation into more accurate results. There are many methods proposed in the literature trying to take into account additional information of objects in order to provide better results [1-11]. One of the first attempts for object-based interpolation has been made by Goshtasby et al [1]. Using a gradient magnitude based approach, corresponding points between consecutive slices are found and then the linear interpolation is applied in order to find the in-between slices. An important assumption of this work is that the difference between consecutive slices is small, so they restrict their search for finding correspondence points to small neighborhoods. It is obvious that this assumption is not true in many cases. To reduce the blurriness of edges, some more recent approaches have been studied, including the column fitting interpolation [2], shape-based method [3], morphology-based method [6], and feature-guided shape interpolation method [7]. A comprehensive summary of common methods (both intensity-based and object-based) for slice interpolation was described in [4, 5].

An increasingly important group of approaches for image interpolation (object-based) are based on image registration. Using the well-known free form deformation non-rigid registration method by Rueckert [8], Penny et al. [9] proposed a registration based method for slice interpolation. Another registration based method was given by Frakes et al. [10] by using a modified version of control grid interpolation (CGI). More recently, Xu et al. [11] described a multi-resolution registration based method for slice interpolation. In general, registration-based slice interpolation methods are guided by two important assumptions. First, the consecutive slices contain similar anatomical features. Second, the registration method is capable of finding the appropriate transformation map to match these similar features. Violation of any of these assumptions results in false correspondence maps, which leads to incorrect interpolation results.

In the present paper, a novel method is developed for slice interpolation by taking into account the well-known curvature-based registration [12, 13]. With a modified version of the registration method and an assumption of having linear movement between corresponding points in given slices, a displacement field is computed and the in-between slice is interpolated using a simple averaging of the registration results. The detail of the proposed method is given in Section 2, followed by some experimental results along with quantitative and qualitative evaluations of the method in Section 3. The conclusion is given in Section 4.

2   Method

Given two images, reference R and template T, image registration is to find a spatial transformation such that the transformed template matches the reference, subject to a suitable distance measure (forward registration) [12]. This transformation can range from a simple translation to more sophisticated non-rigid free form deformations, dependent on the subject and goal of registration. Also depending on the method, registration can be based on matching a set of feature points (landmarks) or been applied directly on image gray values. Here the latter case is of interest. Usually most of the registration methods can be formulated in term of a variational formulation, using a joint functional as follows [12]:

$$E[\mathbf{u}] = D[R,T;\mathbf{u}] + \alpha S \qquad (1)$$

where E is the energy functional, D represents a distance measure (external force) and S represents the rate of smoothness of $\mathbf{u}$ (internal force). The parameter α is used to balance the two terms. In this functional, $\mathbf{u}$ should be found such that the joint functional is minimized. This model is called single direction model because the reference image is fixed and only the template image is moving. This causes asymmetry in the results in such a way that if we fix the template image and move the reference image to match the template image (backward registration) the result may not be exactly opposite to that of the forward registration. For this reason, this model is modified to be used in the context of image slice interpolation by changing the formulation to the following:

$$E[\mathbf{u}] = D[R_1(\mathbf{x}-\mathbf{u}), R_2(\mathbf{x}+\mathbf{u})] + \alpha S \qquad (2)$$

where $R_1, R_2 : \Omega \rightarrow \Re$ are the two images provided as input and $\Omega := [0,1]^2$ is the domain of images, $\mathbf{x}$ is the grid of image values and $\mathbf{u}$ is the displacement values for each grid point. Please note that in Equation (2), it is assumed that the slice to be interpolated, denoted by R, is in the middle of the given images. If R is an arbitrary slice between R_1 and R_2, then we first need to compute the distances from R to R_1 and R_2, denoted by d_1 and d_2 respectively. Then we calculate the ratio $r = d_1 /(d_1 + d_2)$, and the following equation should be considered for interpolating R:

$$E[\mathbf{u}] = D[R_1(\mathbf{x}-r\mathbf{u}), R_2(\mathbf{x}+(1-r)\mathbf{u})] + \alpha S \qquad (3)$$

Without loss of generality, we shall consider Equation (2) in the current paper for image slice interpolation. In this case $r=0.5$ but since the coefficient will be the same for both of the images and practically doesn't affect the process of optimization it is considered to be 1 for simplicity of representation in the rest of the paper. Fig.1 illustrates the idea behind considering linear displacements between corresponding points that is utilized here for slice interpolation.

Several distance measures for D have been proposed in the literature, including the Sum of Squared Differences (SSD), Mutual Information (MI), Normalized Mutual Information (NMI), Cross Correlation (CC) and Normalized Gradient Fields (NGF) [14].

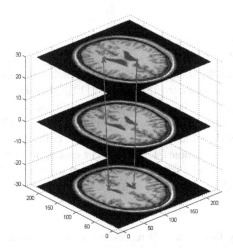

Fig. 1. An illustration of linear displacements between corresponding points utilized in this paper. The main goal is to use the top and bottom slice to reconstruct the in-between slice.

Here SSD is used as distance measure, and the above formulation can be rewritten as:

$$D[R_1(\mathbf{x}-\mathbf{u}), R_2(\mathbf{x}+\mathbf{u})] = \frac{1}{2} \mid R_1(\mathbf{x}-\mathbf{u}) - R_2(\mathbf{x}+\mathbf{u}) \mid_{L_2}^2$$
$$= \frac{1}{2} \int_{\Omega} (R_1(\mathbf{x}-\mathbf{u}(\mathbf{x})) - R_2(\mathbf{x}+\mathbf{u}(\mathbf{x})))^2 dx \tag{4}$$

For the smoothness term S, several common choices are available, such as elastic, fluid, demon, diffusion and curvature registration [12]. Here the curvature approach is used, in which the smoothness term is as follows:

$$S[\mathbf{u}] = \frac{1}{2} \sum_{l=1}^{2} \int_{\Omega} (\Delta u_l)^2 \tag{5}$$

where Δ is the curvature operator and the summation is computed over two dimensions of image and the integral is computed inside the domain of images. As stated in [12], using curvature for smoothness, the need for an additional linear affine pre-registration step can be eliminated. Also it should be mentioned that the curvature operator S^{curv} is defined by $S^{curv} = S^{diff} * S^{diff}$, where "*" represents convolution and S^{diff} is the discrete Laplace operator for 2D images.

In order to minimize the above joint functional in (3), the Gateaux derivative of $E[\mathbf{u}]$ is computed. Making it equal to zero to find the minimum point, an Euler-Lagrange PDE equation can be obtained as:

$$f(\mathbf{x}, \mathbf{u}(\mathbf{x})) + \alpha A^{curv}[\mathbf{u}](\mathbf{x}) = 0 \tag{6}$$

where

$$A^{curv}[\mathbf{u}] = \Delta^2 \mathbf{u}$$

$$f(\mathbf{x}, \mathbf{u}(\mathbf{x})) = (R_2(\mathbf{x}+\mathbf{u}) - R_1(\mathbf{x}-\mathbf{u})).(\nabla R_1(\mathbf{x}-\mathbf{u}) + \nabla R_2(\mathbf{x}+\mathbf{u}))$$

To solve this PDE, a time-stepping iteration method is considered as follows:

$$\partial_t u^{k+1}(\mathbf{x},t) = f(\mathbf{x},u^k(\mathbf{x},t)) + \alpha A^{curv}[u^{k+1}](\mathbf{x},t), k \geq 0 \tag{7}$$

with $u^0 = 0$. Using a finite difference approximation of the derivative with time step τ and also collecting the grid points with respect to a lexicographical ordering, one can derive a discretized version of (7) as follows:

$$(I_n + \alpha\tau A^{curv})\vec{U}_l^{(k+1)} = \vec{U}_l^{(k)} + \tau\vec{F}_l^{(k)}, l = 1,2. \tag{8}$$

where l is the parameter representing the dimension index. Following the same approach as in [12, 13], the optimization process can be done by exploiting Discrete Cosine Transform (DCT).

Assuming slices have the size of $m \times n$, the set of coefficients d_{j_1,j_2} are computed as follows:

$$d_{j_1,j_2} = -4 + 2\cos\frac{(j_1-1)\pi}{m} + 2\cos\frac{(j_2-1)\pi}{n} \tag{9}$$

where $j_1 = 1,2,...,m, j_2 = 1,2,...,n$. Defining $G = DCT[\vec{U}_l^{(k)} + \tau\vec{F}_l^{(k)}]$ for $l = 1,2$, DCT being the discrete cosine transform, we can have:

$$\vec{U}_l^{(k+1)} = IDCT[V] \tag{10}$$

where $V_{j_1,j_2} = G_{j_1,j_2}[1 + \tau\alpha d^2_{j_1,j_2}]^{-1}$ and IDCT is the inverse discrete cosine transform. For further detail the reader is referred to [12, 13]. After finishing the optimization process, a simple averaging of the two transformed input images provides us with the missing in-between slice. Table 1 summarizes the algorithm for curvature registration based slice interpolation method.

3   Results and Discussion

To validate the proposed method for slice interpolation in medical images, several tests have been conducted. The results of the proposed method are compared with two other methods, in both subjective and objective aspects. As a metric, Mean Squared Difference (MSD) is used for comparison.

Assuming I_{org} and I_{rec} as original image and reconstructed image respectively, with the size of $m \times n$, MSD is defined as follows:

$$MSD = \frac{1}{m \times n}\sum_{i=1}^{m}\sum_{j=1}^{n}(I_{org}(i,j) - I_{rec}(i,j))^2 \tag{9}$$

Table 1. Curvature registration based slice interpolation algorithm

---

Initilization

$$\tau, \alpha, X, U^0 = 0, d_{j_1, j_2}$$

for $k = 0,1,\ldots.$

    % computing forces

$$F_l^{(k)} = (R_2(X + U^k) - R_1(X - U^k)).(\nabla R_1(X - U^k) + \nabla R_2(X + U^k))$$

    % solving the linear system

    for $l = 1,2$

$$G = DCT[\vec{U}_l^{(k)} + \tau \vec{F}_l^{(k)}]$$

        for $j_1 = 1,\ldots,m, \quad j_2 = 1,\ldots,n$

$$V_{j_1, j_2} = G_{j_1, j_2}[1 + \tau \alpha d^2_{j_1, j_2}]^{-1},$$

        end

$$\vec{U}_l^{(k+1)} = IDCT[V],$$

    end,

end.

Interpolation

    Result $= (R_1(X - U^{final}) + R_2(X + U^{final}))/2$

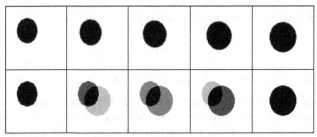

Fig. 2. Top row: results of slice interpolation with proposed method. Bottom row: results of slice interpolation with linear interpolation method.

In the first test, a pair of synthetic images of two circles is used. In the first and last column of Fig. 2 the input images to the algorithms can be seen. Not only the location but also the size of the circle is changed. The goal is to place 3 in-between slices to show the gradual changes of the shape and location of the circle. The results of proposed method and linear interpolation method are presented in the second, third and fourth columns of Fig. 2. As expected the proposed registration based method is able to correctly track the movement of the circle between two slices. Also from the images it can be seen that the transformation can be modeled as an affine transformation which using curvature registration based method it is perfectly estimated.

For the second test, three consecutive slices as in Fig.3 (a) are used. Taking the first and third slices as inputs, the in-between slice is reconstructed by using both linear interpolation and the proposed method. Fig.3 (b) shows the interpolation results using the two methods (top row) as well as the computed difference images (bottom row) with respect to the original image. The computed MSDs are 84.20 and 52.52 for linear and proposed methods respectively. Fig.3 (c) gives a close-up of the results.

Fig.3 (d) gives the optimized displacement fields for both horizontal and vertical directions. Bright and dark shades represent positive and negative displacement values respectively, while gray shades are for displacements near zero.

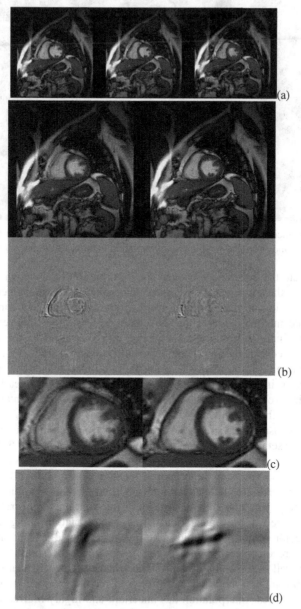

Fig. 3. (a) Three consecutive slices. The first and third images are used for interpolation with parameters set as: $\tau = 0.03, \alpha = 100$ (b) Top row: results of interpolation for linear, non-modified and proposed methods respectively. Bottom row: difference images for the results. (c) Close-up of the results of linear and proposed method. (d) Optimized displacement fields in horizontal and vertical directions

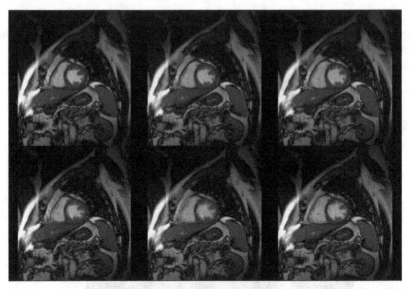

Fig. 4. Results of placing 3 slices between two input slices (first and third slices from Fig.2 (a)) using proposed method (Top row) and linear interpolation method (Bottom row)

As can be seen, the difference between slices is due to the movement of the heart near the center of these images. Using linear interpolation, the movement of heart is not captured, resulting in blurred edges in the interpolated slice. By comparison, the registration-based method captures the movement well and the final result is highly similar to the original one (middle image in Fig. 3 (a)). As a result, the MSD error is significantly reduced and the interpolation result is much sharper. Fig. 4 represents the results of placing 3 in-between slices for the two input images for both proposed method and linear interpolation method. The movement of the heart is perfectly tracked using the proposed registration based method while linear interpolation method cannot capture this movement.

To further demonstrate the strength of the proposed method, the same procedure is applied to another set containing three brain images as shown in Fig. 5 (a). Using the first and third slice, the interpolation results are produced. Besides the linear interpolation, we also compare the proposed method with a non-modified curvature registration based technique, here called non-modified method. For this method, after registering the reference and moving images using curvature registration [12] and finding the optimized displacement fields, linear interpolation along the computed displacement vector of corresponding points in the reference and moving images is implemented to reconstruct the in-between slice. Fig.5 (b) shows the results of interpolation as well as the computed difference images. The MSDs are 71.65, 45.36 and 42.72 for linear, non-modified and proposed methods respectively. As can be seen, the result of linear interpolation has uncertain and highly blurred edges. Result of non-modified method is significantly better than linear interpolation, in terms of MSD but due to nonlinear nature of image registration and optimization process, we still have blurred edges. In comparison, the proposed method gives much sharper edges. This becomes more obvious in the difference images where blurred edges cause widened regions of dissimilarity. Also, it should be mentioned that, in the non-modified method, only one of the images is moving. As a result, more iterations of optimization are needed for convergence, and thus more computational time is required. Fig.5 (c) gives a close-up of the results for better comparison.

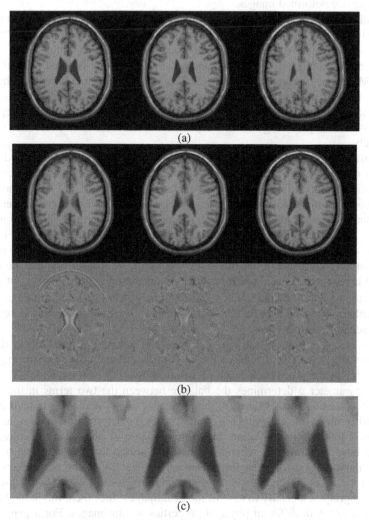

Fig. 5. (a) Three consecutive slices. The first and third images are used for interpolation with parameters set as: $\tau = 0.05, \alpha = 100$ (b) Top row: results of interpolation for linear, non-modified and proposed methods respectively. Bottom row: difference images for the results. (c) Close-up of the results of linear, non-modified and proposed method respectively.

Based on Fig. 5, the effect of moving both images simultaneously in the proposed method in comparison to moving only one of the images in the non-modifed method is obvious. Moving both images, not only reduces the computational time needed for the convergence, but also can prevent the algorithm from getting trapped in local minima which is caused because of large displacements between corresponding points (See Fig.5 (c) for the comparison of the methods); also the integration of linear displacement between corresponding points in the process of optimization reduces the need for additional linear interpolation after registration to a simple averaging between the two deformed images.

A similar test is conducted for the entire brain image database, containing 79 images with the size of 217×181. For interpolation of each evenly numbered slice, a pair of two consecutive slices with odd numberes is used and the reconstructed images are compared with the corresponding slices from the original database. The average MSDs are presented in Table 2. The number in parantheses for the non-modified method represents the improvement percentage with respect to linear interpolation method. The numbers in parantheses for the proposed method represent the improvement percentage with respect to linear and non-modified method respectively.

In terms of computational time, excluding the linear interpolation method which obviously takes less time than the other two, the proposed algorithm outperforms the non-modified method. The algorithm is implemented using MATLAB without any specific code optimization procedure. The average time for the proposed method to produce the in-between image is about 40 seconds while for the non-modified method it is about 50 seconds. This is due to the fact that only one of the images is moving which makes it more time consuming for convergence. The optimization process stops when the improvement in SSD is less than 0.01 %. Also to produce the results presented here, τ and α are fixed for the whole database ($\tau = 0.05, \alpha = 100$). Of course since τ is the time step of the iterative scheme, the process of finding the best value can be further optimized using a line search method to ensure faster and more robust convergence in fewer iterations.

For the smoothness term, the curvature operator penalizes oscillation in the displacement field [12]. Also it reduces the need for additional affine transformation in the beginning of the process of image registration (See Fig.1 for example). The regularization parameter α determines the balance between the two terms in the energy functional. Choosing small values for the parameter causes non-smooth displacement in the final results while choosing big values makes the deformation more rigid which is not useful for slice interpolation due to deformation of objects in the consecutive slices. To have a deformable registration between slices, there should be a trade-off between smoothness of the transformation and the rigidity of the movements. Here the value for α is set intuitively and the same for all the tests provided here which may not be appropriate, especially in case of medical images since there might be different objects (organs) with different physical properties within images. For a general discussion on this subject the reader is referred to [15].

Another thing that may come to mind is that the improvement is not significant compared to the results of the non-modified method. But as it is obvious from the results, by integrating the idea of linear movement between corresponding points in the process of optimization better results can be achieved. However, even in the non-modified method, a linear interpolation is needed between the corresponding points in order to reconstruct the in-between slice. Also it should be mentioned that one of the main assumptions of using registration based methods for slice interpolation is that the objects within the input slices can deform or move, but they cannot disappear. In other words, if from one slice to another the object disappears the result of registration based interpolation is unpredictable. This is not an assumption that can be completely preserved when the input data is a stack of medical images. Overall, the proposed registration based method, can manage to improve the results more than 2.5% percent when compared with the non-modified version (See Table 2). Of course there is room for improvement both in computational time and quality of the final image.

Table 2. Comparison of the average MSDs for brain image database

Method	Linear	Non-modified	Proposed
MSD	118.7652	56.0765 (52.78%)	**54.6450** (53.99%, 2.56%)

4   Conclusion

In this paper, a new registration-based slice interpolation method is proposed. A modified version of curvature registration method has been used with the assumption of linear displacements between corresponding points in two input images. The obtained displacement fields for the two input images are utilized to produce the missing in-between slice. In comparison to both linear interpolation and the non-modified registration-based method, the proposed method produces lower MSD values and less blurred/uncertain edges. The current implementation was performed in MATLAB without any code optimization procedure. An ongoing effort is to implement the algorithm in C/C++, which is expected to consume much less computational time. Part of our future work will be an extension of the linear displacements between images into higher order polynomial formulation that involves more than two adjacent slices.

References

1. Goshtasby, A., Turner, D.A., Ackerman, L.V.: Matching of tomographic slices for interpolation. IEEE Trans. on Medical Imaging 11(4), 507–516 (1992)
2. Higgins, W.E., Orlick, C.J., Ledell, B.E.: Nonlinear filtering approach to 3-D gray-scale image interpolation. IEEE Trans. on Medical Imaging 15(4), 580–587 (1996)
3. Grevera, G.J., Udupa, J.K.: Shape-based interpolation of multidimensional grey-level images. IEEE Trans. on Medical Imaging 15(6), 881–892 (1996)
4. Grevera, G.J., Udupa, J.K.: An objective comparison of 3-D image interpolation methods. IEEE Transactions on Medical Imaging 17(4), 642–652 (1998)
5. Grevera, G.J., Udupa, J.K., Miki, Y.: A task-specific evaluation of three-dimensional image interpolation techniques. IEEE Trans. on Medical Imaging 18(2), 137–143 (1999)
6. Lee, T.Y., Wang, W.H.: Morphology-based three-dimensional interpolation. IEEE Trans. on Medical Imaging 19(7), 711–721 (2000)
7. Lee, T.-Y., Lin, C.-H.: Feature-guided shape-based image interpolation. IEEE Transactions on Medical Imaging 21(12), 1479–1489 (2002)
8. Rueckert, D., Sonoda, L.I., Hayes, C., Hill, D.L., Leach, M.O., Hawkes, D.J.: Nonrigid registration using free-form deformations: application to breast MR images. IEEE Trans. on Medical Imaging 18(8), 712–721 (1999)

9. Penney, G.P., Schnabel, J.A., Rueckert, D., Viergever, M.A., Niessen, W.J.: Registration-based interpolation. IEEE Trans. on Medical Imaging 23(7), 922–926 (2004)
10. Frakes, D.H., Dasi, L.P., Pekkan, K., Kitajima, H.D., Sundareswaran, K., Yoganathan, A.P., Smith, M.J.T.: A new method for registration-based medical image interpolation. IEEE Trans. on Medical Imaging 27(3), 370–377 (2008)
11. Leng, J., Xu, G., Zhang, Y.: Medical image interpolation based on multi-resolution registration. Computers & Mathematics with Applications 66(1), 1–18 (2013)
12. Fischer, B., Modersitzki, J.: A unified approach to fast image registration and a new curvature based registration technique. Linear Algebra and its Applications 380, 107–124 (2004)
13. Modersitzki, J.: Numerical Methods for Image Registration. Numerical Mathematics and Scientific Computation. Oxford University Press, USA (2004)
14. Modersitzki, J.: FAIR: flexible algorithms for image registration, vol. 6. SIAM (2009)
15. Kilmer, M.E., O'Leary, D.P.: Choosing regularization parameters in iterative methods for ill-posed problems. SIAM Journal on Matrix Analysis and Applications 22(4) (2001)

Well-Posed Gaussian-Like Models
for Image Denoising and Sharpening

Xiangtuan Xiong[1], Xinge Li[2], and Guoliang Xu[2,*]

[1] Department of Mathematics, Northwest Normal University,
Lanzhou, Gansu, China
[2] LSEC, ICMSEC, Academy of Mathematics and Systems Science,
Chinese Academy of Sciences, Beijing, China
xuguo@lsec.cc.ac.cn

Abstract. It is well-known that Gaussian filter is the most important model in image denoising. However, the inverse of the Gaussian model for image sharpening is seriously ill-posed. In this paper, we propose several variations of the Gaussian model, which are derived from the varied diffusion equations. Explicit forms for these models (filters) are given in the Fourier space, which facilitate the usage of these models in the image processing. Each of the proposed models has its own distinct feature and plays the role of the image denoising as the Gaussian filter. Furthermore, the inverse problem of the varied diffusion equations are well-posed. Some image denoising and sharpening experiments are conducted showing that the modified models yield more desirable results.

Keywords: Gaussian-like models, image denoising, image sharpening, diffusion equations.

1 Introduction

Noise characterized by Gaussian-like distribution is very often encountered in acquired digital images. It may occur in various practical situations, such as the film grain noise. Gaussian noise can be removed by using both linear and non-linear filtering techniques. There are many techniques which we cannot give here an exhaustive survey. Let us refer to the references [1-5] and therein. Gaussian filter is efficient in smoothing the noise but has the disadvantage of blurring image edges [6]. There are many other linear filtering methods for denoising. These filtering methods tend to blur an image, because pixel intensity values that are significantly higher or lower than the surrounding neighborhood would "smear" across the area. Because of this blurring, linear filters are seldom used in practice for noise reduction; they are, however, often used as the basis for nonlinear noise reduction filters.

The problem of image diffusion plays a key role in image denoising application. Recall that the problem of image diffusion consists of designing a suitable

---

* Corresponding author.

Y.J. Zhang and J.M.R.S. Tavares (Eds.): CompIMAGE 2014, LNCS 8641, pp. 81–94, 2014.
© Springer International Publishing Switzerland 2014

differential operator A on a suitable function space H(e.g. $L^2(\Omega)$, where $\Omega \in \mathbb{R}^2$ denotes the image domain) of images, in other words, the following functional differential equation is considered:

$$\frac{du}{dt} = Au, u(0) = u_0, \ t > 0, \tag{1.1}$$

where u_0 is the initial image to be processed. Depending on the choice of the operator A, the one-parameter family $\{u(t)\}_{t>0}$ may correspond to successively smoothed versions of the initial image u_0. A classical choice for A is the Laplace operator [7], [8], which leads to the equation

$$\frac{du}{dt} = \Delta u, u(0) = u_0, \ t > 0. \tag{1.2}$$

The one-parameter family obtained in this way corresponds to successively blurred versions of the initial image u_0, where the blurring achieved is equivalent to convolving the image with Gaussian kernels of successively increasing variance. The key drawback of the heat equation for denoising purpose is that it blurs out important image structure as well. The procedure of using the classical heat equation is also called isotropic diffusion.

In this paper, we propose several linear PDE-based models for noise removal by modifying the heat diffusion model. Explicit formulas for these models are derived that facilitate the usage of these models in image denoising. From these new models, one can also devise the methods for image sharpening by running these modified heat equations backward in time. Comparative experiments with the classical Gaussian model are conducted. The results show that the new models behave as good as the Gaussian model for image denoising, but much better than the Gaussian model for image sharpening.

The outline of this paper is as follows. In Section 2 we present some modified diffusion equations. The corresponding backward models for image sharpening are given in section 3. In section 4, some numerical results are presented. Section 5 concludes the paper with a summary.

2   Modified Isotropic Diffusion

Consider a noised image defined on $\Omega \subset \mathbb{R}^2$ and let $u_0 = u_0(x, y)$, $(x, y) \in \Omega$, be the intensity of the observed image. The standard way to denoising u_0 is to look for a function u which has the form of

$$u(x, y) = (G * u_0)(x, y), \tag{2.1}$$

where the operator G is the filter kernel, and $*$ is the convolution operator. In the standard heat denoising procedure, the denoised image is given by

$$u(x, y, t) = (G_t * u_0)(x, y) = \int_\Omega G_t(x - r, y - s)u_0(r, s)drds, \quad t > 0, \tag{2.2}$$

where G_t is the Gaussian kernel

$$G_t(x, y) = \frac{1}{4\pi t} e^{-\frac{x^2+y^2}{4t}}, \quad (x, y) \in \mathbb{R}^2, \quad t > 0. \tag{2.3}$$

In this case, $u = u(x, y, t)$ is the solution to the heat equation

$$\begin{cases} \frac{\partial u}{\partial t} - \Delta u = 0, & in \ \mathbb{R}^2 \times (0, \infty), \\ u(x, y, 0) = u_0(x, y). \end{cases} \tag{2.4}$$

The main disadvantage of this classical procedure is that the denoising operator $Ku_0 = G_t * u_0$ has no localization property. In order to overcome this difficulty, we shall modify the heat equation by different methods. In the following, we present four linear models for the denoising problem.

Model 1. *Biharmonic equation.*

Consider the following problem involves biharmonic operator:

$$\begin{cases} \frac{\partial u}{\partial t} = \Delta u + \varepsilon \Delta^2 u, & in \ \mathbb{R}^2 \times (0, \infty), \\ u(x, y, 0) = u_0(x, y), \end{cases} \tag{2.5}$$

where ε is a small positive parameter. Consider the kernel $K_1 = K_1(x, y, t)$ defined by Equation (2.5), that is

$$\begin{cases} \frac{\partial K_1}{\partial t} = \Delta K_1 + \varepsilon \Delta^2 K_1, & in \ \mathbb{R}^2 \times (0, \infty), \\ K_1(x, y, 0) = \delta, \end{cases} \tag{2.6}$$

where δ is the Dirac function in $\mathbb{R}^2$ concentrated in 0. By virtue of Fourier transform $\hat{K}_1(\xi, \eta, t)$ of $K_1(x, y, t)$, Equation (2.6) can be rewritten as

$$\begin{cases} \frac{\partial \hat{K}_1}{\partial t} = -(\xi^2 + \eta^2)\hat{K}_1 + \varepsilon[\xi^4 + 2\xi^2\eta^2 + \eta^4]\hat{K}_1, & in \ \mathbb{R}^2 \times (0, \infty), \\ \hat{K}_1(\xi, \eta, 0) = 1. \end{cases} \tag{2.7}$$

Equation (2.7) has the solution

$$\hat{K}_1(\xi, \eta, t) = e^{[\varepsilon(\xi^4 + 2\xi^2\eta^2 + \eta^4) - (\xi^2 + \eta^2)]t}. \tag{2.8}$$

Therefore, the solution of Equation (2.5) has the following representation

$$u(x, y, t) = K_1(x, y, t) * u_0(x, y) = \int_{\mathbb{R}^2} K_1(x - r, y - s, t)u_0(r, s)drds. \tag{2.9}$$

Equivalently, in the Fourier domain

$$\hat{u}(\xi, \eta, t) = \hat{K}_1(\xi, \eta, t)\hat{u}_0(\xi, \eta), \ \forall (\xi, \eta) \in \mathbb{R}^2, \ t \geq 0, \tag{2.10}$$

where $\hat{u}(\cdot, \cdot, t)$ is the Fourier transform of $u(\cdot, \cdot, t)$. Fig. 2.1 shows the curves of the one-dimensional filter for different ε's and $t = 8$.

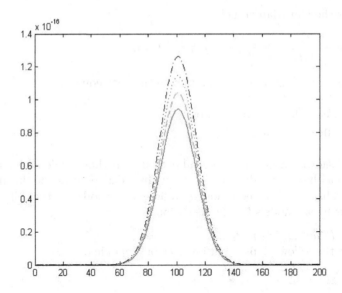

Fig. 2.1. Full line: $\varepsilon = 0.0$; Dash line: $\varepsilon = 0.001$; Dotted line: $\varepsilon = 0.002$; Dash and dot line: $\varepsilon = 0.003$;

Model 2. *Pseudo-parabolic equation.*

Consider the following pseudo-parabolic problem:

$$\begin{cases} \frac{\partial u}{\partial t} - \Delta u - \varepsilon \Delta \frac{\partial u}{\partial t} = 0, \text{ in } \mathbb{R}^2 \times (0, \infty), \\ u(x, y, 0) = u_0(x, y). \end{cases} \tag{2.11}$$

Now we consider the kernel $K_2 = K_2(x, y, t)$ defined by Equation (2.11), that is

$$\begin{cases} \frac{\partial K_2}{\partial t} - \Delta K_2 - \varepsilon \Delta \frac{\partial K_2}{\partial t} = 0, \text{ in } \mathbb{R}^2 \times (0, \infty), \\ K_2(x, y, 0) = \delta. \end{cases} \tag{2.12}$$

Equation (2.12) has the solution

$$\hat{K}_2(\xi, \eta, t) = e^{-\frac{\xi^2 + \eta^2}{1 + \varepsilon(\xi^2 + \eta^2)} t}. \tag{2.13}$$

By virtue of Fourier transform $\hat{K}_2(\xi, \eta, t)$ of $K_2(x, y, t)$, the solution for (2.11) can be formulated as

$$\hat{u}(\xi, \eta, t) = \hat{K}_2(\xi, \eta, t)\hat{u}_0(\xi, \eta), \forall (\xi, \eta) \in \mathbb{R}^2, t \geq 0, \tag{2.14}$$

where $\hat{u}(\cdot, \cdot, t)$ is the Fourier transform of $u(\cdot, \cdot, t)$. Fig. 2.2 shows the curves of the one-dimensional filter for different ε's and $t = 8$.

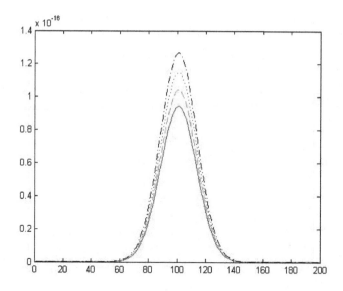

Fig. 2.2. Full line: $\varepsilon = 0.0$; Dash line: $\varepsilon = 0.001$; Dotted line: $\varepsilon = 0.002$; Dash and dot line: $\varepsilon = 0.003$;

Model 3. *Hyperbolic equation*

Consider the following hyperbolic problem:

$$\begin{cases} \frac{\partial u}{\partial t} - \Delta u + \varepsilon \frac{\partial^2 u}{\partial t^2} = 0, \; in \; \mathbb{R}^2 \times (0, \infty), \\ u(x, y, 0) = u_0(x, y), \\ \frac{\partial u}{\partial t}(x, y, 0) = 0. \end{cases} \tag{2.15}$$

Let $K_3 = K_3(x, y, t)$ be the kernel defined by Equation (2.15), that is

$$\begin{cases} \frac{\partial K_3}{\partial t} - \Delta K_3 + \varepsilon \frac{\partial^2 K_3}{\partial t^2} = 0, \; in \; \mathbb{R}^2 \times (0, \infty), \\ K_3(x, y, 0) = \delta, \\ \frac{\partial K_3}{\partial t}(x, y, 0) = 0. \end{cases} \tag{2.16}$$

Equation (2.16) has the solution

$$\hat{K}_3(\xi, \eta, t) = \begin{cases} e^{-\frac{t}{2\varepsilon}} \cos\left[\left(\frac{\xi^2 + \eta^2}{\varepsilon} - \frac{1}{4\varepsilon^2}\right)^{\frac{1}{2}} t\right] & if \; \xi^2 + \eta^2 > \frac{1}{4\varepsilon}, \\ e^{-\frac{t}{2\varepsilon}} \cosh\left[\left(-\frac{\xi^2 + \eta^2}{\varepsilon} + \frac{1}{4\varepsilon^2}\right)^{\frac{1}{2}} t\right] & if \; \xi^2 + \eta^2 \le \frac{1}{4\varepsilon}. \end{cases} \tag{2.17}$$

Using Fourier transform $\hat{K}_3(\xi, \eta, t)$ of $K_3(x, y, t)$, the solution for (2.15) can be formulated as

$$\hat{u}(\xi, \eta, t) = \hat{K}_3(\xi, \eta, t)\hat{u}_0(\xi, \eta), \; \forall (\xi, \eta) \in \mathbb{R}^2, \; t \ge 0, \tag{2.18}$$

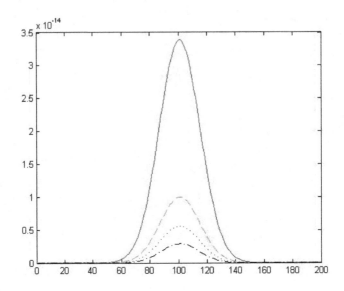

Fig. 2.3. Full line: $\varepsilon = 0.0$; Dash line: $\varepsilon = 0.01$; Dotted line: $\varepsilon = 0.02$; Dash and dot line: $\varepsilon = 0.03$;

where $\hat{u}(\cdot, \cdot, t)$ is the Fourier transform of $u(\cdot, \cdot, t)$. Fig. 2.3 shows the curves of the one-dimensional filter for different ε's and $t = 10$.

A similar problem has been discussed in [9].

Model 4. *Quasi-boundary problem of the diffusion equation*

Consider the following quasi-boundary problem:

$$\begin{cases} \frac{\partial u}{\partial t} - \Delta u = 0, & in \quad \mathbb{R}^2 \times (0, \infty), \\ u(x, y, 0) + \varepsilon u(x, y, T) = u_0(x, y). \ T > 0 \end{cases} \tag{2.19}$$

By virtue of Fourier transform, we have

$$\begin{cases} \frac{\partial \hat{u}}{\partial t} = -(\xi^2 + \eta^2)\hat{u}, & in \quad \mathbb{R}^2 \times (0, \infty), \\ \hat{u}(\xi, \eta, 0) + \varepsilon \hat{u}(\xi, \eta, T) = \hat{u_0}(\xi, \eta), \ T > 0, \end{cases} \tag{2.20}$$

where $u(x, y, T)$ is used as the denoised image on u_0. Thus the solution for (2.19) can be formulated as

$$\hat{u}(\xi, \eta, t) = \hat{K}_4(\xi, \eta, t)\hat{u_0}(\xi, \eta), \ \forall (\xi, \eta) \in \mathbb{R}^2, \ t \geq 0, \tag{2.21}$$

where $\hat{K}_4(\xi, \eta, t)$ is given by

$$\hat{K}_4(\xi, \eta, t) = \frac{e^{-(\xi^2 + \eta^2)t}}{1 + \varepsilon e^{-(\xi^2 + \eta^2)T}}. \tag{2.22}$$

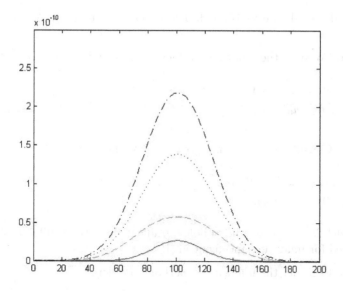

Fig. 2.4. Full line: $\varepsilon = 0.0$; Dash line: $\varepsilon = 0.001$; Dotted line: $\varepsilon = 0.002$; Dash and dot line: $\varepsilon = 0.003$;

Fig. 2.4 shows the curves of the one-dimensional filter for different ε's and $t = T = 14$.

We have describe four variations of the heat equation. For the existence of solutions for these Cauchy problems, the conclusion is that all of them have weak solution. Specifically, we have the following result [9] for Model 3 (for other models, we have the same conclusion):

Theorem 2.1. *Assume that $u_0 \in L^2(\mathbb{R}^2)$. Then equation (2.15) has a unique weak solution $u(x, y, t)$ which is continuous in t with values in $L^2(\mathbb{R}^2)$.*

3   Backward of the Modified Diffusion Equations

It is well-known that the most basic approach for image sharpening is to run the classical heat equation in the backward direction on a given image u_0, i.e., consider

$$\frac{du}{dt} = -\Delta u, u(0) = u_0, \ t > 0. \tag{3.1}$$

However the above problem is ill-posed. The ill-posedness comes from the instability of the problem (3.1). By introducing the regularization parameter ε, the modified models are well-posed. These modified models are reproduced as follows:

Model 1a. Consider the following problem involves biharmonic operator:

$$\begin{cases} \frac{\partial u}{\partial t} + \Delta u - \varepsilon \Delta^2 u = 0, \ in \ \mathbb{R}^2 \times (0, \infty), \\ u(x, y, 0) = u_0(x, y). \end{cases} \tag{3.2}$$

Model 2a. Consider the following pseudo-parabolic problem:

$$\begin{cases} \frac{\partial u}{\partial t} + \Delta u - \varepsilon \Delta \frac{\partial u}{\partial t} = 0, \ in \ \mathbb{R}^2 \times (0, \infty), \\ u(x, y, 0) = u_0(x, y). \end{cases} \tag{3.3}$$

For Model 2a, based on the Sobolev gradient flow, the similar problem has been devised for image enhancement in [10].

Model 3a. Consider the following hyperbolic problem:

$$\begin{cases} \frac{\partial u}{\partial t} + \Delta u - \varepsilon \frac{\partial^2 u}{\partial t^2} = 0, \ in \ \mathbb{R}^2 \times (0, \infty), \\ u(x, y, 0) = u_0(x, y). \\ \frac{\partial u}{\partial t}(x, y, 0) = 0. \end{cases} \tag{3.4}$$

Model 4a. Consider the following quasi-boundary problem:

$$\begin{cases} \frac{\partial u}{\partial t} + \Delta u = 0, \qquad\qquad in \qquad \mathbb{R}^2 \times (0, \infty), \\ u(x, y, 0) + \varepsilon u(x, y, T) = u_0(x, y), \ T > 0. \end{cases} \tag{3.5}$$

Thus, our proposed Models 1-4 can run in the forward direction for image smoothing and in the reverse direction for image sharpening. Now we show that these models are well-posed. For example, we can establish the stability for Model 4a. First we present the following lemma.

Lemma 3.1. *Let* $0 < t < T$, *then*

$$\sup_{s > 0} \frac{e^{st}}{1 + \varepsilon e^{sT}} \leq \varepsilon^{-\frac{t}{T}}. \tag{3.6}$$

The proof of the lemma can be found in [11].

Theorem 3.1. *The solution of problem (3.5) continuously depends on the data* u_0 *if the parameter* ε *is selected appropriately.*

Proof. We prove the following conclusion: Let $u_{0,1}$ and $u_{0,2}$ be any two initial datum satisfying $\|u_{0,1} - u_{0,2}\| \leq \delta$, and $u_\delta^{\varepsilon,1}(\cdot, t)$ and $u_\delta^{\varepsilon,2}(\cdot, t)$ the corresponding solutions, respectively, with $\varepsilon = O(\delta)$. Then $\|u_\delta^{\varepsilon,1} - u_\delta^{\varepsilon,2}\| \to 0$, as $\delta \to 0$. In fact, by Parseval identity, we have

$$\left\| u_\delta^{\varepsilon,1} - u_\delta^{\varepsilon,2} \right\| = \left\| \widehat{u_\delta^{\varepsilon,1}} - \widehat{u_\delta^{\varepsilon,2}} \right\|$$

$$= \left\| \frac{e^{(\xi^2+\eta^2)t}}{1 + \varepsilon e^{(\xi^2+\eta^2)T}} \left(\widehat{u_{0,1}} - \widehat{u_{0,2}} \right) \right\|$$

$$\leq \sup_{(\xi,\eta)\in\mathbb{R}^2} \left| \frac{e^{(\xi^2+\eta^2)t}}{1 + \varepsilon e^{(\xi^2+\eta^2)T}} \right| \delta.$$

Using the inequality (3.6), we have

$$\left\| u_\delta^{\varepsilon,1} - u_\delta^{\varepsilon,2} \right\| \leq \delta \varepsilon^{-\frac{t}{T}}.$$

Hence if $\varepsilon = O(\delta)$ and $t > 0$, we have

$$\| u_\delta^{\varepsilon,1} - u_\delta^{\varepsilon,2} \| \to 0, \text{ for } \delta \to 0.$$

Hence the theorem is proved.   □

4   Experimental Results

In this section we give some experimental results of the proposed models for image denoising and image sharpening. The restoration quality is measured by the *peak signal-to noise ratio* (PSNR) and the *ratio* α of the restored image and the noisy image, which are defined as

$$\text{PSNR} = 10 \log_{10} \left(\frac{MN}{\sum_{i=1}^{M} \sum_{j=1}^{N} (g_{ij} - h_{ij})^2} \right),$$

$$\alpha = \frac{\text{PSNR of the restored image}}{\text{PSNR of the noisy image}},$$

where g is the original image with size $M \times N$, h denotes the compared image, and the unit of PSNR is decibel (dB).

4.1   Image Denoising

We implement the proposed four models by FFT algorithms. The noisy images were created by a built-in function *imnoise* in Matlab. We used Gaussian white noise with mean 0 and variance 0.013. Fig. 4.1 and Fig. 4.2 show the noisy image (a) affected by Gaussian noise, the result produced by Gaussian filter (b), the results produced by Model 1-4 (c)–(f). The data in Table 4.1 and Table 4.2 show the PSNR and the ratio α of the denoised images. Both the figures in Fig. 4.1, Fig. 4.2 and the data in the Table 4.1, Table 4.2 reveal that the results of using these four models are slightly better than (similar to) the result of using the Gaussian model.

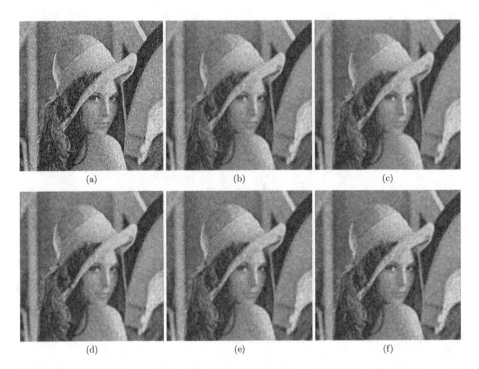

Fig. 4.1. (a) Noisy image; (b) Gaussian filter with $t = 0.000007$; (c) Model 1 with $\varepsilon = 1e\text{-}7, t = 0.000008$; (d) Model 2 with $\varepsilon = 1e\text{-}6, t = 0.000009$; (e) Model 3 with $\varepsilon = 1e\text{-}2, t = 0.6$; (f) Model 4 with $\varepsilon = 1e\text{-}7, T = t = 0.000008$

Table 4.1. A PSNR analysis of the results produced by Models 1–4 when $\sigma = 0.013$

Denoising methods	PSNR	Ratio α
Gaussian denoising	26.540187952987782	1.400387304939815
Biharmonic denoising	26.540553390812221	1.400406587187966
Pseudo-parabolic denoising	26.545284364512106	1.400656215996966
Hyperbolic denoising	26.713080030783942	1.409509918212158
Quasi-boundary denoising	26.534919545311311	1.400109318542716

4.2   Image Sharpening

We implement the Models 1a–4a by FFT algorithms. Now the total noise $n(x, y)$ is added to $u_0(x, y)$ by setting

$$n(x_j, y_k) = \sigma \, r_{jk} \max\{u_0(x_j, y_k)\},$$

where σ denotes the noise level and r_{jk} is a random number drawn from a uniform distribution in the range $[0, 1]$. The blurred and noisy image $u_{0,\delta}(x, y) = u_0(x, y) + n(x, y)$ is the input of the deblurring algorithms. In numerical experiment, we used $\sigma = 0.01$, corresponding to 1% noise.

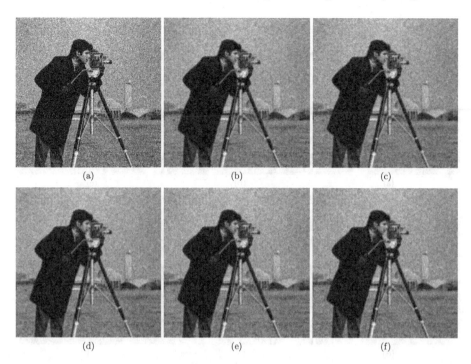

Fig. 4.2. (a) Noisy image; (b) Gaussian filter with $t = 0.000005$; (c) Model 1 with $\varepsilon = 1e\text{-}7, t = 0.000005$; (d) Model 2 with $\varepsilon = 1e\text{-}7, t = 0.000005$; (e) Model 3 with $\varepsilon = 1e\text{-}2, t = 0.38$; (f) Model 4 with $\varepsilon = 1e\text{-}3, T = t = 0.000005$.

The original images were artificially blurred by convolution with a point spread function $p(x, y)$ whose Fourier transform is given by $e^{-t(\xi^2 + \eta^2)}$ with $t = 0.00001$. The results produced by the four models are shown as Fig. 4.3 and Fig. 4.4. The results produced by equation (3.5) where we used the $u(x, y, t)$ as the restored images with $t = 0.00001, T = 0.00003, \varepsilon = 0.00001, t = 0.00001, T = 0.00003, \varepsilon = 0$ are shown as (e) and (f). We can see that when $\varepsilon = 0$, Model 4a is the backward diffusion equation which is ill-posed. The data in Table 4.3 and Table 4.4 show the PSNR and the ratio α of the sharpen images.

From these experiments, we can see that the Model 1a–4a can be used for image sharpening. Model 4a gives the most desirable result. Then the next best

Table 4.2. A PSNR analysis of the results produced by Models 1–4 when $\sigma = 0.013$

Denoising methods	PSNR	Ratio α
Gaussian denoising	24.656801842929241	1.280768517325952
Biharmonic denoising	24.666679924884129	1.281281622653235
Pseudo-parabolic denoising	24.666235401110018	1.281258532389595
Hyperbolic denoising	24.738312631968221	1.285002499214136
Quasi-boundary denoising	24.657568659372121	1.280808348702497

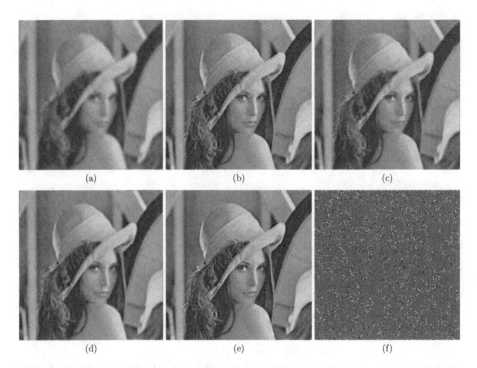

Fig. 4.3. (a) Blurry and noisy image; (b) Model 1a with $\varepsilon = 1e\text{-}6, t = 0.000009$; (c) Model 2a with $\varepsilon = 1e\text{-}9, t = 0.000002$; (d) Model 3a with $\varepsilon = 1e\text{-}9, t = 0.25$; (e) Model 4a with $\varepsilon = 1e\text{-}4, t = 0.00001, T = 0.00003$; (f) Model 4a with $\varepsilon = 0, t = 0.00001, T = 0.00003$

Table 4.3. A PSNR analysis of the results produced by Models 1a–4a when $t = 0.00001$

Sharpening methods	PSNR	Ratio α
Biharmonic Sharpening	31.282961043768719	1.111317438934098
Pseudo-parabolic Sharpening	28.741967970792675	1.021049452145440
Hyperbolic Sharpening	28.751418706894299	1.021385186599279
Quasi-boundary Sharpening	33.094153967774766	1.175659502938391
Backward diffusion Sharpening	-28.788621250083338	-1.022706795348554

result is given by Model 1a, followed by Model 3a and Model 2a. The results from Model 2a and Model 3a are very similar, and it is hard to tell the difference from the figures. The Gaussian model leads to meaningless result.

5   Conclusion

By modifying the classical heat equation, some new image processing procedures have been provided in this paper. These proposed image processing methods work successfully for images which affected by the Gaussian noise. The forward

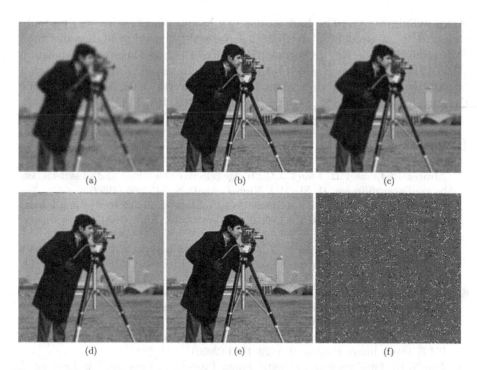

Fig. 4.4. (a) Blurry and noisy image; (b) Model 1a with $\varepsilon = 1e\text{-}6, t = 0.00001$; (c) Model 2a with $\varepsilon = 1e\text{-}9, t = 0.000002$; (d) Model 3a with $\varepsilon = 1e\text{-}9, t = 0.32$; (e) Model 4a with $\varepsilon = 1e\text{-}4, t = 0.00001, T = 0.00003$; (f) Model 4a with $\varepsilon = 0, t = 0.00001, T = 0.00003$

Table 4.4. A PSNR analysis of the results produced by Models 1a–4a when $t = 0.00001$

Sharpening methods	PSNR	Ratio α
Biharmonic Sharpening	28.214870088277660	1.124041782053958
Pseudo-parabolic Sharpening	25.655530230161659	1.022081187303828
Hyperbolic Sharpening	26.038350279607826	1.037332213774591
Quasi-boundary Sharpening	29.544977398930715	1.177031435634203
Backward diffusion Sharpening	-30.411212090741060	-1.211541039386162

applications of these models for image denoising are as good as (sometimes better) the Gaussian filter. The backward application of these models are much more stable than inverse of the Gaussian model. Therefore, we believe that the provided denoising and sharpening methods could be very useful in many image analysis applications. In the future, we intend to do some research on the features of these proposed kernels and extend our image processing methods to nonlinear models.

Acknowledgments. The first author (X. Xiong) of this work was partially supported by a grant from the National Natural Science Foundation of China (No. 11001223), the Key (Keygrant) Project of Chinese Ministry of Education (No. 212179). The second and third authors (X. Li and G. Xu) were supported in part by NSFC under the grants 11101401 and 81173663, NSFC Funds for Creative Research Groups of China (grant No. 11021101, 11321061).

References

1. Alvarez, L., Lions, P.L., Morel, J.M.: Image selective smoothing and edge detection by nonlinear diffusion. II, SIAM J. Numer. Anal. 29, 845–866 (1992)
2. Aubert, G., Kornprobst, P.: Mathematical Problems in Image Processing: Partial Differential Equations and the Calculus of Variations. Appl. Math. Sci. Springer, New York (2006)
3. Gilboa, G., Sochen, N., Zeevi, Y.Y.: Forward-and-backward diffusion processes for adaptive image enhancement and denoising. IEEE Trans. Image Process. 11, 689–703 (2002)
4. Lysaker, M., Lundervold, A., Tai, X.C.: Noise removal using fourth-order partial differential equations with applications to medical magnetic resonance images in space and time. IEEE Trans. Image Process. 12, 1579–1590 (2003)
5. You, Y., Kaveh, M.: Fourth-order partial differential equations for noise removal. IEEE Trans. Image Process. 9, 1723–1730 (2000)
6. Jain, A.K.: Fundamentals of Digital Image Processing. Prentice Hall, Englewood Cliffs (1989)
7. Witkin, A.: Scale-space filtering. In: Proceedings of the Internatinal Joint Conference on Artificial Intelligence, Karlsruhe, West Germany, pp. 1019–1021 (1983)
8. Witkin, A.: Scale-space filtering: A new approach to multi-scale description. In: Proceeding of the IEEE International Conference on Acoustics, Speech, and Signal Processing, vol. 9, pp. 153–159. IEEE Computer Society Press, Piscataway (1984)
9. Barbu, T.: Novel linear image denoising approach based on a modified Gaussian filter kernel. Numer. Func. Anal. Optimz. 33(11), 1269–1279 (2012)
10. Calder, J., Mansouri, A., Yezzi, A.: Image diffusion and sharpening via Sobolev gradient flows. SIAM J. Imaging. Sci. 3(4), 981–1014 (2010)
11. Xiong, X.T.: A regularization method for a Cauchy problem of the Helmholtz equation. J. Comput. Appl. Math. 233, 1723–1732 (2010)

Pattern Classes in Retinal Fundus Images Based on Function Norms

Isabel N. Figueiredo[1], Júlio S. Neves[1], Susana Moura[1],
Carlos Manta Oliveira[2], and João Diogo Ramos[2]

[1] CMUC, Dep. of Mathematics, University of Coimbra, Portugal
[2] Critical Health, S.A., Coimbra, Portugal

Abstract. Retinal fundus images are widely used for screening, diagnosis and prognosis purposes in ophthalmology. Additionally these can also be used in retinal identification/recognition systems, for identification/authentication of an identity. In this paper the aim is to explain how norms in function spaces can be used to set up, automatically, classes of different retinal fundus images. These classifications rely on crucial and unique retinal features, such as the vascular network, whose location and measurement are appropriately quantified by weighted norms in function spaces. These quantifications can be understood as retinal pattern assessments and used for improving the efficiency and speed of retinal identification/recognition frameworks. The proposed methods are evaluated in a large dataset of retinal fundus images, and, besides being very fast, they achieve a reduction of the search in the dataset (for identification/recognition purposes), by 70% on average.

Keywords: Weighted function norms, Retinal fundus images, Vessel network.

1 Introduction

The retina is an anatomic structure of the human eye, essential for the process of human vision. It translates the incoming light, *i.e.* the optical images, into electrical impulses that are processed in the brain [1].

Retinal fundus photography is a non-invasive imaging technique, where the retinal tissues are projected into the two-dimensional imaging plane, by using reflected light. Thus it is a process, that provides a two-dimensional image, such that the image intensities are proportional to a reflected quantity of light in the retinal tissues. In the last 160 years retinal fundus images have been systematically used by clinicians and eye specialists for screening, managing and monitoring different diseases (see also [2] for an automated and ongoing diabetic retinopathy screening program: *Retmarker*®).

On the other hand, it is known that some human retina features, related to texture, size, location, and pigmentation of different retinal structures vary a lot from individual to individual. Furthermore, retinal vascular network is itself a unique structure to each individual. The awareness of this fact was first stated

Y.J. Zhang and J.M.R.S. Tavares (Eds.): CompIMAGE 2014, LNCS 8641, pp. 95–105, 2014.

in [3], where it is reported that every retina contains a unique blood vessel pattern. Subsequently in [4] it is conducted a study, that concludes that even among identical twins the blood vessel patterns are different and unique. Therefore, retinal identification/recognition procedures (see for instance [9, 10]) are valuable instruments in biometric information (as *e.g.* fingerprint or facial recognitions). It is certainly not the most practical solution for traditional identification applications, such as access control. Notwithstanding, with the emergence of EHR (Electronic Health Records) and as equipments are becoming increasingly affordable, the automatic assessment of who a retinal picture belongs to, allows for automation of processes and reduction of errors. To achieve this assessment, several authors have proposed image registration methods with high efficacy (see for example the works [11–13]). However these methods would require a 1 to 1 comparison between the new image and each image in the database. The work herein proposes not an alternative to these methods, but rather a previous step before those methods, which reduces the required number of images to be searched.

In this paper it is described a methodology for defining pattern classes in retinal fundus images, based on particular function norms, which have shown the ability to locate and measure efficiently the retinal vascular network. The main contributions of the present work rely on a combination of particular methods and mathematical techniques, which involve three major steps : i) the extraction of the vessel network, by using the green channel of the original retinal fundus image, with curvelets for denoising [5] and wavelets for vessel extraction/segmentation [6]; ii) appropriate definitions of function (weighted) norms, that applied to the images derived in i) measure the vessel network distribution along the eye; finally, iii) the use of suitable minimum distance classifiers for designing the pattern classes [7]. This work focuses on points ii) and iii). Starting by the extraction of the vessel network, we first derive a procedure, based on suitable weighted function norms, that is able to automatically identify if the new image belongs either to the left or to the right eye. Subsequently, having the dataset split into left or right eye images, a classification of the dataset into pattern classes is performed, again using particular weighted function norms that quantify the vessel network distribution along the eye, by emphasizing the features in some parts of the eye.

For a better understanding of the relevance of the work developed in this paper assume now that we have a large dataset of retinal fundus images separated into classes, each class corresponding to images of the same patient's eye. In the context of retinal identification/recognition systems the goal is to develop an efficient automatic procedure, that assigns a new incoming image to the correct class, or that creates a new class, if the new image belongs to a new patient. This was precisely our main motivation for developing the present work. We describe in this paper an automatic and very fast methodology that performs an unsupervised design of pattern classes of retinal fundus images, aiming at reducing the search and speed up the process of retinal identification/recognition.

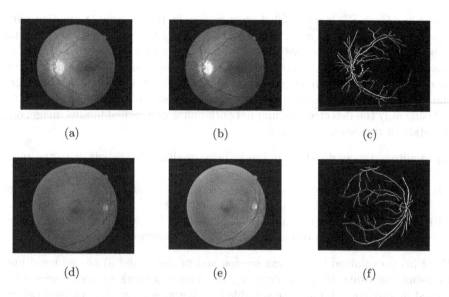

(a)   (b)   (c)

(d)   (e)   (f)

Fig. 1. (a), (d) Original retinal fundus images (Critical Health & AIBILI). (b), (e) Denoised green channels. (c), (f) Vessel networks extracted from (b), (e).

After this introduction, the layout of the paper consists of a description of the methodology in Sections 2 and 3, including the particular weighted function norms used and the proposed pattern classification approach, then the results obtained for a large dataset are presented in Section 4, and finally some conclusions and outlook.

2   Vessel Network Location and Measurement

In this section we explain how weighted function norms are used for measuring the size of the vessel network as well as its distribution along the image.

For extracting the vessels, firstly, the green channel is denoised, by using fast discrete curvelets transforms [5], and then the vessel network is obtained, from this denoised green channel, using wavelets and employing the same method as in [6] (see Figure 1).

Hereafter we assume that a given grayscale (or scalar) image I can be represented by a function (also denoted by I) defined on the rectangle $\Omega = [-0.5, 0.5] \times [-0.5, 0.5]$ of R^2 representing the pixel domain of the image $I : \Omega \subset R^2 \to R$. We also denote by $x = (x_1, x_2)$ any arbitrary point in Ω. Moreover we denote by $L^1_\omega(\Omega)$ the real-valued function spaces endowed with the norm $\|.\|_{L^1_\omega}$. These spaces consist of Lebesgue measurable functions $f : \Omega \to R$, such that [8]

$$\|f\|_{L^1_\omega} := \int_\Omega |f(x)|\, \omega(x)\, dx < \infty, \tag{1}$$

where $\omega : \Omega \to R_0^+$ is a so-called positive weight (a measurable function with $w(x) > 0$ for all $x \in \Omega$ a.e.). When $\omega \equiv 1$, then $L_\omega^1(\Omega) = L^1(\Omega)$ is the usual Lebesgue space. The positive weight function ω can be defined in a variety of ways, and it has several advantages over the weight $\omega \equiv 1$. In particular it can be chosen, in order to enhance relevant features of the function f, for instance, the location of the highest values of f or the distribution of the values of f in Ω.

Using only the detected vascular network image of a retinal fundus image, our intention in this work is threefold:

i) to automatically decide if an image belongs either to the left or to the right eye;
ii) subsequently, to quantify the vessel network distribution along the eye by emphasizing the features in some parts of the eye;
iii) and finally to use the previous information for designing retinal fundus classes to be used in retinal identification/recognition frameworks.

Point iii) is explained in the next section and points i) and ii) are achieved just by using the value $\|I\|_{L_\omega^1}$ (I denoting the vessel network (scalar) image of a retinal fundus image), for some suitable positive weights w, as explained below. In fact by choosing the following function

$$w(x_1, x_2) := 1 + \alpha x_1 + \beta x_1^2 + \gamma x_2^2 \tag{2}$$

for defining a weight, then when used in $\|I\|_{L_\omega^1}$ (see (1)), it reinforces the left or right part of the eye (depending on a negative or positive α, respectively) and the locations closer to the inner part or to the border of the image (depending on the values of β and γ). We clarify now these properties for five important particular cases of (2).

The weight $w_r(x_1, x_2) := 1 + 2x_1$ enhances the features from the right hand side of the image, while $w_l(x_1, x_2) := 1 - 2x_1$ intensifies the features from the left hand side. Therefore, these two weights are extremely suited for distinguishing images having the optic disk on the right from those that have the optic disk on the left.

On the other hand, there are other weights that enable other type of assessment of the vessel expansion in the image. For example, the radial weight $w_1(x_1, x_2) := 1 + x_1^2 + x_2^2$ emphasizes the vessels (if available) in the outer center part of the image (part close to the border), giving an idea of how long the vessels are away from the center. The radial weight $w_2(x_1, x_2) := 1 - x_1^2 - x_2^2$ intensifies the features in the inner center part of the image (part far from the border) and provides the information on how the vessels spread around the center. The weight $w_3(x_1, x_2) := 1 - 2x_2^2$ strengthens horizontal strips in the center of the image, and therefore supplies the information on how long the vessels stretch horizontally.

We illustrate now, just for two particular images, the importance of the function norms (with the weights w_l, w_r, w_1, w_2, w_3), in assessing automatically some features of the vessels, without the need of visualizing the images. Let us denote by I_l and I_r the images (c) and (f) of Figure 1, respectively. Clearly, for

I_l the vessels are concentrated more on the left side of the image, while for I_r the vessels are distributed more to the right. Therefore, $\|I_l\|_{L^1_{\omega_l}}$ should be bigger than $\|I_l\|_{L^1_{\omega_r}}$, and $\|I_r\|_{L^1_{\omega_r}}$ should be bigger than $\|I_r\|_{L^1_{\omega_l}}$, where w_l and w_r are the left and right weights defined before. Moreover, when we compare the vessel network of I_l and I_r, the image I_r has more long vessels along a horizontal central strip, more vessels in the inner center as well as in the outer center of the image. Therefore, $\|I_r\|_{L^1_{\omega_i}}$ should be bigger than $\|I_l\|_{L^1_{\omega_i}}$, where ω_i, $i = 1, 2, 3$, are the other weights defined above. In fact, the following values for the weighted norms of I_r and I_l, with the previous five weights, confirm all these aspects.

Spliting Left/Right eye

$$\|I_l\|_{L^1_{\omega_l}} = 0.051466, \quad \|I_l\|_{L^1_{\omega_r}} = 0.034193,$$

$$\|I_r\|_{L^1_{\omega_l}} = 0.035542, \quad \|I_r\|_{L^1_{\omega_r}} = 0.053381.$$

Assessment of vessels expansion

$$\|I_l\|_{L^1_{\omega_1}} = 0.045885, \quad \|I_l\|_{L^1_{\omega_2}} = 0.039774, \quad \|I_l\|_{L^1_{\omega_3}} = 0.039058,$$

$$\|I_r\|_{L^1_{\omega_1}} = 0.048681, \quad \|I_r\|_{L^1_{\omega_2}} = 0.040242, \quad \|I_r\|_{L^1_{\omega_3}} = 0.039481.$$

3   Vascular Pattern Classes

In the first place, images from the left eye should be separated from those from the right eye (a broad pattern classification), and only afterwards a more fine pattern classification is performed, separately, for both the left eye and the right eye images. This section explains how these (broad and fine) pattern classifications can be automatically performed, by using the weighted norms.

3.1   Left and Right Eye Separation

Consider a given dataset of vessel network images, corresponding to different patients, and containing images from the left and right eyes. As observed, and illustrated in the previous section, the weights ω_l and ω_r can be used to assess if an image corresponds to the left and right eye. For an image I, representing the vessel network, the automatic decision is made by comparing the values of $\|I\|_{L^1_{\omega_l}}$ and $\|I\|_{L^1_{\omega_r}}$. The biggest value determines to which eye the image belongs to :

$$\text{if} \quad \|I\|_{L^1_{\omega_l}} < \|I\|_{L^1_{\omega_r}} \longrightarrow I \text{ is a right eye image,}$$

$$\text{if} \quad \|I\|_{L^1_{\omega_r}} < \|I\|_{L^1_{\omega_l}} \longrightarrow I \text{ is a left eye image.}$$

In this way two sub-datasets, the left and right eye datasets are automatically created. Then each sub-dataset can be partitioned into classes as described in the following section.

3.2 Eye Pattern Classes

We describe now how the previous weighted function norms, associated with the weights ω_1, ω_2, and ω_3, can be used for designing pattern classes in retinal fundus images (either from the left or the right eye) and explain an approach for recognition technique, based on matching and the minimum distance classifier, very similar to the method described in [7], Chapter 12.

We represent each retinal class by a prototype pattern (which is a function norm, in our case) and an unknown pattern (an unknown norm, in our case) is assigned to the closest class, corresponding to the minimizer of the (Euclidean) distance between the unknown and each prototype pattern. In order to explain how the pattern classes are built let us denote by $\|.\|$ any of the norms $\|.\|_{L^1_{\omega_i}}$, for $i = 1, 2, 3$, introduced in the previous section and proceed as follows:

i) Consider a given dataset of vessel network images, corresponding to N patients, and containing only images from the left eye (for a dataset with right eye images the procedure is similar). We also assume that a large number of patients have more than one image in the dataset. We first gathered the images in classes, where one class is identified with a patient (more precisely, a patient left eye in this case), and contains only images of that patient. Remark that this gathering requires *a priori* knowledge: the set of images belonging to each patient is known. These classes are denoted by C_j, $j = 1, \ldots, N$. That is, for patient j

$$C_j := \{I_j^1, \ldots, I_j^{n_j}\}$$

where n_j is the total number of images of patient j in the dataset, and I_j^i (for $i = 1, \ldots, n_j$) represents an image, existent in the dataset and belonging to patient j. Moreover for each $j = 1, \ldots, N$, let

$$\max_j := \text{maximum of } \|.\| \text{ in } C_j$$

$$\min_j := \text{minimum of } \|.\| \text{ in } C_j$$

$$m_j \quad := (\min_j + \max_j)/2$$

$$\Delta_j \quad := \begin{cases} \max_j - \min_j & \text{if } \max_j \neq \min_j \\ \text{maximum} \{\max_i - \min_i : i = 1, \ldots, N\} & \text{if } \max_j = \min_j. \end{cases}$$

We also define for each patient j the interval

$$[\min_j, \max_j] = [m_j - th\, \Delta_j, m_j + th\, \Delta_j], \quad \text{with} \quad th = 1/2,$$

and observe that the norms of the images of patient j (that is of class C_j) belong to $[\min_j, \max_j]$.

ii) After defining the classes, now an automatic classification criterium is needed to assign an unknown image to a certain class (or group of classes) existing in the dataset. We propose to extend slightly the class C_j to a new enlarged class denoted by EC_j (meaning enlarged class C_j), to allow inclusion of new incoming images of the same patient j, whose norms tend to deviate a little bit from the values represented in the interval $[\min_j, \max_j]$. Therefore, when the norm of an image is within $[m_j - th\,\Delta_j, m_j + th\,\Delta_j]$, for a fixed $th > 1/2$, the image is assigned to the class EC_j. Thus one image may belong to more than one class, belonging to the dataset, or to none. If it does not belong to any a new class should be created. We remark that th should be slightly larger than $1/2$, because $1/2$ is the lowest value which assures $C_j \subseteq EC_j$ (in fact, from i) above, $C_j = EC_j$ if $th = 1/2$). In addition, we should increase th in order to enlarge the classes but in such a way that the number of intersections between the classes EC_j would not increase drastically. These intersections are quantified by the average, denoted by $\overline{\cap C}$, of the percentages $p_{\cap C_j}$ of classes EC_i, $i \neq j$, that intersect a given class EC_j. We remark that the lowest value of $\overline{\cap C}$ is attained when $th = 1/2$.

iii) Moreover, and finally, in order to evaluate the dimension of each class, we calculate the average, denoted by $\overline{\#C}$, of the percentages $p_{\#C_j}$ of images that belong to the class EC_j (percentages with respect to the total number of images in the dataset).

Summarizing, this approach is an unsupervised method (whose automatic descriptors rely on weighted function norms of the vascular network) for designing pattern classes of retinal fundus images. For a (left eye or right eye) dataset, the values

$$\overline{\cap C}, \quad p_{\cap C_j} \quad \text{and} \quad \overline{\#C}, \quad p_{\#C_j}$$

represent the gathering of patients and the number of images in each class, respectively. In particular, if we consider these pattern classes in the context of retinal identification/recognition systems, the numbers $\overline{\cap C}$ and $p_{\cap C_j}$ give the information about the amount of search reduction that can be achieved in a large dataset. In the next section we apply this approach to a large dataset for illustrating and concretizing the efficient properties of these quantities.

We also emphasize that this pattern classification is done only once for a given dataset. It is not repeated each time for a new incoming image. Therefore, the time required for defining the classes is not included in the time required for evaluating whether a new incoming image belongs to an existing class, of the dataset, or if it originates a new one (see the end of section 4 for the information concerning the execution time in the experimental tests).

4   Experimental Results

Here the classification proposed in this paper, and its ability to clearly differentiate pattern classes of retinal images, is evaluated.

We use a proprietary dataset (owned by Critical Health, Portugal, http://www.critical-health.com/, and the research institute AIBILI - Association for Innovation and Biomedical Research on Light and Image - Portugal, http://www.aibili.pt/), which includes images from an ongoing diabetic retinopathy screening program [2]. This dataset contains 1505 retinal fundus images: 757 right eye images of 192 patients (with 1 to 5 images per patient) and 748 left eye images of 190 patients (with 2 to 5 images per patient). Each image has the optic disk in the field of view of the image. We have performed 2 different experimental tests.

Test 1 - In this experiment we start from a manual splitting of the images into left eye and right eye, creating two sub-datasets (the right eye and the left eye sub-datasets). Then we performed a classification of each sub-dataset into pattern classes with a threshold $th = 0.51$ (see Section 3) and using the weighted norms $\|.\|_{L^1_{\omega_i}}$ with the weights ω_i, $i = 1, 2, 3$, discussed before. This gives a precise information of how the vessels are spread in the eye.

Test 2 - In this second experiment we use a cascade method with two steps.

Cascade Step 1 - Here the goal consists in assessing the ability of the weighted function norms of the vessel network in automatically deciding whether the image corresponds to the left or right eye. For this end we have used the weights ω_l and ω_r considered before. In this dataset, there were only 6 misclassified images (2 are from the left eye and 4 from the right eye, corresponding to 4 different patients), that come from images where the vessels expand significantly to the opposite side of the optical disk. This shows a very low failure rate of only 0.4%, with respect to the total number of images (1505).

Cascade Step 2 - In this second step, after the splitting obtained in Step 1, a classification of the right eye and left eye sub-datasets into pattern classes is performed (like in Test 1, but now the misclassified images were included).

The Tables 1 to 3 display the results, for all the left eye images of the dataset, of our pattern classification with the 3 norms $\|.\|_{L^1_{\omega_i}}$ with the weights ω_i, $i = 1, 2, 3$. Results for right eye images are nearly identical. The figures on the left columns are for the first test (manual splitting, without any cascade) and the figures on the right columns are for the second test (cascade method) including the misclassified images (and, consequently 4 new classes were created with one image per class).

Now, we comment on the information provided by these tables. For instance, in Table 1 for Test 1 and the norm $\| \cdot \|_{L^1_{\omega_3}}$, the result $\overline{\cap C} = 27.55\%$ means that, on average, each class intersects about 27.55% of the total number of classes. This means that in the context of retinal identification/recognition frameworks, the dataset is reduced in 72% on average. Similarly, $p_{\cap C_j}(> 60\%) = 0.53\%$ indicates that only 0.53% of the classes intersects more than 60% of the total number of classes, and $p_{\cap C_j}(\leq 30\%) = 54.21\%$ means that 54.21% of the classes intersects at most 30% of the total number of classes. On the other hand, the result $\overline{\#C} = 15.5\%$ signifies that, on average, each class contains 15.5% of the total number of images in the dataset. Moreover, $p_{\#C_j}(\leq 30\%) = 86.32\%$, means that 86.32% of the classes have at most 30% of the total number of images in the dataset, and $p_{\#C_j}(> 50\%) = 1.58\%$ tells that only 1.58% of the classes have more than 50% of the total number of images.

In Table 2, the value $p_{\cap C_j} = 19.07\%$ means that, for Test 2 and norm $\| \cdot \|_{L^1_{\omega_2}}$, 19.07% of the classes intersect a minimum of 20% and a maximum of 30%

Table 1. Vascular network norms (left eye)

I (vessel network image)	$\|I\|_{L^1_{\omega_1}}$		$\|I\|_{L^1_{\omega_2}}$		$\|I\|_{L^1_{\omega_3}}$	
% for:	Test 1	Test 2	Test 1	Test 2	Test 1	Test 2
$\overline{\cap C}$ (%)	30.11	31.52	27.75	29.31	27.55	26.66
$p_{\cap C_j}$ (> 60%)	1.58	2.58	0.53	2.06	0.53	1.03
$p_{\cap C_j}$ (≤ 30%)	48.95	47.94	53.68	53.09	54.21	51.55
$p_{\cap C_j}$ (≤ 50%)	86.84	85.97	92.63	90.72	92.11	90.72
$\overline{\#C}$ (%)	16.80	17.4	15.5	16.1	15.5	16.0
$p_{\#C_j}$ (> 50%)	2.11	3.09	2.11	3.09	1.58	1.55
$p_{\#C_j}$ (≤ 20%)	64.74	63.92	70.53	69.59	69.47	68.56
$p_{\#C_j}$ (≤ 30%)	83.16	81.96	86.32	85.05	86.32	85.57

Table 2. Left Eye Frequency Classes from Table 1, for $\|\cdot\|_{L^1_{\omega_2}}$

Frequency Classes	$p_{\cap C_j}$		$p_{\#C_j}$	
% for:	Test 1	Test 2	Test 1	Test 2
]0%, 20%]	38.42	34.02	70.53	69.59
]20%, 30%]	15.26	19.07	15.79	15.46
]30%, 40%]	24.21	22.68	8.42	8.25
]40%, 50%]	14.74	14.95	3.16	3.61
]50%, 60%]	6.84	7.22	2.11	3.09
]60%, 70%]	0	0.52	0	0
]70%, 100%]	0.53	1.55	0	0

of the total number of classes of the dataset. In this same Table 2, the value $p_{\#C_j} = 8.25\%$ shows that, for Test 2 and norm $\|\cdot\|_{L^1_{\omega_2}}$, 8.25% of the classes have a total number of images that is between 30% and 40% of the total number of images of the dataset. For Table 3, the interpretation is the same as for Table 2, the only difference is that now the norm is $\|\cdot\|_{L^1_{\omega_3}}$.

Finally we stress that these methods are extremely fast. All the implementations of the models and norms are done in MATLAB® R2012a (The Mathworks, Inc. [14]), on an iMac computer with a 2.93 GHz Intel Core 2 Duo processor and 4 GB of RAM, running OS X 10.9.1. In particular, either Test 1 or the cascade,

Table 3. Left Eye Frequency Classes from Table 1, for $\| \cdot \|_{L^1_{\omega_3}}$

Frequency Classes	$p_{\cap C_j}$		$p_{\# C_j}$	
% for:	Test 1	Test 2	Test 1	Test 2
]0%, 20%]	36.84	35.05	69.47	68.56
]20%, 30%]	17.37	16.49	16.84	17.01
]30%, 40%]	24.21	24.74	7.37	8.25
]40%, 50%]	13.68	14.43	4.74	4.64
]50%, 60%]	7.37	8.25	1.58	1.55
]60%, 70%]	0	0.52	0	0
]70%, 100%]	0.53	0.52	0	0

in Test 2, is performed in fraction of seconds: about 0.1 seconds in each step of
the cascade, for each frame.

5   Conclusion

The methodologies proposed in this paper aim at a pattern classification on retinal fundus image. They rely on the computation of appropriate function norms
of the corresponding retinal vessel network images. The results suggest that
the weighted norms of the vessel network are valuable descriptors for defining
pattern classes.

Nevertheless, the success of the proposed methods depend on a good extraction of the vessel network. In particular, we cannot expect good results with
images such that the optic disk is not in the field of view of the image, or images
with very bad quality. We remark that, in our study, no alignment of the original
images was performed, otherwise even better results would be expected.

In addition we can also make these methods more efficient. In effect, since
each norm measures a particular feature of each image, it is natural to consider
the influence of several function norms simultaneously, for improving the pattern
classification. For instance, let EC_j^1 and EC_j^2 be the classes obtained by using the
function norms with weights ω_1 and ω_2, respectively, and let $EC_j = EC_j^1 \cap EC_j^2$
be the intersection of these two classes. Then, for this new (intersection) classes
we have obtained the following values for Test 1: $\overline{\cap C} = 24.76\%$, $p_{\cap C_j}(\leq 30\%)$
$= 58.42\%$, $\overline{\# C} = 11.8\%$, $p_{\# C_j}(\leq 20\%) = 81.05\%$ which, as expected, are better
results than those displayed in Table 1, for single weighted norms.

The most important scientific contribution of this paper is a cascade method
proposed for pattern classification, based on the weighted function norms. The
correspondent results show that it is possible, in a large database, and in the

context of retinal identification/recognition to reduce the search to a subset of nearly seventy percent (70%) of the existing classes (each class being a different patient).

Finally the main direct potential real-world application, of the classification proposed in this work, is the acceleration of retinal identification/recognition systems, which will be treated in a separate work. In addition, the consideration of other key retinal features, such as the geometric or texture components of the image, deserve further research and will be postponed to a future work.

Acknowledgments. This work was partially supported by the research project PTDC/MAT-NAN/0593/2012 and by CMUC and FCT (Portugal), through European program COMPETE/FEDER. The authors would also like to thank Dr. Gonçalo Quadros for having proposed the study of the interesting and challenging retina topic.

References

1. Abràmoff, M., Garvin, M., Sonka, M.: Retinal imaging and image analysis. IEEE Reviews in Biomedical Engineering 3, 169–208 (2010)
2. Oliveira, C.M., Cristóvão, L.M., Ribeiro, M.L., Abreu, J.R.: Improved automated screening of diabetic retinopathy. Ophthalmologica 226, 191–197 (2011)
3. Simon, G., Goldstein, I.: A new scientific method of identification. Journal of Medicine 35, 901–906 (1935)
4. Tower, P.: The fundus oculi in monozygotic twins: report of six pairs of identical twins. Archives of Ophthalmology 35, 225–239 (1955)
5. Candes, E., Demanet, L., Donoho, D., Ying, L.: Fast discrete curvelet transforms. Multiscale Modeling & Simulation 5, 861–899 (2006)
6. Bankhead, P., Scholfield, C., McGeown, J., Curtis, T.: Fast retinal vessel detection and measurement using wavelets and edge location refinement. PloS One 7, e32435 (2012)
7. Gonzalez, R.C., Woods, R.E.: Digital Image Processing, 3rd edn. Prentice-Hall, Inc., NJ (2006)
8. Bennett, C., Sharpley, R.: Interpolation of Operators. Academic Press (1988)
9. Zibran, M.F.: Eye Based Authentication: Iris and Retina Recognition. Technical Report# 2011-04, University of Saskatchewan (2009)
10. Sukumaran, S., Punithavalli, M.: Retina recognition based on fractal dimension. International Journal of Computer Science and Network Security 9(10), 66–70 (2009)
11. Zheng, J., Tian, J., Deng, K., Dai, X., Zhang, X., Xu, M.: Salient feature region: a new method for retinal image registration. IEEE Transactions on Information Technology in Biomedicine 15(2), 221–232 (2011)
12. Wei, L., Pan, L., Lin, L., Lu, L.: The retinal image registration based on scale invariant feature. In: 2010 3rd International Conference on Biomedical Engineering and Informatics (BMEI), vol. 2, pp. 639–643. IEEE (October 2010)
13. Xiao, D., Vignarajan, J., Lock, J., Frost, S., Tay-Kearney, M.L., Kanagasingam, Y.: Retinal image registration and comparison for clinical decision support. The Australasian Medical Journal 5(9), 507 (2012)
14. THE MATHWORKS, INC., http://www.matlab.com

Identification of Distinct Blood Vessels in Retinal Fundus Images

Nilanjana Dutta Roy[1], Milan Someswar[1], Harshit Dalmia[1],
and Arindam Biswas[2]

[1] Department of Computer Science and Engineering,
Institute of Engineering and Management, Kolkata, India
{nilanjanaduttaroy,milansomeswar,harshitdalmia}@gmail.com
[2] Department of Information Technology,
Indian Institute of Engineering Science and Technology, Shibpur, India
barindam@gmail.com

Abstract. Many retinal diseases could be characterized by regular tracking of retinal nerves (blood vessels). Identification of each distinct nerve of human retina in ophthalmology plays a vital role for the diagnosis of diabetes, cardiovascular disease etc. In the proposed work, each retinal nerve is identified and colored distinctly. This approach may help the ophthalmologists and scientists to keep track of individual parts of a retinal nerve since it is identified distinctly. Moreover, this work plays an important role in preparing the binary template for retinal authentication system. Experimental results show encouraging outputs.

Keywords: fundus image, opthalmology, distinct nerve coloring, nerve tracking, authentication system.

1 Introduction

The blood vessels in any retinal image are considered as an important indicator for diagnosing some diseases such as diabetes, hypertension, and arteriosclerosis. Typically ophthalmologists use the characteristics of vessels like caliber, color, tortuosity to diagnose and plan a treatment for patients. For example, the images, one shown in Fig. 1, taken by retinal camera, are usually unevenly, non-uniformly illuminated, and poorly contrasted. It can be prohibitive and time consuming for an ophthalmologist to diagnose on the basis of these images. To ease this process, many algorithms were developed to segment blood vessels in retinal images. Ocular fundus images tell us about retinal, ophthalmic, and even systemic diseases. The retinal images, widely used by the ophthalmologists, play an important role in the detection and diagnosis of many eye diseases [1].

Several diseases such as glaucoma, diabetic retinopathy, and macular degeneration are very serious in nature which are the most common causes of blindness if they are not detected in early stage [2]. Symptoms of many retinopathies are related to morphological features of the retinal vascular tree [3]. The clinical procedure of diagnostic for retinopathy is based on an attentive evaluation of the

Y.J. Zhang and J.M.R.S. Tavares (Eds.): CompIMAGE 2014, LNCS 8641, pp. 106–114, 2014.

main features of the retinal vessel structure, obtained from fundus camera images. Traditionally, the vascular tree is analyzed manually by a time-consuming process that demands both training and skill. Furthermore, manual detection of blood vessels is very difficult since the blood vessels in a retinal image are complicated in structure and have low contrast. Therefore, an automatic analysis of fundus images would be of immense help to the ophthalmologist due to the large number of patients.

The human retina has potential to reveal important information about retinal, ophthalmic, and even systemic diseases such as diabetes, hypertension, and arteriosclerosis [4]. Retinal imaging is increasingly being used in large scale, population based studies for detection of glaucoma, diabetic retinopathy, age-related macular degeneration, and cardiovascular disease [5]. The analysis of the relationship between the change in retinal blood vessel features and their linkage with retinal and systemic disease triggers timely detection and treatment while a disease is still in the early stages. Besides implementation of large scale screening programs, the automated analysis of retinal vasculature can assist in evaluation of retinopathy of prematurity, foveal avascular region detection, arteriolar narrowing, the relationship between vessel tortuosity and hypertensive retinopathy, computer-assisted laser surgery, retinal image registration and mosaic synthesis, and biometric identification [6]. Automated segmentation of the retinal vasculature would be valuable in reducing the cost associated with trained human graders and removes the systemic error and inconsistency induced by manual grading. The medical community in general considers automatic retinal vasculature quantification as the first step in the development of a computer assisted ophthalmic diagnostic system. However, the automated segmentation of retinal blood vessels is a complicated task due to the variation in vessel width, the presence of central vessel reflex, uneven illumination, lack of image contrast, and inclusion of noise during image acquisition. The main objective of this paper is to color the different nerve branches originating out from the root with different colors, which makes it easier to track nerves and it makes traversal easier in a particular path.

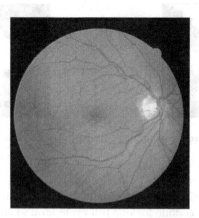

Fig. 1. A retinal image from the DRIVE database

2   Proposed Method

We have taken the retinal fundus image from DRIVE database [17] as the input of our algorithm. By applying the different steps of the given algorithm, the results have been generated.

Input: Vessel Segmented Binary Fundus Image
Output: Distinctly colored retinal nerves

Step 1. Consider retinal fundus images as input from DRIVE [17] database.

Step 2. Preprocessing on the image is done starting from the left most top corner of the fundus image till the right bottom corner of the image.

   Step 2.1 [Optic disc detection]. While traversing, the area in the image having maximum concentration of white pixels in the black background within a certain window is detected as root of the vessel tree or Optic disc.

      Step 2.1.1. We use the property of circle to color the central root. Suppose we have a circle with its center at (x_1,y_1) and radius r, For all points which satisfy the equation

$$(x\text{-}x_1)^2+(y-y_1)^2\text{-}r^2 < 0$$

we can safely conclude that the point clearly lies within the circle which represents the root of the nerve image.

   Step 2.2 [Bifurcation point/crossover points detected]. For a particular window scanning, the non-vascular regions are considered. If the number of non-vascular regions (black regions) is equal to 3, color the region red, indicating bifurcation, or else if the number of non-vascular regions is greater than 3, color the region blue, indicating crossover [18].

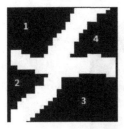   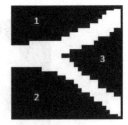

Fig. 2. Detected as crossover point   **Fig. 3.** Detected as bifurcation point

Step 3. For each pixel window in the fundus image, do the following

   Step 3.1. Traversal is done for one full cycle around the surface of the circle which has been detected as optic disc. While traversing around the surface, refer Fig. 4

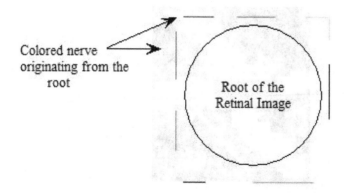

Colored nerve originating from the root

Root of the Retinal Image

All the nerves protruding out from the root in cyclic traversal of minimum row-1 are colored distinctly

Fig. 4. Nerve Beginnings Distinctly Colored

Step 3.1.1 from two rows above the root to row=0, we are checking its 3 neighborhood pixels in row+1 to determine its color. Hence we assign a color to all pixels based on its neighborhood color

Step 3.1.2 from two columns left of the root to column=0 and check its 3 neighborhood pixels in column+1 to determine its color. Hence we assign a color to all pixels based on its neighborhood color

Step 3.1.3 from two rows below the root to row=height and check its 3 neighborhood pixels in row-1 to determine its color. Hence we assign a color to all pixels based on its neighborhood color

Step 3.1.4 from two columns right of the root to column=width and check its 3 neighborhood pixels in column-1 to determine its color. Hence we assign a color to all pixels based on its neighborhood.

Step 3.2. We repeat then the above steps 3-4 times and by applying the logic of Depth First Search (limited), the colors are spread throughout the same nerve.

Step 3.2.1 if any Bifurcation point appears, spread the colors throughout it.

Step 3.2.2 if any crossover point appears, then spread the colors only through the nerve showing a tendency to go towards the same direction. The direction is considered based on the logic that, in case any Crossover point detected, a checking is done to see the angular difference between the nerves. Any two nerves, making an angle approximately 180° (threshold value is fixed) between them, are considered as the same nerve.

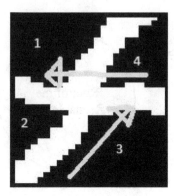

Fig. 5. Showing which direction to follow

Step 4. Now all the nodes have been traversed and the color of each pixel has been determined. The output is then saved into an image buffer in the required format.

Step 5. The algorithm has thus created the output image having nerves colored distinctly.

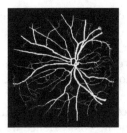

Fig. 6. Input:(original fundus image)   **Fig. 7.** Output:(each set of nerves colored)

2.1 Analysis

The root detection is a simple algorithm in which we search for the most concentrated part of the image with white pixels setting a certain window size, since it is known that the root is more concentrated and thin nerves protrude out from it thus making it the most concentrated region in the input image.

The proposed algorithm of nerve coloring is very effective in the sense that the decision of the color is based on the previous row/column, so once a previous row/column is assigned a color, it becomes easier for the next row because all it has to do is that to look at its neighborhood pixels.

Regarding the Time Complexity, to find the window we need to traverse through the whole 2-D array of pixels representing the input images, next to color minimum row-1 in cyclic order we need one iteration. Next we have have a nested loop for traversing the image from minimum row-2 to 0th row, this is again a $O(n^2)$task, for each pixel we now do search for the row below it and perform Depth Limited Search till a certain extent(Depth First Search has $O(n^2)$ complexity for adjacency matrix representation), now we perform this search for each white pixel, hence it is upper bounded by $O(n^4)$, the fact that number of white pixels are at max half so the complexity is easily within the $O(n^4)$ bound(assuming height=width=n here).

For constructing the circle we can use the Digital Circle drawing algorithm or use the properties of circles to color the central root. Suppose we have a circle with its center at (x_1,y_1) and radius r. For all points which satisfy the equation

$$(x\text{-}x_1)^2+(y-y_1)^2\text{-}r^2 < 0 \ ,$$

we can safely conclude that the point clearly lies within the circle which represents the root of the nerve image.

The fact that we use the adjacent row/column as reference helps us removing tedious searching by Depth First Search because if its nearby pixel is already colored it assigns the color then to itself, thus reducing one call which may end up being close to $O(1)$, but in some points which do not have a pixel below exactly colored(i.e. it is black, because if it was white it would have already been colored in the previous iteration) in those cases the Depth First Search(implemented in a Depth Limited Manner) will lead to at maximum $O(n^2)$ time. Hence overall if we see from an amortized aspect in cases where we do $O(1)$ work we are basically saving on time which can be utilized later which may lead to reduction in the average time taken for the pixel to become easily less than $O(n^2)$.Hence we conclude that the upper bound is not a tight upper bound and the exact upper bound will be clearly less than the $O(n^2)$ bound proposed.

Thus the proposed algorithm solves the problem of coloring the nerves distinctly, repeating Depth Limited Search for 3-4 iterations ensures coloring of all points, the reason why it has been said small is because we are using Depth Limited Search, so for larger dead parts once the Depth Limit is over it returns the control back to the main function, this was the main reason for deploying Depth Limited Search, it also obviously amortizes the cost also which is another advantage.

Nerve coloring is useful in the sense that we are able to track individual nerves and when a crossover occurs only one of the crossing over nerves color continues further down the branch. The algorithm helps us to identify the nerves properly hence it makes it easier to view an image to see the distinct nerves (It may be very tedious for anyone to see the nerve with a naked eye and follow it to track it in an image with only white pixels).

3   Experimental Results

The test results have been generated on gcc compiler running on a machine with 1 GB RAM and Dual Core 3.0 GHz processor. In the below images we see that all the nerves have been distinctly colored and the algorithm is successful in detecting the root also.

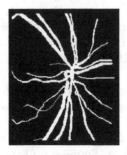

Fig. 8. Input Image 1

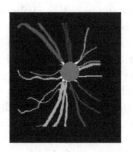

Fig. 9. Output Image 1

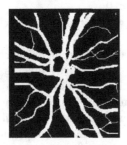

Fig. 10. Input Image 2

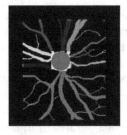

Fig. 11. Output Image 2

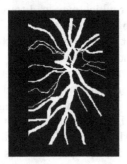

Fig. 12. Input Image 3

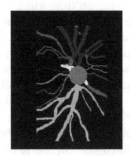

Fig. 13. Output Image 3

4   Conclusion

The nerve coloring algorithm proposed by us is successful in providing the desired result. This could help doctors/opticians to track the nerves easily, therefore it reduces their job of tracking each nerve while examining a retinal image. Since while tracking, the color indicates it is the same nerve. Knowledge on blood vessel location can be useful for evaluation of retinopathy prematurity [7], arteriolar narrowing [8,9] , vessel tortuosity to characterize hypertensive retinopathy [10], vessel diameter measurement to diagnose hypertension and cardiovascular diseases, and computer assisted laser surgery. Also, the vascular tree can be used as valuable information for retina based authentication and to locate other fundus features such as the fovea and the optic disc.

References

1. Rawi, M.A., Qutaishat, M., Arrar, M.: An improved matched filter for blood vessel detection of digital retinal images. Computers in Biology and Medicine 37(2), 262–267 (2007)
2. Riveron, E.F., Guimeras, N.G.: Extraction of blood vessels in ophthalmic color images of human retinas. In: Martínez-Trinidad, J.F., Carrasco Ochoa, J.A., Kittler, J. (eds.) CIARP 2006. LNCS, vol. 4225, pp. 118–126. Springer, Heidelberg (2006)
3. Stanton, A.V., Wasan, B., Cerutti, A., Ford, S., Marsh, R., Sever, P.P., Thom, S.A., Hughes, A.D.: Vascular network changes in the retina with age and hypertension. Journal of Hypertension 13, 17241728 (1995)
4. Bernardes, R., Serranho, P., Lobo, C.: Digital Ocular Fundus Imaging: A Review. Ophthalmologica 226(4), 161–181 (2011)
5. Abrmoff, M.D., Garvin, M.K., Sonka, M.: Retinal Imaging and Image Analysis. IEEE Reviews in Biomedical Engineering 3, 169–208 (2010)
6. Fraz, M.M., Remagnino, P., Hoppe, A., et al.: An Ensemble Classification-Based Approach Applied to Retinal Blood Vessel Segmentation. IEEE Transactions on Biomedical Engineering 59(9), 2538–2548 (2012)
7. Heneghan, C., Flynn, J., OKeefe, M., Cahill, M.: Characterization of changes in blood vessel width and tortuosity in retinopathy of prematurity using image analysis. Med. Image Anal. 6, 407–429 (2002)
8. Grisan, E., Ruggeri, A.: A divide and impera strategy for the automatic classification of retinal vessels into arteries and veins. In: Proc. 25th Int. Conf. IEEE Eng. Med. Biol. Soc., pp. 890–893 (2003)
9. Hatanaka, Y., Fujita, H., Aoyama, M., Uchida, H., Yamamoto, T.: Auto- mated analysis of the distributions and geometries of blood vessels on retinal fundus images. In: Proc. SPIE Med. Imag. 2004: Image Process., vol. 5370, pp. 1621–1628 (2004)
10. Foracchia, M., Grisan, E., Ruggeri, A.: Extraction and quantitative description of vessel features in hypertensive retinopathy fundus images. In: Book Abstracts 2nd Int. Workshop Comput. Asst. Fundus Image Anal (2001)
11. Lowell, J., Hunter, A., Steel, D., Basu, A., Ryder, R., Kennedy, R.L.: Measurement of retinal vessel widths from fundus images based on 2- D modeling. IEEE Trans. Med. Imag. 23(10), 1196–1204 (2004)
12. Becker, D.E., Can, A., Turner, J.N., Tanenbaum, H.L., Roysam, B.: Image processing algorithms for retinal montage, synthesis, mapping and real-time location determination. IEEE Trans. Biomed. Eng. 45(1), 115–118 (1998)
13. Shen, H., Roysam, B., Stewart, C.V., Turner, J.N., Tanenbaum, H.L.: Optimal scheduling of tracing computations for real-time vascular landmark extraction from retinal fundus images. IEEE Trans.Inf. Technol. Biomed. 5, 77–91 (2001)
14. Hoover, A., Goldbaum, M.: Locating the optic nerve in a retinal image using the fuzzy convergence of the blood vessels. IEEE Trans. Med. Imag. 22(8), 951958 (2003)
15. Siddalingaswamy, P.C., Prabhu, K.G.: Automatic localization and boundary detection of optic disc using implicit active contours. International Journal of Computer Applications 1, 1–5 (2010)

16. Aquino, A., Gegndez-Arias, M.E., Marn, D.: Automated optic disc detection in retinal images of patients with diabetic retinopathy and risk of macular edema. International Journal of Biological and Life Sciences 8(2), 87–92 (2012)
17. The DRIVE database, Image sciences institute, university medical center utrecht, The Netherlands (2007), http://www.isi.uu.nl/Research/Databases/DRIVE/ (last accessed on July 7, 2007)
18. Saha, S., Roy, N.D.: Automatic Detection of bifurcation points in retinal fundus images. International Journal of Latest Research in Science and Technology 2(2), 105–108 (2013), http://www.mnkjournals.com/ijlrst.htm ISSN (Online): 2278-5299

Segmentation of Two-Phase Flow: A Free Representation for Levet Set Method with a Priori Knowledge

Mauren Louise Sguario, Lucia Valeria Ramos de Arruda, Iuri Nack Buss, and Henderson Cari Nascimento

Federal Technological University of Parana, Curitiba, Parana, Brazil
{mlsguario,vlarruda}@utfpr.edu.br
http://www.utfpr.edu.br

Abstract. In this paper, the segmentation approaches based on active contours-based model were united. The result is a new approach which improves the average freely previously trained format, using the method of contour active for Level Set. In this case, there is no restriction evolution of the interface as other approaches that use the junction active contours and prior knowledge. This approach was chosen for the correct identification of the form of gas bubbles in gas-liquid two-phase flow. The main objective of this work is to provide a system of validation for the various approaches of flow instrumentation widely used. The promising results indicate that the system of image segmentation by the proposed approach gives good results and can be used as an efficient method of validation to other existing approaches.

Keywords: Priori Shape, Level Set Method, Two-phase flow.

1 Introduction

The study of two-phase flow has important applications in a growing number of areas, including transportation of oil and gas, nuclear power and chemical processing. Reliable measurements about the respective distribution of the phases in the pipeline, including the void fraction and classification of standards in the flow, for example, are crucial for accurate modeling of two-phase systems.

Image processing techniques consist in a powerful tool to study the phenomena of two-phase flow and they are typically non-intrusive and relatively simple to design and implement. In regard to the horizontal flow of air-water, focus of this paper, several approaches aim to extract the gas bubbles from the flow images basically using simple image processing operations.

Shi et al. [1] suggests an approach based on threshold in order to segment air bubbles, but the method may be highly sensitive to the presence of noise and low lighting conditions. Dihn et al. [2] apply an approach of background subtraction followed by boundary detection in a binary image, which also has drawbacks for poor lighting or noise.

Y.J. Zhang and J.M.R.S. Tavares (Eds.): CompIMAGE 2014, LNCS 8641, pp. 115–132, 2014.
© Springer International Publishing Switzerland 2014

Recently, the Hough Transform was used to detect objects with circular shape, however, the approximation by spherical shapes cannot be generalized to the several flow standards [3]. In Hanafizadeh and colleagues (2011) the images were pre-processed by the filter of the average and the background subtraction algorithm was applied to the images of the vertical two-phase flow of gas-liquid. This approach allows the reduction of noise caused by the image acquisition process. Then, these authors used an iterative thresholding and morphological math techniques as morphological closing, which resulted in the separation of gas bubbles. However, it was observed that in some cases there were joints and unnecessary separations [4].

Although there are extensive experimental studies about this issue, the automatic image analysis to identify and measure parameters of two-phase flows is very limited. Thus, this paper proposes a new approach for gas bubbles segmentation in horizontal two-phase flow of gas-liquid (air-water) to provide a system to identify the shape of the slug pattern (vide 2.1). For this purpose, an extension of digital images segmentation approach based on active contours, or snakes approach, and an extension of shape model were joint. The goal is to segment the gas bubbles in images of horizontal two-phase flow of gas-liquid by extending the *Level Set* approach by incorporating the previously trained gas bubble shape information, which will be responsible for the evolution of the initial curve. Thus, a model of the object shape is obtained from a set of training images, where the shape is defined by the Point Distribution Model - PDM [5]). The result is a new approach that freely evolves the previously trained average shape, using the method of active contour by Level Set. In this case, there is no restriction on the evolution of the interface as in other approaches that use the combination of active contours and prior knowledge. The proposed model is tested and validated on image segmentation horizontal two-phase flow of gas-liquid in slug pattern and compared to the active shape model approach with prior knowledge [5] and to the approach of Level Set method without prior knowledge [6].

This paper is organized as follows: the Section 2.1 describes the basic characteristics of the two-phase slug flow that are necessary to understand the shape model. In the Section 2.2, a brief review of some image segmentation methods based on prior knowledge is presented. Then in the Section 3 the proposed approach based on active contours and prior knowledge is detailed. The qualitative and quantitative results will be presented in Section 4. Concluding remarks and future perspectives of this research are proposed in Section 5.

2   Background and Related Studies

2.1   Slug Flow

Among the patterns of flow, the slug pattern has been studied individually since 1969 [7], being one of the most frequent patterns in industrial applications. It is an intermittent flow whose characteristics vary in space and time. It is characterized by a range of liquid pistons followed by a large elongated bubble, and it may have dispersed bubbles or not depending on the velocity of the phases.

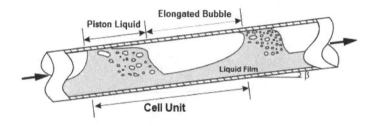

Fig. 1. Representation of a unit cell in horizontal gas-liquid slug flow as well as the liquid film, the elongated bubble and the liquid piston

Wallis, 1969 [7] introduces the concept of a unit cell as illustrated in Figure 1, which graphically represents the model in slug flow. It is possible to observe in the figure the liquid piston and its adjacent elongated bubble and several dispersed bubbles in the respective liquid film. With the description and analysis of the behavior of a unit cell, all the properties of slug flow along a pipeline can be provided. This pattern is considered in this paper for the extraction of the average shape of the elongated bubble, which will allow the study of the flow properties.

2.2 Studies Related to Segmentation Based on Prior Knowledge

In this section, a review of some approaches of segmentation based on active contours and prior information about the object shape will be presented. Some approaches, although promising, do not have widespread use typically due to results obtained in uncontrolled environments, where there is a greater presence of noise and low lighting, which may consequently lead to lack in accuracy in the final segmentations. In many applications, it is possible to obtain prior knowledge about the object shape whose location is wanted and incorporate this knowledge to mold the segmentation, representing an improvement in their performance.

This prior knowledge may be used in conjunction with active contours approaches (*snakes*), which were originally introduced by Kass, Witkins and Terzopoulos in 1987 [8]. The basic idea is based on local contours deformation obtained from functional energy minimization. This energy is defined such that its minimum value is reached on the contours of the target object whose segment is wanted. Depending on the shape of the contour representation, the deformable models can be classified as parametric and geometric models. An equation of movement is set to conduct the initial contour to the boundaries of the structure. The procedure can be understood as a curve evolution model. The deformable parametric models are related to the active contours approach [8] whereas the geometric models are based on the *Level Set* method by Osher and Sethian, 1988 [9]. In the first case the contours are sampled as discrete points and they are tracked according to their respective equation of movement.

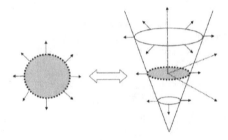

Fig. 2. Principle of *Level Set* method. The figure to the left shows only the expansion of a circumference, and the figure at the right illustrates the circumference such as the level zero curve of a larger function. (Based on [11]).

The equation of movement for this model can be derived by functional or dynamics energy forces. The definition of functional energy has two parts: internal energy and external energy.

The internal energy aims to maintain the smoothness and the contour regularity and it is generally defined by the geometric contour properties like length, area and curvature. The external energy aims to conduct the contour to the correct position and its definition is based on the image information [10].

The deformable geometric models are based on *Level Set* [9]. They were initially proposed to process the topological changes during the curve evolution. The main idea of *Level Set* method consists in representing a determined interface as the level zero interface of a bigger function (called *Level Set* function). This formulation, which can be seen in Figure 2 for the two-dimensional case, leads to an efficient and versatile representation of curve evolution. The gray region on the figure illustrates the level zero of *Level Set* function.

The previously described approaches were not developed for the use of prior knowledge, however, prior knowledge was recently incorporated in the methods. And the (*Active Shape Model - ASM* [5]) was developed to use prior information. To this end, it creates a statistical model of the objects shape that deforms iteratively in order to meet an example of the object in a new image. The model was developed by Tim Cootes and Chris Taylor in 1995 [5]. The forms are limited by PDM (*Point Distribution Models*). The point distribution model is a model that represents the average geometric shape and some statistical shapes of geometrical variation inferred by a training shapes set.

In order to find the best position of each point, an alternative is to focus on the edges, or set a statistical model about what is expected to the point. The methodology suggests the use of the Mahalanobis distance to detect a better position for each referential point. It is also known as intelligent snakes method [12], since it is analogous to an active contour model which regards the constraints of the explicit shape. The prior knowledge of the object of interest aims the development of accurate and automatic computational tools. In this case the average shape is obtained in statistical models and the possible variations are inserted into the set of training data. Getting this prior knowledge requires a good set of images with manual annotation of training data from the object of interest. The performance of the statistical model is influenced by the size of the set of training data and the complexity of the anatomical variation of the object of interest [13].

Shortly after the initial presentation of deformable models by Kass et al. [8], Terzopoulos et al. extend the concept to 3D application [14]. In Delingette and Epidarte [15] is introduced the deformable simplex mesh, which provides a stable internal energy that can be easily customized to deform toward a specific shape. Using a different approach, McInerney and Terzopoulos [16] presents a method to implement changes in the topology of deformable surfaces. After nearly two decades of deformable models, several review papers on this subject have been published [17], [18], [19]. Osher and Sethian introduced the *Level Set* method [9], however, Malladi et al. [20] apply the idea in digital images, where they present a representation of the implicit shape and apply it with the regional specificities or based on the edges of objects. Tsai et al. [21] propose an implementation for segmentation by *Level Set* that is oriented by optimization directly on the linear subspace created by principal components.

Rousson and Paragios [22] present a new approach that builds a shape model directly on the *Level Set* space using a collection of samples. This model is used as basis to introduce a priori shape vigorously, being constructed by a variably framework that explores the information about the *level set* representation. They also add a new energy term that proposes meet the local variability. Recently, El Hadji S. Diop and Valrie Burdin [23] combine Mumford-Shahs techniques and active contours with prior knowledge of shape.

The study that comes closest to this approach was developed by Leventon et al., in 2000 [24] who proposed the integration of a set of deformable shapes during the *level set* evolution. The priori shapes were obtained by defining a probability distribution over the variations of the training set elements. The proposed shape model was based on a Principal Component Analysis (PCA), which was then applied to a function of signed distance built with the training set, consisting of contours of the segmented object. Then, at each step of the proposed segmentation algorithm, *level set* locally evolved thanks to the intrinsic image characteristics such as gradients and curvature, but the evolution is also guided by the maximum estimates of the previous position of the shape.

Although the existing methods are very powerful in solving problems of object detection, there is still a need to develop new approaches due to the complexity and particularity of the problems found in practical situations. Especially in segmentation of the gas bubbles in gas-liquid two-phase flow the shape may vary and in this case the prior information about the shape is important, however, the free evolution of the curve to the boundary of the image must be allowed.

In the next section, the proposed segmentation approach is presented.

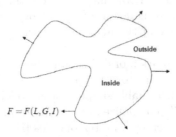

Fig. 3. Propagating with velocity F (Based on [11])

3   Proposed Approach

3.1   Level Set

The principle of active contours models (*snakes*) is to evolve a curve (interface), subject to constraints of a given image u_0 in order to detect the different objects in the scene. Ideally, it starts with a curve around the object to be detected (segmented) and the curve then moves toward its normal and the boundaries of the object. This movement is related to the speed F given by a function that may depend on local properties L (determined by local geometrical information such as curvature), global G (determined by the shape and positioning of the curve) and independent I (those that do not depend on the shape of the curve, like the velocity of a fluid under such curve) [25].

Given a hyper surface $(N-1)$-dimensional closed, $\Gamma(t=0)$, the aim is to propose an Eulerian formulation (where the coordinate system remains fixed) for the propagation of $\Gamma(t)$ in the direction of its normal according to a velocity function, F, which can be written as [11]:

$$F = F(L, G, I),\tag{1}$$

The figure 3 shows na example of the interface propagation as a function of the velocity F.

The main idea of the Level Set method consists in incorporate such interface as the zero Level Set of a function ϕ. We have $\phi(x, t = 0)$, where x is a point in $\Re^N$ defined by [25]:

$$\phi(x, t = 0) = \pm d,\tag{2}$$

where d is the distance from x to $\Gamma(t=0)$, and the plus (minus) sign is chosen if the point x is out of (into) the initial hyper surface $\Gamma(t=0)$. Thereby, we have the initial function $\phi(x, t = 0) : \Re^N \to \Re$ with the following properties:

$$\Gamma(t = 0) = \{x | \phi(x, t = 0) = 0\}.\tag{3}$$

At this point, we need to define how to adjust the value of ϕ for other instants of time in order to correctly represent the spread of the curve. Thereby, we must define an equation for the function $\phi(x, t)$ such that its Level Set, $\phi = 0$, contains the incorporation of spread of $\Gamma(t)$. To this end, we assume that $x(t)$ is the path of a point on the interface that is being propagated, that is, $x(t = 0)$ is a point of $\Gamma(t = 0)$ and $\dot{x}(t).n = F(x(t))$, where $\dot{x}(t)$ is the vector normal to the interface at $x(t)$ and $n = \nabla\phi/|\nabla\phi|$. The requirement that the zero Level Set function of ϕ should correspond to hyper surface means [25]:

$$\phi(x(t), t) = 0. \tag{4}$$

By the chain rule:

$$\phi_t + \nabla\phi(x(t), t).\dot{x}(t) = 0. \tag{5}$$

Since F provides the velocity in the normal direction outside, then $\dot{x}(t).N = F$. Thus, we obtain an equation of evolution for ϕ, we can see it as follows:

$$\phi_t + F|\nabla\phi| = 0, \tag{6}$$

given $\phi(x, t = 0)$ [25] (See [25] about the complete formulation of the interface evolution).

3.2   Priori Shape Definition

The definition of the average shape of the object of interest used in this paper is based on the Active Shape Model approach. The Active Shape Model developed by Tim Cootes and Chris Taylor in 1995 [5] is a statistical model of the objects shape that deform in an iterative manner, in order to find an example of the object in a new image. The shape is limited by the Point Distribution Model. In this case the statistical shape model will vary only for shapes observed in a set of labeled training examples. This shape is represented by a set of points (controlled by the shape model). The algorithm shall learn the standard shape based on training. Such shape is obtained by manual marking of points that delimit the base shape. The marked points should systematically occupy the same specific region of each training images, otherwise the model will fail to accurately capture the particular variations of each specific image part [5].

The manual step of marking the points defines a data taking, or coordinates taking, from points that are considered by specialists as limits for the observed shape. Thereby, the manual marking of several distinct images is required, representing all small possible variations of the objects of interest. However, at the end of the training series an amount of intercepted shapes of different images of the same formation is taken, which must be converted to a single final pattern after processing the data that has to be able to include and recognize images from the same phenomenon, but distinct from those used during the training series.

The standard shape modeling by the PDM method is the statistical evaluation of the coordinates provided by the training points. To compare series of points or equivalent vectors from different images they need to be aligned in relation to a group of coordinate axes. The alignment can be obtained by resizing, rotating or translating the shapes until they are more similar to each other.

The alignment of the points is a prerequisite in order to obtain statistical values that describe the standard shape. There is a superposition of equivalent points as well as the formation of clouds and diffuse points when all the points marked next to the average standard shape are aligned and overlapped. As these reference markings are partially correlated and do not move independently, the points distribution model (PDM) seeks a variation pattern of coordinates within this diffuse points zone or clouds [5].

Basically, the PDM method sets the points cloud as an allowed domain for formations. Considering them as ellipsoids by using the orthogonal transformation process, calculated by applying Principal Components Analysis (PCA), providing a varying model of coordinates, or a region to which the movement of the shape is allowed when compared with the standard.

Finally, the final model obtained by manual training will be unique for each shape, endowed with parameters that make it flexible to be used in the recognition and segmentation of images that have the features and shape that must be located. Figure 5 (b) illustrates, as an example, the final shape model of one species of heron obtained by the point distribution model.

3.3   Free Level Set Priori Shape

After the definition of the average shape, it is necessary to consider an image that contains an object similar in shape to a sample in the training set. So the goal is to recognize the area in the image that corresponds to this object. Thus, the model shape is then defined as the initial curve (marker) for evolution of *Level Set* [6].

Thereby, the shape model is built using a representation of the points distribution model [5] (as described above) and then it is defined as the initial curve (marker) for the variable *Level Set* evolution [6] adapted. In image segmentation, active contours are dynamic curves that move toward the boundaries of the object. To achieve this goal, it is explicitly set an external energy that can move the curve of level zero toward the object boundaries. Consider I as an image and g is the boundary indicator function defined by:

$$g = \frac{1}{1 + |\nabla(G_\sigma * I)|^2} \tag{7}$$

where G_σ is the Gaussiano kernel with standard deviation σ. An external energy is defined for a function $\phi(x, y)$ as follows:

$$\varepsilon_{g,\lambda,v}(\phi) = \lambda L_g(\phi) + v A_g(\phi) \tag{8}$$

Where $\lambda > 0$ and v are constants and terms $L_g(\phi)$ and $A_g(\phi)$ are defined by:

$$L_g(\phi) = \int_\Omega g\delta(\phi)|\nabla\phi|dxdy \tag{9}$$

and

$$A_g(\phi) = \int_\Omega gH(-\phi)dxdy \tag{10}$$

respectively, where δ is the one-variable Dirac function and H is a *Heaviside* function [6].

So the following total functional energy is defined:

$$\varepsilon(\phi) = \mu P(\phi) + \varepsilon_{g,\lambda,v}(\phi) \tag{11}$$

The external energy $\varepsilon_{g,\lambda,v}$ drives the zero *level set* against the boundaries of the object, whereas the internal energy $\mu P(\phi)$ penalizes the deviation of ϕ from a signed distance function during its evolution.

To understand the geometric meaning of the energy $L_g(\phi)$, suppose that the zero *level set* of ϕ can be represented by a differentiable parameterized curve $C(p)$, $p \in [0,1]$. The functional energy $L_g(\phi)$ em (9) calculates the length of the level zero curve of ϕ in conformal metrics $ds = g(C(p))|C'(p)|dp$.

The functional energy $A_g(\phi)$ in (9) is introduced to accelerate the evolution of the curve. Note that when the function g is constant with value 1, the functional energy (9) is the area of region $\Omega_\phi^- = \{(x,y)|\phi(x,y) < 0\}$. The functional energy $A_g(\phi)$ in (9) can be seen as a weighted area of Ω_ϕ^-. The coefficient v of A_g may be positive or negative depending on the relative position of the initial contour of the object of interest. For example, if the initial contours are placed outside the object, the coefficient v must have a positive value, so that the contours can shrink faster. But if the initial contours are placed inside the object, the coefficient v must be negative to accelerate the expansion of the contours.

So, the initial marker, represented by the prior knowledge is incorporated to the functional energy at each iteration as follows:

$$u(t+1) = u(t) + delt * (\lambda L_g(\phi) + vA_g(\phi) + \mu P(0)) \tag{12}$$

where *delt* is the time step and $u(t)$ is obtained by the prior trained shape which is at the same time defined as initial marker. In this case, the proposed approach creates a framework consisting of four energy terms. The first three $(\lambda L_g(\phi) + vA_g(\phi) + \mu P(0))$ introduced in [6] and the last $u(t)$ based on the representation of object shape model proposed here.

Figure 4 (b) illustrates the result of segmentation using the proposed approach in Li et.al [6] without prior knowledge and the Figure 4 (d) shows the result of segmentation using the approach here proposed. The goal is to segment the cell nucleus, in this case a monocyte. We notice from the previously defined knowledge that the evolution of the initial curve evolves more efficiently.

Figure 5 shows the evolution of ϕ according to Equation (12). Figure 5 (a) illustrates the initial *level set* function obtained by the average shape and its zero level curve is shown in Figure 5 (b). Figure 5 (c) is obtained from the final segmentation after 300 iterations.

The basic algorithm of the proposed approach is described below:

This approach has several desirable aspects such as the possibility to use more than one initial marker (due to topological properties of the *Level Set*

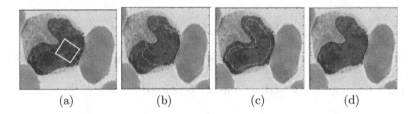

Fig. 4. Segmentation result: (a) initial marker, (b) Segmentation result in Li et. al [6], (c) prior trained shape and (d) result of segmentation using the approach here proposed

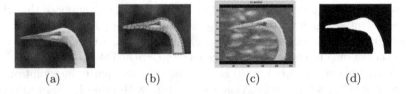

Fig. 5. Segmentation using *Free Level Set Priori Shape*: (a) original image, (b) average shape definition by the points distribution model, (c) evolution of the initial curve, (d) segmentation result

method, the regions defined by these markers will merge), the ease of extension to extract three-dimensional shapes and low sensitivity to noise. The approach also allows the automatic handling of the possible topological changes often observed in practice situations [6]. Moreover, the approach proposes the initial curve evolution (shape model), without restrictions imposed by shape.

4 Results and Discussion

In this section, the results obtained by segmentation using the proposed approach are compared to those obtained by segmentation approaches based on *Level Set* without prior knowledge [6] and Active Shape Model of incorporation of prior information in [5]. In addition, the quantitative results are also provided in order to evaluate the segmentation.

Algorithm 1. Algorithm to image segmentation.

1: get the average shape of the object using the point distribution model;
2: given a new input image I;
3: set a marker (or initial curve) inside or outside the region, from the average trained shape;
4: evolve the marker until obtaining the velocity function F reduced to approximately zero.

In this research, the following parameters were used: $\lambda = 5.0$, $v = 3.5$, $\mu = 0,04$, evolution curve varying from 150 to 350 iterations, $\lambda_2 = 5.0$ and the step of $delt = 1$. These values were set to maintain a stable evolution of the curve, thus preventing that the boundaries of the object are overcome.

4.1   Images of Air-Water Two-Phase Flow

Initially a model for representing the shapes of gas bubbles in gas-liquid two-phase flow in slugging, as in the example shown in Figure 7 (j, k e l) was prepared. The goal is to build a model that describes the typical shape, using the examples in Figure 7 as a training set. The database consists of 20 images for training and 30 for testing, for each shape shown in Figure 7, totalizing 60 images for training and 90 test images. Therefore, the representation is extracted from each example as a set of labeled points, calculating the average positions of the points and the main shapes in which the points of each example tend to vary from the average. It is important to mention that in some images of two-phase flow overlapping parts may occur, in which case there is a greater presence of droplets of gas through the bubble in slugging, which is common in practical situations. Also, the capture of images from the digital camera generates a set of frames to represent a complete bubble, divided as follows: initial part of the gas bubble (denoted as nose), central part of the gas bubble (denoted as body) and final part of the gas bubble (denoted as tail), which may or may not have dispersed bubbles in a liquid medium. In this case, three different types of structures in flow images are considered: first, the images of the nose of the gas bubble (Figure 6 a, b e c); then images of the body of the gas bubble (Figure 6 d, e e f) and at last images of the tail of the gas bubble (Figure 6 g, h e i). It is worth noting that the presence of droplets is an inherent characteristic of the highest displacement velocity of the gas bubbles, so at low velocities this phenomenon will not occur. The selected points are around the boundary, as shown in Figure Figura 7 (j, k and l) for each structure. It must be done for each shape in the training set.

The labeling of points is important. Each marked point is a specific part of the object or of its boundary. If the labeling is incorrect, with one point placed at different locations in each shape of training, the method does not capture the variability of shape reliably. In the shown example, the points were manually placed in each one of 20 images for each part (nose, Figure 7 (a, b and c), body, Figure 7 (d, e and f) and tail, Figure 7 (g, h and i)).

The points are manually placed only during the training phase, it is not necessary to find these points in advance when the models are used in segmentation of new images. See [5] for details on the alignment of data in the training set.

The proposed approach was evaluated on images of the gas-liquid two-phase flow in slugging in order to segment the gas bubbles. The results are shown in Figure 9 (j, k, and l), and as expected, they are superior to those made by Li et. als approach [6] in classical active contours, Figure 9 (d, e and f) and by Cootes [5] in ASM approach, Figure 9 (g, h and i). The free evolution without imposing of shape is particularly useful due to variation of some tail shapes of gas bubbles. Note in Figure 8 the variation of the shape of the final part of the

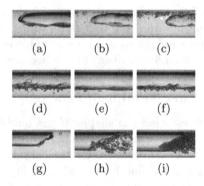

Fig. 6. Detachment of gas droplets in liquid medium: (a, b and c) droplets in the nose of the gas bubble, (d, e and f) droplets in the body of the gas bubble, (g, h and i) droplets in the tail of the gas bubble

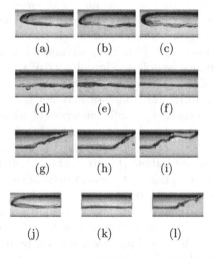

Fig. 7. Representation of database (a, b, c) shape of the nose of the gas bubble (d, e and f) shape of the body of the gas bubble (g, h and i) shape of the tail of the gas bubble (j, k and l) and points marked for the definition of the average shape

gas bubbles (tail) in two-phase flow in slugging. To overcome this limitation, it is required the use of an average shape large enough to be inserted outside the bubble and thus evolve to a stop at the boundaries.

One advantage of the proposed approach to be highlighted is the fact that the object is segmented in 150 iterations, whereas in Li et. al. [6] 350 iterations were necessary and in Cootes [5] 50 iterations, however, its computational cost is higher, making the proposed approach fast in the execution process.

The results presented in Figure 9 illustrate the importance of prior information about the shape of the segmented object in the segmentation process. On the

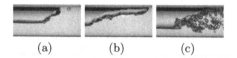

(a)   (b)   (c)

Fig. 8. Variation in the tail of the two-phase flow in slugging for different velocities of the gas bubble

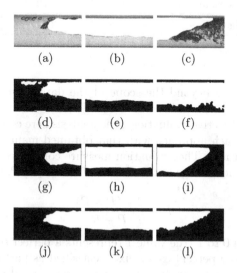

(a)   (b)   (c)

(d)   (e)   (f)

(g)   (h)   (i)

(j)   (k)   (l)

Fig. 9. Segmentation results: (a, b and c) Ground-Truth, (d, e and f) Li et. al [6], (g, h and i) Active Shape Model [5], (j, k and l) Free Level Set Priori Shape

other hand, incorporating priori shape to the segmentation help the evolution of the curve discarding those pixels with similar intensity values that, however, do not belong to the object of interest. However, in case where many dispersed bubbles appear in the image, the bubble cannot be correctly restored by the approaches of Li et al. (2006) and Cootes [5]; especially the nose and tail of the bubble (Figure 9 d, e, f, g, h and i) compared to the proposed segmentation model (Figure 9 j, k and l).

4.2   Evaluation of Segmentations

This last section is dedicated to the quantitative evaluation of the segmentation results obtained with the proposed approach and the methods proposed in Li et. al. [6] and Cootes [5]. The evaluation of the results of segmentation obtained using algorithms is a challenge because it is difficult to reach an agreed set of test provided by ground-truth images. This occurrence is due to the fact that the manual segmentation of images is a laborious task and often subjective. Moreover, the specialist often tends to add to his segmentations, semantic

Table 1. Comparative result by F-Measure, set of 30 images of the nose of the gas bubble

Approach for Segmentation	F-Measure Score
ASM	0,68
Li et. al	0,70
Level Free	0,74

considerations that are beyond the scope of the data driven by segmentation algorithms [26].

Aiming reduce subjective evaluations, the analysis here compares the segmentation results from each approach with that obtained manually by the specialist (called ground-truth). The evaluation measure considered is the *F-measure*, which is the harmonic average of the indices of precision, P, and recall, R [26]:

$$F = \frac{2 \times (P \times R)}{P + R} \qquad (13)$$

where F varies from 0 to 1 (the value 1 represents a perfect segmentation). The accuracy indicates the percentage of pixels classified as part of the object that are actually relevant, while recall is the proportion of total pixels belonging to the object that were correctly classified [27].

The segmentation of the gas bubbles present in the two-phase flow is not an easy task, especially for the slug pattern in which there are droplets of gas in liquid medium. Moreover, from the three formats studied here (nose, body and tail), two (nose and tail) have variations in shape and size, making it difficult to automate steps such as extraction of markers. Another complicating aspect is related to the non-controlled environment for the acquisition of images, which results in images with low contrast between the boundary and the background, for example. The results of segmentation of each shape are evaluated in next section.

4.3   Base with Images Representing the Bubble Nose

Table 1 shows the average *F-Measure* index calculated considering for measures of precision calculation and recall, only the pixels belonging to the segmented region that best approximates the object of interest.

Note that the proposed approach leads to superior results. These numbers reflect the advantage of obtaining prior information about the object to be segmented. We note that the approach of Cootes [5] leads to lower results mainly due to restriction imposed by the average shape whereas the proposed approach has better response in the free evolution of the initial curve.

Table 2. Comparative Result by F-Measure, set of 30 images of the body of the gas bubble

Approach for Segmentation	F-Measure Score
ASM	0,92
Li et. al	0,98
Level Free	0,99

Table 3. Comparative Result by F-Measure, set of 30 images of the tail of the gas bubble

Approach for Segmentation	F-Measure Score
ASM	0,86
Li et. al	0,81
Level Free	0,91

4.4 Base with Images Representing the Bubble Body

Table 2 shows the average *F-Measure* index for the body of the gas bubbles. Again, the proposed approach presents the best values and in this case, the restriction of the shape was less efficient than the free evolution of the curve, both in the proposed approach with variation as in the approach of Li et. al. [6]. It is noteworthy that in this format, all results are promising since the segmentation process is simpler.

4.5 Base with Images Representing the Bubble Tail

Table 3 presents the average *F-Measure* index for the tail of gas bubbles. Note that the proposed approach leads to superior results again. These numbers reflect the advantage of obtaining prior information mainly in images that have many dispersed bubbles. It is noted that the approach of Li et al. al. [6] leads to lower results mainly because the intensities of gray levels resemble the gray levels of the object of interest, which makes the proposed approach advantageous since it considers the values of intensity, however, taking into account the previously trained shape.

5 Conclusion

This paper proposes a new image segmentation approach that is based on active contours and formulated from a *level set* approach. Although existing methods are very powerful in solving problems of object detection, there is still a need to develop new approaches due to complexity and particularity of the problems found in practical situations, especially in low-contrast images in the intensities of gray levels.

As shown in the numerical results in Section 4, the classical active contours methods were not so good in segmentation of complex structures such as those found in two-phase flow images presented here. In this study, we opted for the prior representation of the object as an additional information that can easily lead the segmentation to the wanted object, such that the zero level set is also guided not only by the characteristics of the image, but also by a set of a priori shapes, and it is incorporated into the sequence as a variable formulation of the segmentation problem.

The additional term is projected not to interfere in the important property of the signed distance function developed by Li et. al. [6], which is necessary to ensure a good evolution of the initial curve.

The initial marker is represented by prior knowledge and incorporated into the functional energy at each iteration. It is obtained by the difference between the prior trained shape, which is at the same time as initial marker and the curve evolving in time u_t. In this case, the proposed approach creates a framework consisting of four energy terms. The first three $(\lambda L_g(\phi) + v A_g(\phi) + \mu P(0))$ introduced in Li et al. al. [6] and the last u_t based on the representation of object shape model proposed here.

The robustness and efficiency of the approach are presented in Section 4 in pictures of real gas-liquid two-phase flow (Section 4.3), along with quantitative evaluations of the results of segmentation, which were reported in Tables 1, 2 and 3. Both qualitative and quantitative results confirm the good performance of the proposed algorithm.

The segmentation of gas-liquid two-phase flow presents the problem of bubbles dispersed in the liquid because the intensities of gray levels in question generate superposition of bubble in slugging in some regions. However, segmentation performed by the proposed approach was superior to the compared approaches, and it is really promising. Indeed, most of the problems of occlusion and/or overlap are solved. Future researches include decrease in the restriction imposed by the priori shape and 3D representation of two-phase flow, as well as inclusion of other flow patterns.

References

1. Shi, L., Zhou, Z., Ren, R.: Parameter measurements of two-phase bubbly flow using digital image processing, pp. 3858–3861 (2004)
2. Tri, B.S.K., Dinh, B., Choi, T.-S.: Application of image processing techniques to air/water two-phase flow. In: Proc. SPIE 3808, pp. 725–730 (1999)
3. Galindo, E., Larralde-Corona, C.P., Brito, T.: Development of advanced image analysis techniques for the in situ characterization of multiphase dispersions occurring in bioreactors. Journal of Biotechnology 116(3), 261–270 (2005)

4. Hanafizadeh, P., Ghanbarzadeh, S., Saidi, M.H.: Visual technique for detection of gas liquid two phase flow regime in the airlift pump. Journal of Petroleum Science and Engineering 75(3-4), 327–335 (2011)

5. Cootes, T.F., Taylor, C.J., Cooper, D.H., Graham, J.: Active shape models-their training and application. Computer Vision and Image Understanding 61(1), 38–59 (1995)

6. Chunming Li, C.G., Xu, C., Fox, M.: Level set evolution without re-initialization: A new variational formulation. In: IEEE Computer Society Conference on Computer Vision and Pattern Recognition, vol. 1, pp. 430–436 (2005)

7. Wallis, G.B.: One-dimensional two-phase flow. McGraw-Hill (1969)

8. Kass, M., Witkin, A., Terzopoulos, D.: Snakes: Active contour models. International Journal of Computer Vision 1(4), 321–331 (1987)

9. Osher, S., Sethian, J.A.: Fronts propagating with curvature-dependent speed: algorithms based on hamilton-jacobi formulations. Journal of Computational Physics 79(1), 12–49 (1988)

10. Ma, Z., da Silva Tavares, J.M.R., Jorge, R.M.N.J.: A review on the current segmentation algorithms for medical images. In: IMAGAPP 2009 (2009)

11. Sethian, A.J.: Level set methods: An act of violence. American Scientist (1996)

12. Cootes, T., Baldock, E., Graham, J.: An introduction to active shape models. Image Processing and Analysis, 223–248 (2000)

13. Tomoshige, S., Oost, E., Shimizu, A., Watanabe, H., Nawano, S.: A conditional statistical shape model with integrated error estimation of the conditions; application to liver segmentation in non-contrast {CT} images. Medical Image Analysis 18(1), 130–143 (2014),
http://www.sciencedirect.com/science/article/pii/S1361841513001473

14. Terzopoulos, D., Witkin, A., Kass, M.: Constraints on deformable models: Recovering 3d shape and nongrid motion. Artif. Intell. 36(1), 91–123 (1988),
http://dx.doi.org/10.1016/0004-3702(88)90080-X

15. Delingette, H., Epidaure, P.: Simplex meshes: a general representation for 3d shape reconstruction. Tech. Rep. (1994)

16. Mcinerney, T., Terzopoulos, D.: Topology adaptive deformable surfaces for medical image volume segmentation. IEEE Transactions on Medical Imaging 18, 840–850 (1999)

17. McInerney, T., Terzopoulos, D.: Deformable models in medical image analysis: a survey. Medical Image Analysis 1(2), 91–108 (1996),
http://www.sciencedirect.com/science/article/pii/S1361841596800077

18. Jain, A.K., Zhong, Y., Dubuisson-Jolly, M.-P.: Deformable template models: A review. Signal Processing 71(2), 109–129 (1998),
http://www.sciencedirect.com/science/article/pii/S016516849800139X

19. Montagnat, J., Delingette, H., Ayache, N.: A review of deformable surfaces: Topology, geometry and deformation. Image and Vision Computing 19, 1023–1040 (2001)

20. Malladi, R., Sethian, J.A., Vemuri, B.C.: Shape modeling with front propagation: A level set approach. IEEE Trans. Pattern Anal. Mach. Intell. 17(2), 158–175 (1995),
http://dx.doi.org/10.1109/34.368173, doi:10.1109/34.368173

21. Tsai, A., Yezzi, A., Wells, W., Tempany, C., Tucker, D., Fan, A., Grimson, W.E., Willsky, A.: A shape-based approach to the segmentation of medical imagery using level sets. IEEE Trans. Med. Imag., 137–154 (2003)

22. Rousson, M., Paragios, N.: Shape priors for level set representations (2004)

23. Diop, E.H.S., Burdin, V.: Bi-planar image segmentation based on variational geo-
    metrical active contours with shape priors. Medical Image Analysis 17(2), 165–181
    (2013),
    http://www.sciencedirect.com/science/article/pii/S1361841512001351
24. Leventon, M.E., Grimson, Faugeras, O.: Statistical shape influence in geodesic
    active contours. In: Proceedings of the IEEE Conference on Computer Vision and
    Pattern Recognition, vol. 1, pp. 316–323 (2000),
    http://dx.doi.org/10.1109/cvpr.2000.855835
25. Sethian, J.A.: Level Set Methods and Fast Marching Methods. Cambridge UPress
    (1999)
26. Alpert, S., Galun, M., Basri, R., Brandt, A.: Image segmentation by probabilistic
    bottom-up aggregation and cue integration. In: Proceedings of the IEEE Confer-
    ence on Computer Vision and Pattern Recognition (June 2007)
27. Dorini, L.B.: Transformação de imagens baseadas em morfologia matemática,
    Ph.D. dissertation, Unicamp - Universidade Estadual de Campinas, Campinas
    (2009)

Analysis and Segmentation of a Three-Dimensional X-ray Computed Tomography Image of a Textile Composite

Ilya Straumit*, Stepan V. Lomov, and Martine Wevers

Department of Metallurgy and Materials Engineering (MTM), KU Leuven, Belgium
straumit.ilya@mtm.kuleuven.be

Abstract. Microfocus X-ray computed tomography allows obtaining highly detailed three-dimensional images of inspected objects. Regarding textile composites, resolution of this technique is enough to distinguish individual fibres. For the purpose of modelling, the micro-CT image of a composite must be segmented in order to separate materials components. This paper presents results of application of structure tensor and first-order statistics to compose a feature vector and segment the image. Results show that, depending on the choice of the variables used in the segmentation, the image can be segmented into the matrix, yarns and voids (pores) domains, or into the domains of matrix and yarns of different primary orientation.

1 Introduction

Microfocus X-ray computed tomography (micro-CT) is a non-destructive evaluation technique that allows obtaining three-dimensional image of internal structure of inspected object. It finds application in many areas including material science, where it is indispensable for studying geometry of reinforcement in composite materials. Mechanical properties of composites are determined by the distribution and orientation of its constituents. Modern micro-CT systems can achieve resolution of the image down to 0.5 μm, which, compared to the diameter of carbon (7 μm) or glass (12 μm) fibre, is enough to distinguish individual fibres inside the yarns of the textile reinforcement. This highly-detailed volumetric information can serve as a solid experimental basis for the modelling of material structure. In order to achieve this, high-level information that can be used to construct a model must be extracted from the micro-CT data.

The most common method of modelling in mechanics and material science is finite element modelling, which is used to calculate stresses and evaluate strength of mechanical structures. In biomechanics, a connection between micro-CT and finite element modelling has been established in order to evaluate strength and predict damage modes of bones and bone implants [1,2]. The models created in these studies have isotropic properties of constituent materials. In the case of composite materials, where the reinforcement is usually anisotropic, the information about orientation is also required.

---

* Corresponding author.

Y.J. Zhang and J.M.R.S. Tavares (Eds.): CompIMAGE 2014, LNCS 8641, pp. 133–142, 2014.
© Springer International Publishing Switzerland 2014

One of the first image processing techniques to extract orientation of fibres was manual measurement of elliptic cross-sections of individual fibres in microscopic images [3]. The angle of inclination of a fibre was estimated from the eccentricity of the cross-section. It was shown that this method has significant systematic error for fibres approximately perpendicular to the image plane [4]. The Mean Intercept Length method involves segmentation of the image and counting of the number of intersections of a line with the boundaries of segmented domains. An ellipse is then fitted and primary directions are calculated from the lines of different orientations [5]. Recently, another method has been proposed for the orientation analysis in composites, which uses structure tensor [6].

Structure tensor is a technique used in the image processing area. In several studies, it was applied for edge detection in potential field data [7], anisotropy and orientation analysis of brain microstructure from microscopic images [8], anisotropy analysis of micro-CT images of trabecular bone [9], as an additional term in the active contour model of image segmentation [10].

Besides information about orientations, a segmentation of the material domain into its components is required for modelling. Components of a composite material usually have different density and elemental composition. Due to this, in the micro-CT image they have different average grey value. Another parameter that distinguishes them is anisotropy. The reinforcement, which consists of fibres, has different structure in the micro-CT image. In this study, a measure of anisotropy is formulated on the basis of structure tensor. Along with average grey value and first-order statistics, it is used for segmentation of the image with k-means algorithm. The outcome of this procedure is a voxel-based model for permeability or mechanical simulations.

2   Feature Variables

Each variable at a given point is calculated from the neighbourhood W of the point, which is defined as follows:

$$W(\bar{p}) : \forall \{\bar{x}\}(|x_1 - p_1| \leq w_r, |x_2 - p_2| \leq w_r, |x_3 - p_3| \leq w_r) \tag{1}$$

where $\bar{p}$ is the current calculation point and w_r is the size of the calculation window. The structure tensor is a matrix of first-order derivatives of the three-dimensional image I:

$$S'(r) = \begin{bmatrix} \left(\frac{\partial I}{\partial x}\right)^2 & \frac{\partial I}{\partial x}\frac{\partial I}{\partial y} & \frac{\partial I}{\partial x}\frac{\partial I}{\partial z} \\ & \left(\frac{\partial I}{\partial y}\right)^2 & \frac{\partial I}{\partial y}\frac{\partial I}{\partial z} \\ sym & & \left(\frac{\partial I}{\partial z}\right)^2 \end{bmatrix} \tag{2}$$

The value used as a feature variable is obtained by integration of the structure tensor over the neighbourhood of a current calculation point:

$$S(p) = \int_{W(p)} S'(r)dr \tag{3}$$

Eigenvalue decomposition of the structure tensor gives three eigenvalues $\lambda_1 \leq \lambda_2 \leq \lambda_3$ and three eigenvectors $\{v_1, v_2, v_3\}$. Two measures of anisotropy are defined on the basis of the eigenvalues of the structure tensor:

$$\beta = \begin{cases} \frac{\lambda_3 - \lambda_1}{\lambda_3} & \text{if } \lambda_3 > 0, \\ 0 & \text{if } \lambda_3 = 0. \end{cases} \tag{4}$$

and

$$\gamma = \begin{cases} \frac{\lambda_2 - \lambda_1}{\lambda_3} & \text{if } \lambda_3 > 0, \\ 0 & \text{if } \lambda_3 = 0. \end{cases} \tag{5}$$

Further they are referred to as β-anisotropy and γ-anisotropy. The statistical variables are calculated as follows:

$$Mean\ (average\ grey\ value) = \mu = E[x], \tag{6}$$

$$Standard\ deviation = \sigma = \sqrt{E[(x - \mu)^2]}, \tag{7}$$

$$Skewness = \frac{E[(x - \mu)^3]}{\sigma^3}, \tag{8}$$

$$Kurtosis = \frac{E[(x - \mu)^4]}{\sigma^4} \tag{9}$$

Here the expectation operator E works over the set of points inside the neighbourhood W.

3   Implementation

A computer program has been written in C#, which performs calculation of the described feature variables. The program takes as input an image stack or a single *.vol file, containing a 3D micro-CT image. When an image stack is processed, it is first assembled in a single 3D array. Expansion of the dynamic range can also be performed on the image if it has insufficient contrast.

The size of micro-CT images presents a challenge in their processing as it can be quite large. For example, micro-CT images obtained with Nanotom X-ray computed tomography system can have maximum size of 12 GB even with the 8 bit per pixel storage format. For SkyScan-1172 the size can reach 33 GB, and for SkyScan-1272 - 677 GB. Therefore, a micro-CT image often cannot be loaded into the memory entirely and should be processed from the disk. The developed program handles large volumes of the images, reading them by small chunks and processing each chunk in parallel, using all available processors or cores (Fig. 1).

The program is compatible and can be integrated with the Root framework, developed by CERN, which provides functions to create and display histograms. Root is an open source code library written in C++, which has the interpreter

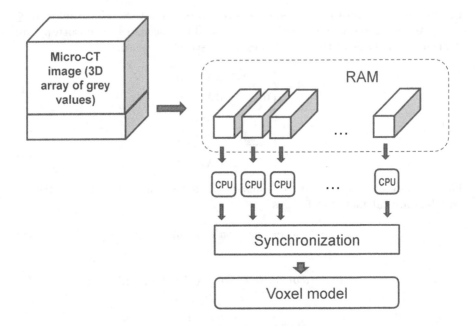

Fig. 1. Processing of the micro-CT images

that can execute C++ code. In VoxTex, the interpreter is called with the pre-generated input files that contain C++ code and raw numerical data. The interpreter is launched as a separate process and persists after termination of the host process. VoxTex has built-in viewer of micro-CT images and derived variables, but it also supports import into the VTK format, which is used to transfer the data into ParaView. ParaView is an open-source multi-platform data visualization application, which provides surface and volume rendering of three-dimensional scalar and vector data.

4   Experimental

A sample of carbon/epoxy 3D-reinforced composite with the size of the cross-section 2.7 mm^2 was used in the study. The sample was scanned with the Nanotom X-ray computed tomography system at KU Leuven. Parameters of the tomographic acquisition are given in the Table 1.

The obtained image (Fig. 2) has dimensions 1264*1336*1998 pixels. It shows matrix, yarns of the three primary directions (warp, weft and Z-yarns), and pore (air). Grey values in the image reflect X-ray attenuation coefficient, which depends on the density and molecular weight of the material. Due to this, air has the lowest grey value. The image also features ring artefacts distortion with the shape of concentric circles, which is caused by the dispersion of sensitivity of the detector pixels.

Table 1. Parameters of the tomographic acquisition

Parameter	Value
Voltage, kV	70
Current, µA	220
Resolution, µm	2.34
Number of projections	5000
Tube mode	1

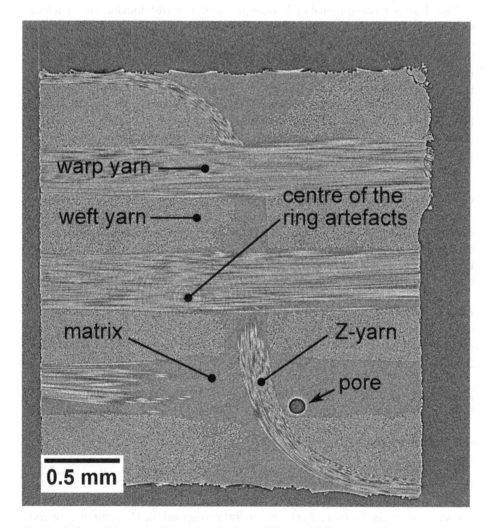

Fig. 2. A slice of the three-dimensional micro-CT image of the carbon/epoxy composite sample with resolution of 2.34 µm

5 Results

Feature variables, derived from the micro-CT image, are shown in Fig. 3. Both β and γ-anisotropy correlate with the yarns. The β-anisotropy has higher level at yarns and more uniform distribution compared with the γ-anisotropy. However, β-anisotropy also detects boundary of the pore. Ring artefacts slightly increase level of the β-anisotropy and decrease level of the γ-anisotropy.

Statistical variables derived from the image are shown in Fig. 3(d,e,f). The distribution of the standard deviation is similar to the β-anisotropy except more emphasized boundary of the pore. The skewness and kurtosis mainly detect boundaries, especially of the pore.

Fig. 4 shows two-dimensional histograms of the distribution of variables: anisotropy versus z-component of the orientation vector (v_z, axis Z is orthogonal to the image plane), and anisotropy versus average grey value. In both histograms three clusters can be distinguished. In the first histogram, the cluster with $v_z \approx 0$ is related to the yarns in the XY plane (plane of the image), and the two clusters with $v_z \approx 1$ are related to the yarns orthogonal to the image (higher β-anisotropy), and to the matrix (lower β-anisotropy). In the second histogram, the cluster with the lowest average grey value (around 107) is related to the air (pores), and the two other clusters are related to the yarns (higher β-anisotropy) and to the matrix (lower β-anisotropy).

Results of the segmentation by various feature variables using k-means algorithm are shown in Fig. 5. Segmentation using z-component of the orientation vector allows for separating yarns of different orientation (Fig. 5 a,b). Usage of β-anisotropy in the segmentation results in lower number of isolated voxels and smoother boundary between domains. However, segmentation with β-anisotropy classifies boundary of the pore as part of the yarn. In both cases, ring artefacts introduce significant distortion in the result of the segmentation, as centre of the artefact structure is recognized as yarn.

Segmentation by the β-anisotropy and average grey value (Fig. 5c) allows separating the three phases present in the image: matrix, yarns and air (pore). The ring artefacts do not affect the result of the segmentation in this case. However, certain amount of isolated voxels is present. Segmentation by the same variables and the number of clusters two (Fig. 5d) produces result of the similar quality.

Segmentation by the standard deviation and average grey value (Fig. 5e,f) produces significantly lower amount of isolated voxels and is not affected by the ring artefacts. However, boundary of the pore is still falsely classified as a part of the yarn.

Fig. 6 shows the segmented 3D images visualized with ParaView.

6 Discussion

The choice of variables to use in the segmentation depends on the desired outcome. Inclusion of a component of the orientation vector allows separating components of the material that have the same characteristics in the micro-CT image, but differ in

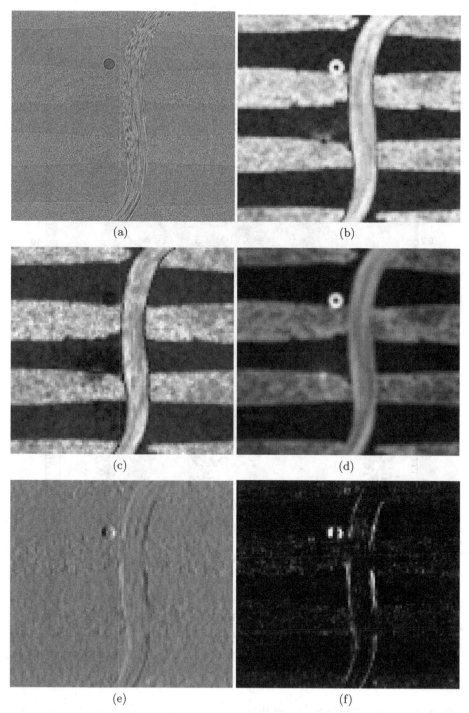

Fig. 3. The original micro-CT image (a) and the feature variables: β-anisotropy (b), γ-anisotropy (c), standard deviation (d), skewness (e) and kurtosis (f)

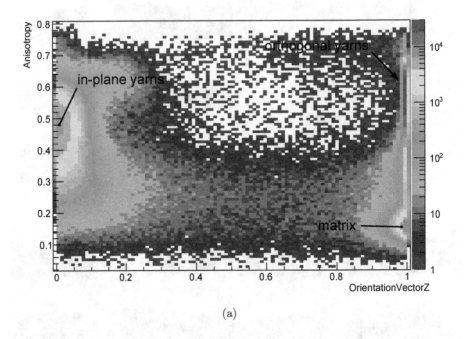

(a)

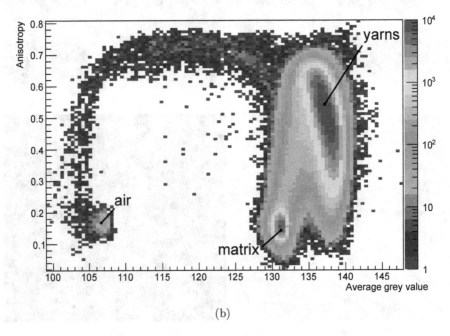

(b)

Fig. 4. Two-dimensional histograms showing distribution of the β-anisotropy versus z-component of the orientation vector (a), and β-anisotropy versus average grey value (b)

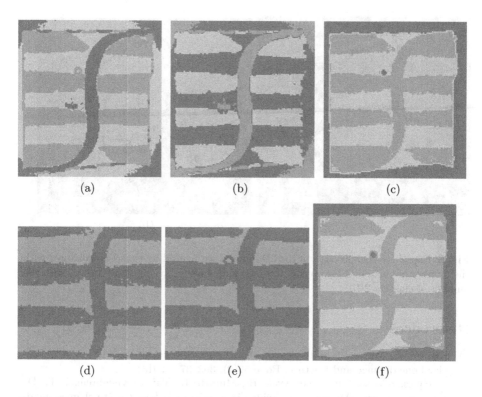

Fig. 5. Results of segmentation of the micro-CT image by different combinations of the feature variables: a - $\{v_z, \beta\text{-anisotropy}\}$; b - $\{v_z, \gamma\text{-anisotropy}\}$; c - $\{\beta\text{-anisotropy},$ average grey value$\}$ with the number of clusters 3; d - $\{\beta\text{-anisotropy},$ average grey value$\}$ with the number of clusters 2; e - $\{$standard deviation, average grey value$\}$; f - $\{$standard deviation, average grey value$\}$ with the number of clusters 3. The number of clusters, where not specified, is 2.

the orientation. This is reasonable when these components have different mechanical properties, which must be taken into account in modelling.

Segmentation by the β-anisotropy and average grey value seems to produce the most correct result, as it is not affected by the ring artefacts and classifies correctly boundary of the pores. When classified incorrectly, for example as yarn, a pore will be reflected in the resulting model not as void, but as a spherical inclusion. Such a non-physical inclusion with the mechanical properties of the yarn can produce significant local distortion in the resulting stress-strain fields.

Acknowledgements. The work is supported by the European Commission, QUICOM project, Grant Agreement No ACP2-GA-2012-314562. The X-ray computed tomography images have been made on the X-ray computed tomography facilities at the KU Leuven, financed by the Hercules Foundation (project AKUL 09/001: Micro- and nano-CT for the hierarchical analysis of materials). The authors would like to thank A.E. Bogdanovich (NCSU, USA) for the provision of the material and for useful discussions of the material's internal structure.

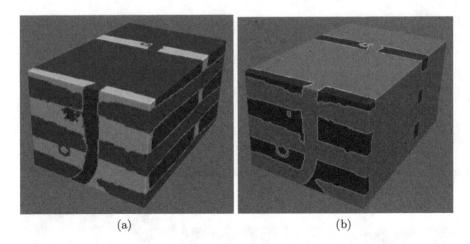

(a)   (b)

Fig. 6. ParaView visualization of the 3D images, segmented by $\{v_z, \beta\text{-anisotropy}\}$ with the number of clusters 3 (a), and by {standard deviation, average grey value} with the number of clusters 2 (b)

References

1. Hambli, R.: Micro-CT finite element model and experimental validation of trabecular bone damage and fracture. Bone 56(2), 363–374 (2013)
2. Jaecques, S.V.N., Van Oosterwyck, H., Muraru, L., Van Cleynenbreugel, T., De Smet, E., Wevers, M., et al.: Individualised, micro CT-based finite element modelling as a tool for biomechanical analysis related to tissue engineering of bone. Biomaterials 25(9), 1683–1696 (2004)
3. Fakirov, S., Fakirova, C.: Direct determination of the orientation of short glass fibers in an injection–moulded polyethylene terephthalate system. Polymer Composites 6, 41–46 (1985)
4. Eberhardt, C., Clarke, A., Vincent, M., Giroud, T., Flouret, S.: Fibre-orientation measurements in short-glass-fibre composites - II: a quantitative error estimate of the 2D image analysis technique. Compos. Sci. Technol. 61(13), 1961–1974 (2001)
5. Tabor, Z.: Equivalence of mean intercept length and gradient fabric tensors - 3d study. Medical Engineering & Physics 34, 598–604 (2012)
6. Straumit, I., Lomov, S., Verpoest, I., Wevers, M.: Determination of the local fibers orientation in a composite material from micro-CT data. In: Proceedings of the Composites Week @ Leuven and TexComp-11 Conference, Leuven, Belgium (2013)
7. Sertcelik, I., Kafadar, O.: Application of edge detection to potential field data using eigenvalue analysis of structure tensor. Journal of Applied Geophysics 84, 86–94 (2012)
8. Matthew, D., Budde, J.A.: Frank, Examining brain microstructure using structure tensor analysis of histological sections. NeuroImage 63, 1–10 (2012)
9. Tabora, Z., Petryniak, R., Latala, Z., Konopkac, T.: The potential of multi-slice computed tomography based quantification of the structural anisotropy of vertebral trabecular bone. Medical Engineering & Physics 35, 7–15 (2013)
10. Ge, Q., Xiao, L., Zhang, J., Wei, Z.H.: An improved region-based model with local statistical features for image segmentation. Pattern Recognition 45, 1578–1590 (2012)

Image Segmentation by Image Analogies

Asma Bellili and Slimane Larabi

USTHB University, Computer Science Department,
BP 32 El Alia, Algiers, Algeria
slarabi@usthb.dz

Abstract. In this paper we propose a new technique for image segmentation based on contour detection using image analogies principle. A set of artificial patterns are used to locate contours of any query image. Each pattern allow the location of contours corresponding to specific intensity variation. Boundaries are extracted based on the properties of located contours. In addition, elementary regions derived from the motion of contours in images are located and combined jointly with the boundaries for image segmentation. Experiments are conducted and the obtained results are presented and discussed.

Keywords: Image Segmentation, Analogies, Contour Detection, Multi-Scale.

1 Introduction

Image segmentation is a preprocessing step whose goal is to express an image in meaningful way and to divide it into spacial regions having some common characteristics. This task which change the representation of an image into something that is easier to analyse is a fundamental process in many computer vision applications.

There are many image segmentation methods proposed in the literature. Many states of the art have been done and published [6] [14] [15] .

A review of the literature in image segmentation indicates that natural images segmentation algorithms can be divided into two categories : Region based and Edge-based approaches. Region based approaches aim to regroup pixels having similar attributes, and the edges-based methods aim to separate regions having dissimilar attributes.

This problem remains an attractive topic for two reasons: the first one is that the results of proposed techniques are still far from what can do the human. The second one is that the segmentation is a critical step for all applications.

Image analogy is a new technique for image processing by example which consist in two steps:

- The first one consist on designating two images (A, A') such that A' is the transformation of A applying a filter.

Y.J. Zhang and J.M.R.S. Tavares (Eds.): CompIMAGE 2014, LNCS 8641, pp. 143–151, 2014.
© Springer International Publishing Switzerland 2014

- Assuming that the transformation between (A, A') is learned, the second step consist to apply to any given image B the same transformation $(A : A')$ giving the image B' [7] [9].

Image analogies has been largely used in different applications such as super resolution [8], texture [2] [3] [5], curves synthesis [11], image colorization, image enhancement and artistic filters [16], [17]. An advantage of image analogies technique is the possibility to learn very complex and non linear image filters such as artistic filters in witch various drawing and painting styles are synthesized based on scanned real world examples [9].

Few works have been devoted for the use of image analogies in image processing. A method for supervised segmentation of medical images is proposed by Lackey and Colagrosso [12] applying directly and naively the algorithm of Hertzmann [9]. This method is applied only to find by analogies the same coloured regions in medical images as those processed by the expert. We notice here that the application of naive way to image segmentation like is made in [12] requires numerous pairs of learned images (A, A') where A is initial image and A' is the segmented image. This is due to the requirement of all lighting conditions in learned images.

S. Larabi and N. M. Robertson proposed a method based on the learning of the expertise of hand draw contours to locate outlines of a query image in the same way that is done for the reference [13]. The result of their approach was a set of images which contains several contours, each one is the result of using of artificial pattern instead of hand drawn contours.

In [4], authors proposed a method based on these contours in order to define and locate the outlines of objects. In this work, we propose a method to extract boundaries of objects and then to segment image in regions. The next section is devoted to a brief review of contour detection by image analogies and the inferred properties. Our method is presented in section 3 followed by the results of experiments conducted on Weizmann data set [1] presented section 4.

2   Contour Detection by Image Analogies and Properties: A Brief Review

The idea is to start from a pair of images (A, A') , A is an initial image and the second one A', identical to A, in addition, contours are hand drawn. The aim was to localize the contours of any other query image B using the expertise learned from the pair (A, A') (see figure 1)[13].

A set of artificial patterns are proposed instead of hand drawn contours in images as learning images (see figure 2). The use of these patterns allow locating fourteen images of contours. Each one is obtained by the corresponding pattern (A, A').

In [4], authors demonstrated that contours in the 14 images of contours located by image analogies technique are moving from one image to another and are more steady around the boundaries of regions. However, for others parts of the image, they are moving fastly (see figure of table 1).

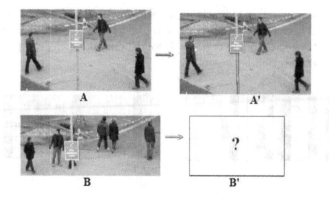

Fig. 1. Contour detection: The main idea [13]

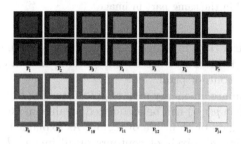

Fig. 2. Artificial patterns used as training images

Table 1. Contours located using a selection of the 14 artificial patterns

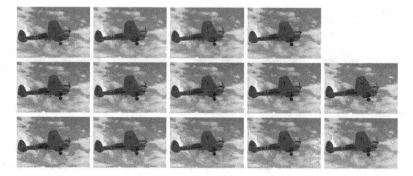

3   Image Segmentation

3.1   Energy Map of Pixels

The stability of a contour is measured from its motion in all images of contours. More the motion of the contour is slow, more it will be considered as the region boundaries [4] (see figure 3).

In this section, we propose firstly an algorithm for measuring the stability of a pixel among all images of contours. A map of energy is created from the images of contours and used to locate regions. Also, depending on the energies of pixels, multi-scale segmentation is presented.

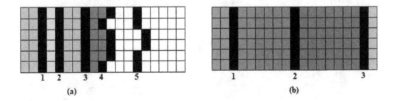

(a)   (b)

Fig. 3. (a)Slow motion of contours located using five successive patterns and reported in the same part in image, (b) Fast motion of contours located using three successive patterns and reported in the same part in image

Let $p_{i,j}^k$ be the pixel (i, j) in image IM_k of contours obtained using the pairs of patterns $P_k, k = 1..14$. There are 14 images IM_k and in each one the pixel $p_{i,j}^k$ may be or not a contour pixel.

Our aim is to compute an energy map of pixels starting from the set of images of contours. Each pixel $p(i, j)$ will be associated a value measuring its appertaining to a border of region or to inside of region. As explained above, around the pixel $p(i, j)$ in the image, pixels of contours of all images $IM_k, k = 1..14$ are moving from the darkest part to the clearest one (see figure 4).

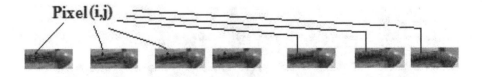

Fig. 4. Appearance of the same pixel (i, j) for different images IM_k of contours

To evaluate the evolution of the contour around $p(i, j)$ in all images of contours $IM_k, k = 1..14$, we consider an area of $((2N + 1) \times (2N + 1))$ pixels. For each pixel p, and for each IM_k, we search the nearest pixels of contours q following the n directions in the defined area. Four directions are considered: Horizontal, vertical and two diagonals directions. The energy of the pixel p is computed using the distances d_k of the nearest contour pixel $q_{i,j}^k$ to p in the image IM_k. The energy E of p is defined by equation 3.1.

$$E = \sum_{k=1}^{k=14} 2^{N-d_k} \qquad (1)$$

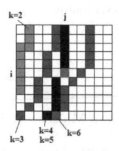

Fig. 5. Search area of contour pixels for all 14 images. Notice the presence of five contours located using five successive patterns $k = 2..6$, two of them pass by $p(i,j)$

More there are pixels q nearest to $p(i,j)$ found in successive images $IM_k, k = 1..14$, more the energy E is highest. However, when there are few (one or zero) pixels q found, this implies that the energy E is very low. For example, $E = 2$ is associated to $p(i,j)$ in case where there is only one pixel contour located at distance $(N-1)$ from the central pixel (i,j). However, when there are five contours pixels located (such that illustrated by figure 5), corresponding to the distances $N-1, 1, 0, 0, 1$ (moving from the left to right), the energy E is then equal to $E = 2^1 + 2^{N-1} + 2^N + 2^N + 2^{N-1}$, for $N = 5$, $E = 98$. This energy is then synonymous of the appertaining of the pixel $p(i,j)$ to the inside or to the border of region. The values of energy computed have similar significance like the result of merging of all images of contours giving largest contours at borders of regions and thinnest elsewhere (see figure 6).

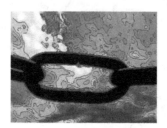

Fig. 6. Result of merging all 14 images of contours

The Algorithm
Begin
-$(IM_k, k=1..14)$ are the images of contours located using the patterns (A^k, A'^k)
-N is the distance defining the search area
-I_m is the map of energies to compute
For each $p(i,j)$ of I_m
Do For each image IM_k

Do search the nearest pixel contour q to $p(i,j)$
d=distance (q,p), if $d < N, E(i,j) = E(i,j) + 2^{N-d}$
EndFor
EndFor
End.

3.2   From Map of Energies to Multi-scale Segmentation

The different values of energy associated to each pixel define the map of energies end noted I_m. We used this map to locate the boundaries of regions at different scales: (high, intermediates and low) which correspond to the four intervals of energy: $[46, 56[$, $[56, 64[$, $[64, 128[$, $[128, \infty]$. For each value of energy, there are pixels of boundaries which are selected, where strong boundaries are associated to high values of energy. Figures of table 2 illustrate for each image the located boundaries at low, intermediate and high scale.

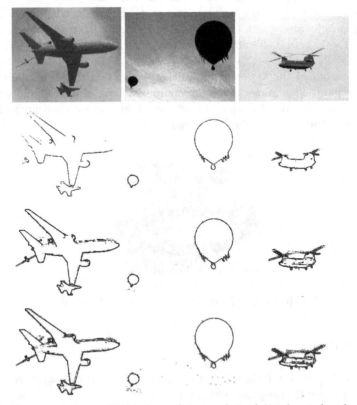

Table 2. For some images of Weizmann data set, boundaries located at low (second row), intermediate (third row) and high (fourth row) scales

Once the boundaries are located, an additional processing is required in order to achieve the segmentation. Elementary regions defined as the areas between contours located using two successive patterns are firstly located and combined jointly with the located boundaries in order to locate regions in image. Figure 7 illustrates these elementary regions where 14 colors are associated to elementary regions obtained using the 14 artificial patterns.

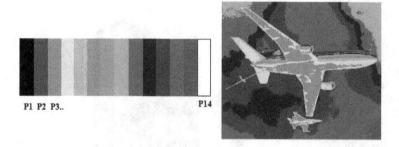

Fig. 7. At the left: the different colors associated to elementary regions located using each one of the 14 patterns. At the right, the result obtained for image from Weizmann data set

4   Results

In this section we present results obtained by applying our method on Weizmann data set. Figures of table 3 show the boundaries detection of images at high scale, the elementary regions located using the 14 patterns and the result of fusion with computed boundaries. Compared to the ground truth data, we achieved a good values of recall and precision (see figure 8).

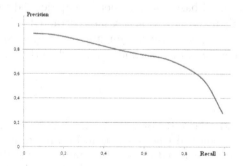

Fig. 8. Evaluation of the results obtained on Weizmann data set

Table 3. For some images of Weizmann data set, boundaries located at high scale, the located elementary regions, the result of fusion process

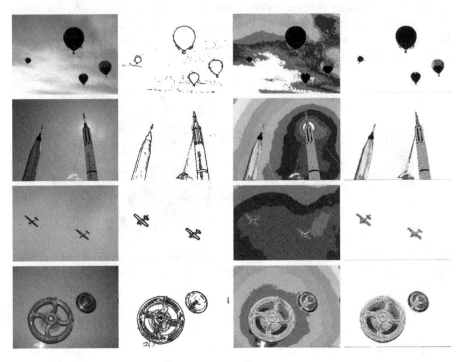

5   Conclusion

In this paper we proposed a new technique for image segmentation based on contour detection using image analogies principle. A set of artificial patterns are used to locate contours in any query image. Each pattern allow the location of contours corresponding to specific intensity variation. Multi-scale boundaries of regions are then extracted based on the energy map derived from the properties of contours located. Elementary regions are also extracted and combined with the boundaries to locate the regions. Experiments are conducted and the obtained results show the efficiency of our method compared to the state of the art.

References

1. Alpert, S., Galun, M., Basri, R., Brandt, A.: Image Segmentation by Probabilistic Bottom-Up Aggregation and Cue Integration. In: Proceedings of the IEEE Conference on Computer Vision and Pattern Recognition (June 2007)
2. Ashikhmin, M.: Synthesizing natural textures. In: Proceedings of 2001 ACM Symposium on Interactive 3D Graphics (2001)
3. Ashikhmin, M.: Fast texture transfer. IEEE Computer Graphics and Applications 23(4), 38–43 (2003)

4. Bellili, A., Larabi, S., Robertson, N.M.: Outlines of objects detection by analogy. In: Wilson, R., Hancock, E., Bors, A., Smith, W. (eds.) CAIP 2013, Part I. LNCS, vol. 8047, pp. 385–392. Springer, Heidelberg (2013)

5. Bhat, P., Ingram, S., Turk, G.: Geometric texture synthesis by example. In: Proceedings of the 2004 Eurographics/ACM SIGGRAPH symposium on Geometry processing, Nice (2004)

6. Cheng, H.D., Jiang, X.H., Sun, Y., Wang, J.L.: Color image segmentation: advances and prospects. In: Pattern Recognition (2001)

7. Cheng, L., Vishwanathan, S., Zhang, X.: Consistent image analogies using semi-supervised learning. In: IEEE Conference on Computer Vision and Pattern Recognition (CVPR), Anchorage (2008)

8. Freeman, W.T., Pasztor, E.C., Carmichael, O.T.: Learning Low-Level Vision. International Journal of Computer Vision 40(1), 25–47 (2000)

9. Hertzmann, A., Jacobs, C., Oliver, N., Curless, B., Salesin, D.: Image analogies. In: Proceedings of the 28th Annual ACM Conference on Computer Graphics and Interactive Techniques, New York (2001)

10. Hertzmann, A., Jacobs, C.E., Oliver, N., Curless, B., Seitz, S.M.: Image analogies. In: SIGGRAPH Conference Proceedings, pp. 327–340 (2001)

11. Hertzmann, A., Oliver, N., Curless, B., Seitz, S.M.: Curve analogies. In: EGRW 2002 Proceedings of the 13th Eurographics Workshop on Rendering, Switzerland (2002)

12. Lackey, J.B., Colagrosso, M.D.: Supervised segmentation of visible human data with image analogies. In: Proceedings of the International Conference on Machine Learning; Models, Technologies and Applications (2004)

13. Larabi, S., Robertson, N.M.: Contour detection by image analogies. In: Bebis, G., et al. (eds.) ISVC 2012, Part II. LNCS, vol. 7432, pp. 430–439. Springer, Heidelberg (2012)

14. Nikhil, R.P., Sankar, K.P.: A review on image segmentation techniques. In: Pattern Recognition (1993)

15. Haralick, R.M., Shapiro: Image segmentation techniques. In: Computer Vision, Graphics and Image Processing (1985)

16. Sykora, D., Burianek, J., Zara, J.: Unsupervised colorization of black-and-white cartoons. In: Proceedings of the 3rd Int. Symp. Non-photorealistic Animation and Rendering, pp. 121–127 (2004)

17. Wang, G., Wong, T., Heng, P.: Deringing cartoons by image analogies. ACM Transactions on Graphics 25(4), 1360–1379 (2006)

Improving Atlas-Based Medical Image Segmentation with a Relaxed Object Search

Renzo Phellan[1], Alexandre X. Falcão[1], and Jayaram Udupa[2]

[1] LIV, Institute of Computing, University of Campinas, Campinas, SP, Brazil
`ra144686@students.ic.unicamp.br, afalcao@ic.unicamp.br`
[2] MIPG, Dept. of Radiology, University of Pennsylvania, Philadelphia, PA, USA
`jay@mail.med.upenn.edu`

Abstract. Medical image segmentation using 3D probabilistic atlases has been actively pursued to avoid the time-consuming involvement of experts in manual object (organ) delineation for quantitative analysis. By mapping a new 3D image onto the reference coordinate system of the atlas, built for some organ of interest, these techniques take a binary decision based on the probability of each voxel to be part of that organ. However, image-based techniques have also been proposed to refine object delineation at the initial position given by the atlas-based segmentation. In this paper, we relax this condition for delineation refinement by moving an atlas based on the prior probability map to search for the organ around that initial position. Our method uses the multi-scale parameter search algorithm with a suitable criterion function to evaluate automatic 3D organ delineations, as obtained by the image foresting transform algorithm in an uncertainty region of the atlas. Experiments with eight organs in CT and MR images have indicated that our method can improve atlas-based segmentation with statistical significance. Moreover, the relaxed object search consistently found the organ with higher accuracy outside the position obtained by the atlas, which reinforces our claim.

Keywords: Medical image segmentation, atlas-based segmentation, image foresting transform, multi-scale parameter search.

1 Introduction

The quantitative analysis of organs in medical imaging applications very often requires a precise definition of their spatial extent (object delineation) in the image. Manual organ delineation by experts is a time-consuming, tedious, and error-prone task, also subjected to inter-observer variability [1]. Moreover, it requires experts with considerable experience in manual delineation [2]. In order to solve this problem, image segmentation methods based on probabilistic atlases have been actively investigated [6, 14, 15].

From a set of training images, containing a given organ of interest, the 3D atlas is built by selecting one image as reference and mapping the remaining ones onto its coordinate system, ideally via affine registration followed by locally-deformable image registration [3, 16]. Several techniques also build multiple atlases for a given organ [17,18], but we will focus our study on the single-atlas case.

Y.J. Zhang and J.M.R.S. Tavares (Eds.): CompIMAGE 2014, LNCS 8641, pp. 152–163, 2014.
© Springer International Publishing Switzerland 2014

The atlas construction requires a careful segmentation of the organ in all training images, which is usually done manually by experts, in a slice-by-slice fashion, but it can also take advantage from interactive segmentation methods [4]. The registration deformation field may be applied to the organ segmentation masks or the training images may be segmented in the reference coordinate system. Those segmentation masks are essentially used to estimate the prior probability of each voxel to be part of that organ in the reference system. By mapping a new image onto the reference system, the techniques take a binary decision, as organ or not-organ, based on those probabilities [1]. They can also refine object delineation at that position by using some image-based technique. In [5], for instance, the delineation refinement technique is a watershed transform. In [6], the atlas-based segmentation is refined by active contours.

In this paper, we propose a relaxed search for the organ around the initial position, as indicated by the 3D atlas-based segmentation, using the Multi-Scale Parameter Search (MSPS) algorithm [7] with a suitable criterion function to evaluate automatic 3D organ delineations obtained by the Image Foresting Transform (IFT) algorithm [8]. The prior probability map (atlas) is thought of as a moving organ appearance model that can translate over the image around its initial position. Seed voxels for the IFT algorithm are estimated inside and outside the atlas (i.e., in regions with prior probability equal to 1 and 0, respectively). The remaining voxels are considered in an uncertainty region, wherein the boundary of the organ is expected to be, when the atlas is placed at the correct position of the organ in the image. For each considered position of the atlas in the image, the internal and external seeds compete among themselves for the voxels in the uncertainty region by offering to them paths in an implicitly-defined image graph. The uncertainty region is then divided into internal and external voxels, such that the object will consist of the internal seeds and all voxels conquered by optimum paths rooted at them. The MSPS algorithm selects the IFT solution which produces the maximum mean arc weight on the IFT graph cut.

A previous work [9] has proposed a similar strategy using the IFT algorithm and exhaustive object search over the entire image in multiple scales, but using a different type of object appearance model, named *cloud*, which relies only on image translations to build and use the model. Given that they do not use neither locally-deformable nor affine image registration, we preferred to constrain our study in atlas-based segmentation.

Section 2 presents the methodology for atlas construction and its use as in the traditional atlas-based segmentation paradigm. The relaxed object search is presented in Section 3 with a short description of the MSPS and IFT algorithms. The analysis of the improvements over the traditional atlas-based segmentation approach is conducted in Section 4. Experiments with eight organs, representing challenging segmentation tasks in CT and MR images, demonstrate that the relaxed object search usually finds a more accurate organ delineation outside the initial atlas position and it can improve atlas-based segmentation with statistical significance. Section 5 states the conclusions and discusses future work.

2   Atlas-Based Image Segmentation

A medical image $\hat{I}$ is a pair (D_I, I) where $D_I \in Z^3$ is the image domain and $I(v) \in Z$ is a scalar value assigned to every voxel $v \in D_I$. Image $\hat{I}$ is said to be binary, when $I(v) \in \{0,1\}$. A probabilistic atlas $\hat{P} = (D_I, P)$ in the same domain presents the prior probability $P(v \in O) \in [0,1]$ of the voxel v be part of a given organ $O \in D_I$, given its position.

For a given medical image training set, we wish to construct a single atlas for each organ of interest, by affine and locally-deformable image registrations. Given that our training sets already come with the original and the binary masks of the organs, as created by experts using manual and interactive segmentation methods, we use those masks to select a reference coordinate system, register all original images into the reference system, and use their respective deformation fields to map their masks. The details about this process and the use of the resulting atlas for segmentation are given next.

2.1   Atlas Construction

Several approaches to build a probabilistic atlas for a given organ select as reference image the one with maximum mean similarity with respect to the other training images [10]. We use the same strategy, but the similarities between their respective binary masks are measured based on the *Average Symmetric Surface Distance* (ASSD) [2]. Other measures, such as Dice Similarity Coefficient (DSC) and Jaccard Coefficient, only give a global simmilarity impression between the binary masks while ASSD is much more sensitive to their local differences.

We used the tool described in [11], whose implementation and binaries are publicly available at http://elastix.isi.uu.nl, for affine registration followed by locally-deformable image registration into the reference coordinate system. We also configured its parameters as suggested in [12]. The resulting deformation fields for the original images are then applied to transform their respective binary masks.

In the reference system, the prior probability $P(v \in O)$ of a voxel v to belong to an organ O is measured as the percentage of times that $I(v) = 1$ at location v in the training binary masks. Let $x = I(v)$ be a random variable. In our case, the conditional probability density $\rho(x \mid v \in O)$ is a Gaussian distribution, whose mean and standard deviation are computed over the intensities of the voxels in O, using all training images. By Bayes's formula, the posterior probability is

$$P(v \in O \mid x) = \frac{P(v \in O)\rho(x \mid v \in O)}{\rho(x)}, \tag{1}$$

where the joint probability density $\rho(x)$ is simply the normalized histogram of the training images.

Figures 1, 2 and 3 illustrate the resulting images that represent the prior probability (atlas), conditional probability density, and posterior probability maps in the reference image domain for one of the objects: the cerebellum in MR-T1 images.

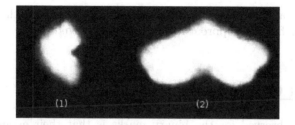

Fig. 1. Prior probability of the cerebellum model: (1) sagittal slice (2) coronal slice

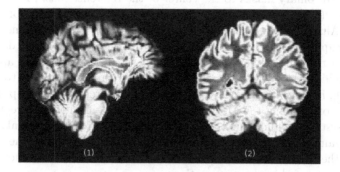

Fig. 2. Conditional probability density of the cerebellum model: (1) sagittal slice (2) coronal slice

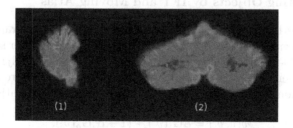

Fig. 3. Posterior probability of the cerebellum model: (1) sagittal slice (2) coronal slice

2.2 Classical Use of the Atlas for Image Segmentation

By applying the same registration scheme to a new image, one can decide if its voxels belong to the organ or to the background by simply thresholding the posterior probability map at 0.5. However, possible registration errors can compromise the accuracy of this approach. This has motivated authors to refine atlas-based object segmentation by image-based techniques [5, 6].

We claim that, if a problem exists due to registration errors, then we should first improve the prior probability map and then use it to search for the object locally, around the position (center of the mask) suggested by the atlas-based segmentation method, rather than only at that position, as in [5, 6]. Moreover, the criterion function for this search can take into account the quality of those delineations. If a more accurate delineation is found outside the initial atlas position, then refinement approaches, such as [5,6], would not be able to provide the best result.

3 Relaxed Object Search

A first aspect observed for the binary masks is that their geometric centers were not at the same position after registration into the reference system. By translating all binary masks to the center of the reference mask, $P(v \in O)$ (the atlas) and $P(v \in O \mid x)$ change, while the other terms in Equation 1 remain the same. Although the same procedure described for classical segmentation in Section 2.2 applies to the corrected atlas, we still wish to refine object delineation.

The prior probability map (atlas) is then used as a moving organ appearance model to guide object delineation by the IFT algorithm [8], similarly to the cloud model in [9]. However, instead of using exhaustive search, we speed up the search process by constraining the MSPS optimization algorithm [7] in a region of the reference system around the initial model position. This region is also learned from the training set by recording the relative positions between the geometric centers of the binary masks and the center of the reference image domain. The details are presented in the next sections.

3.1 Delineating Objects by IFT and Moving Atlas

The image foresting transform (IFT) interprets an image $\hat{I}$ as a graph $(D_I, \mathcal{A})$ by taking an adjacency relation $\mathcal{A} \subset D_I \times D_I$ between its voxels. For segmentation, we use $\mathcal{A}$ as a 26-neighborhood where a voxel v' belongs to the adjacent set $\mathcal{A}(v)$ of a voxel v when $\|v' - v\| \leq \sqrt{3}$. The weight $w(v, v')$ of each arc in $\mathcal{A}$ is given by a combination between local image and global object information.

$$w(v, v') = \alpha G_i(v') + (1 - \alpha) G_o(v'), \tag{2}$$

where $G_i(v')$ is the magnitude of the 3D Sobel's gradient of the original image $\hat{I}$ and $G_o(v')$ is the magnitude of the 3D Sobel's gradient of the conditional probability density map $\rho(x \mid v \in O)$ estimated for image $\hat{I}$ based on its values and the Gaussian distribution learned by training. Note that, we do not need the segmentation of $\hat{I}$ to estimate its $\rho(x \mid v \in O)$. Given that $G_o(v')$ may not be perfect, we observed that the best solution is to combine it with $G_i(v')$. The parameter $0 \leq \alpha \leq 1$ is then found by 2-fold cross validation among the training images.

The arc weights are meant to be higher on the object's border than inside and outside it. At any given position of the atlas in the image, it defines three regions: interior with voxel values 1, exterior with voxel values 0, and uncertainty region $\mathcal{U}$ with values in $(0, 1)$. The interior and exterior voxels are used to define seed sets $\mathcal{S}_i$ and $\mathcal{S}_e$, which must compete for the most closely connected voxels in $\mathcal{U}$. This competition then considers a reduced graph $(D_U, \mathcal{A})$, where $D_U = \mathcal{U} \cup \mathcal{S}_i \cup \mathcal{S}_e$

and a path-cost function $f(\pi_v)$ applied to any path $\pi_v = \langle v_1, v_2, \ldots, v_n \rangle$, $v_n = v$, in the graph, including the trivial ones $\langle v \rangle$ formed by a single voxel.

$$f(\langle v \rangle) = \begin{cases} 0 & \text{if } v \in \mathcal{S}_i \cup \mathcal{S}_e, \\ +\infty & \text{otherwise,} \end{cases}$$

$$f(\langle v_1, v_2, \ldots, v_n \rangle) = \max_{i=1,2,\ldots,n-1} \{w(v_i, v_{i+1})\}. \tag{3}$$

The IFT algorithm then minimizes a cost map

$$C(v) = \min_{\forall \pi_v \in \Pi(\mathcal{U}, \mathcal{A}, v)} \{f(\pi_v)\} \tag{4}$$

by computing an optimum-path forest rooted at $\mathcal{S}_i \cup \mathcal{S}_e$. That is, considering the set $\Pi(\mathcal{U}, \mathcal{A}, v)$ of all possible paths π_v from $\mathcal{S}_i \cup \mathcal{S}_e$ to every voxel $v \in D_{\mathcal{U}}$, the algorithm assigns to v the path π_v^* of minimum cost, such that the object is defined by the union between the interior voxels and the voxels of $\mathcal{U}$ that are rooted in $\mathcal{S}_i$.

   This seed competition process avoids paths that cross the object's border as much as possible due to the design of the path-cost function and minimization of the cost map. The operator can also be sought as an improved watershed transform from internal and external markers, but with gradient formulation, markers, and delineation algorithm different from the one proposed in [5].

3.2   Scoring Candidate Objects

As the atlas translates inside the search region, seeking for a maximum score, a candidate object is fastly obtained by the IFT algorithm constrained in that reduced graph $(D_U, \mathcal{A})$. The candidates O are scored by the mean arc weight along the IFT graph cut.

$$score(O) = \frac{1}{|B_O|} \sum_{\forall(v,v') \in B_O} w(v, v') \tag{5}$$

where $B_O : (v, v') \in \mathcal{A} \backslash v \in O, v' \notin O$.

3.3   Searching for the Best Candidate

The MSPS algorithm further speeds up the search for the best candidate by avoiding delineation in all points of the search region in order to obtain the solution as the candidate O with maximum $score(O)$. The parameters of this algorithm are the three possible translations along x, y, and z. From the initial atlas position and delineation score, the algorithm perturbs the system by displacements along x, y, and z in different scales of the parameter space to avoid local maxima. From the position that holds the maximum score after perturbation, the algorithm repeats the process until no improvement be observed in the score.

By combining the search in different scales, the method performs a broader look at the behavior of the criterion function, which is suitable to deal with the nonconvexity of the problem. The scales are set according to the bounding constraints inherent to the problem. For any position during the search, we applied positive and negative displacements of 1, 5 and 10 voxels along the x, y, and z axes.

4   Evaluation

In this section, we evaluate the improvement of our method, which includes the relaxed object search, over the classical atlas-based segmentation described in Section 2. The experiments involved two datasets: (a) 35 MR-T1 images of the brain with voxel sizes $0.98 \times 0.98 \times 0.98$ mm^3 and their corresponding binary masks for the cerebellum; and (b) 35 CT images of the thorax with voxel sizes $2.5 \times 2.5 \times 2.5$ mm^3 and their corresponding binary masks for the following organs: Right Lung (RPS), Left Lung (LPS), Respiratory System (RS), Pericardial Region (PC), Thoracic Skin (TSkn), Trachea and Bronchi (TB), and Internal Mediastinum (IMS). In the case of PC and TB, however, we had only 25 and 30 binary masks available, respectively. The binary segmentations were obtained by multiple experts using manual and interactive segmentation tools. More details about these datasets can be obtained in [13].

First, Table 1 shows the value of the parameter α for each organ. Then, it indicates the total volume in mm^3 of each image and the volume of the learned search region mentioned in Section 3. As we can see, this region represents a minimum fraction of the total volume of the image, so the search process is effectively accelerated.

Table 1. Values of α and search region

Organ	Alpha (α)	Image Vol. (mm^3)	Search Region Vol. (mm^3)	% of Search Region
C	0.2	5 367 063	30	0.0006
RPS	0.7	631 750 000	5156	0.0008
LPS	0.7	631 750 000	4500	0.0007
RS	0.7	631 750 000	8125	0.0013
PC	0.5	631 750 000	7219	0.0011
TSkn	0.1	631 750 000	2250	0.0004
TB	0.7	631 750 000	7219	0.0011
IMS	0.0	631 750 000	5250	0.0008

The experiments randomly divided the datasets 10 times into 70% for training and 30% for test, for statistical analysis. The results were evaluated by two measures: Dice Similarity Coefficient (DSC) and Average Symmetric Surface Distance (ASSD). DSC has been popular in the literature of atlas-based segmentation [2]. However, pointed out by the authors in [2], it sometimes can over/underestimate the quality of segmentation due to its global characteristic. Therefore, as suggested in [2], we preferred to base our conclusions on both DSC and ASSD. In both cases, we performed a two-tailed Z-test, with a 95% confidence limit. In this case, the critical value for null hypothesis rejection was 1.96.

The results are shown in Tables 2 and 3 for DSC and ASSD, respectively. According to both measures, the relaxed object search of our method can improve the classical atlas-based segmentation with statistical significance for C, LPS, RS and TSkn. Athough DSC indicates that their results are not statistically significant in the case of RPS, ASSD disagrees in favor to our method. According to both measures, the methods perform equivalently for PC and IMS, in which the maximum score was also at the initial atlas position. Finally, our method did not perform better for TB, since the choice of seeds needs to be more carefully done in the case of sparse objects.

Table 2. DSC scores

Organ	Atlas-Based Segm.	With Object Search	# of Images	Z-test	Significant
C	83.93 +/- 4.72	92.41 +/- 0.33	35	10.60	Yes
RPS	95.95 +/- 0.32	95.89 +/- 0.55	35	-0.52	No
LPS	95.75 +/- 0.41	96.10 +/- 0.10	35	4.91	Yes
RS	96.00 +/- 0.33	96.25 +/- 0.79	35	1.76	Yes
PC	90.05 +/- 0.55	90.11 +/- 1.01	25	0.245	No
TSkn	74.30 +/- 0.97	98.28 +/- 0.82	35	111.43	Yes
TB	76.58 +/- 2.89	76.74 +/- 4.12	30	0.18	No
IMS	82.49 +/- 3.34	82.6 +/- 2.98	35	0.14	No

Table 3. ASSD scores in mm

Organ	Atlas-Based Segm.	With Object Search	# of Images	Z-test	Significant
C	4.457 +/- 1.276	2.198 +/- 0.108	35	10.44	Yes
RPS	1.920 +/- 0.251	1.395 +/- 0.278	35	8.296	Yes
LPS	2.119 +/- 0.329	1.348 +/- 0.033	35	13.80	Yes
RS	2.245 +/- 0.289	1.300 +/- 0.225	35	15.28	Yes
PC	2.748 +/- 0.133	2.750 +/- 0.325	25	-0.024	No
TSkn	14.265 +/- 0.301	1.600 +/- 0.700	35	98.35	Yes
TB	1.428 +/- 0.460	3.025 +/- 0.850	30	-9.05	Yes
IMS	4.390 +/- 1.746	4.075 +/- 1.275	35	0.86	No

It is also important to observe that atlas-based segmentation requires about 5 minutes only to register a new image into the atlas coordinate system and the relaxed object search takes about 12 seconds on the same personal computer. Therefore, its additional time is not a problem. The personal computer has an Intel Core i5 2.4 GHz processor and 4 GB of RAM.

We can see in Figures 4 and 5 an example of the segmentation results when using our model and the classical model. The yellow areas represent segmentations of the cerebellum. We can also see, in Figure 6, a 3D rendering of LPS segmentation using both models, as compared to experts' segmentation.

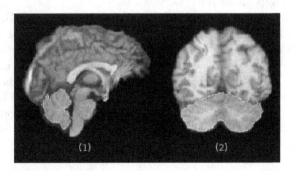

Fig. 4. Segmentation result using our model: (1) sagittal slice (2) coronal slice

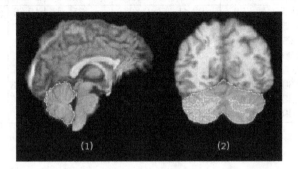

Fig. 5. Segmentation result using the classical model: (1) sagittal slice (2) coronal slice

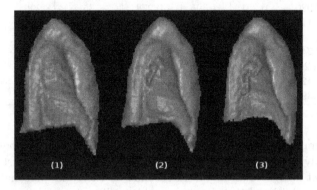

Fig. 6. Segmentation result for LPS using: (1) experts' segmentation (2) our model (3) the classical model

We are showing Figures 7 and 8 in order to illustrate that DSC can omit some local deviations, which can be discovered by using ASSD. Figure 7 has a DSC of 95.13% and a ASSD of 2.70 mm, while Figure 8 has a DSC of 95.44% and a ASSD of 1.48 mm. The white area represents the segmentation error. As we can see, both figures have similar DSC scores, but they exhibit a significative difference, which can be detected by analizyng their ASSD distances.

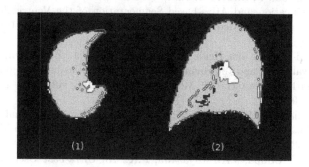

Fig. 7. Segmentation result for RPS using our method: (1) axial slice (2) sagittal slice

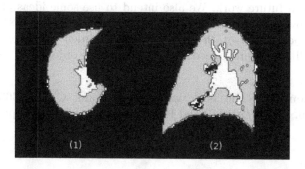

Fig. 8. Segmentation result for RPS using our method: (1) axial slice (2) sagittal slice

5   Conclusion

We have presented a fast and effective solution to correct possible registration errors to improve atlas-based image segmentation. Our method interprets the atlas as a moving object appearance model in order to search for a better object delineation around the initial atlas position. This search is based on the MSPS algorithm [7] and its criterion function evaluates object delineations produced by the IFT algorithm [8] — more specifically, the mean arc weight along the IFT graph cut.

We have validated the method using two datasets of MR and CT images of the brain and thorax, respectively, with a total of eight organs of interest: cerebellum, right lung, left lung, respiratory system, pericardial region, thoracic skin, trachea and bronchi, and internal mediastinum. The relaxed object search could improve the segmentation results with statistical significance for five out of these eight organs, being equivalent to the classical procedure only in the cases of the pericardium region and internal mediastinum.

The proposed approach relies on an optimization algorithm for the search, its criterion function, a delineation algorithm, and a few parameters that are learned by training. These elements can be investigated using other techniques for further improvements in future work. We also intend to use some ideas of the present paper to improve other techniques [9, 13] that build and use a system of object appearance models without the computational burden of image registration. Finally, we will also improve seed selection for sparse objects.

Acknowledgement. The first two authors thank CNPq (303673/2010-9, 479070/2013-0, 131835/2013-0) and FAPESP for the finantial support.

References

[1] Vos, P.C., Išgum, I., Biesbroek, J.M., Velthuis, B.K., Viergever, M.A.: Combined Pixel Classification and Atlas-based Segmentation of the Ventricular System in Brain CT Images. In: Medical Imaging 2013, vol. 8669, pp. 86691O-1–86691O-6 (2013)

[2] Langerak, T.R., Van der Heide, U.A., Kotte, A.N.T.J., Berendsen, F.F., Pluim, J.P.W.: Evaluating and Improving Label Fusion in Atlas-based Segmentation Using the Surface Distance. In: Medical Imaging 2011, vol. 7962, pp. 796226-1–796226-7 (2011)

[3] Park, H., Bland, P.H., Meyer, C.R.: Construction of an Abdominal Probabilistic Atlas and its Application in Segmentation. IEEE Transactions on Medical Imaging 22(4), 483–492 (2003)

[4] Falcão, A.X., Udupa, J.K., Miyazawa, F.K.: An Ultra-Fast User-Steered Image Segmentation Paradigm: Live-Wire-On-The-Fly. IEEE Transactions on Medical Imaging 19(1), 55–62 (2000)

[5] Grau, V., Mewes, A.U.J., Alcañiz, M., Kikinis, R., Warfield, S.K.: Improved Watershed Transform for Medical Image Segmentation Using Prior Information. IEEE Transaction on Medical Imaging 23(4), 447–458 (2004)

[6] Gao, Y., Tannembaum, A.: Combining Atlas and Active Contour for Automatic 3D Medical Image Segmentation. In: ISBI 2011, pp. 1401–1404 (2011)

[7] Chiachia, G., Falcão, A.X., Rocha, A.: Multiscale Parameter Search (MSPS): A Deterministic Approach for Black-box Global Optimization. Technical Report, Institute of Computing, University of Campinas (2011)

[8] Miranda, P.A., Falcão, A.X.: Links Between Image Segmentation Based on Optimum-Path Forest and Minimum Cut in Graph. Journal of Mathematical Imaging and Vision 35(2), 128–142 (2009)

[9] Miranda, P.A.V., Falcão, A.X., Udupa, J.K.: Cloud Bank: A multiple Clouds Model and its use in MR Brain Image Segmentation. In: Proc. of the Sixth IEEE Intl. Symp. on Biomedical Imaging: From Nano to Macro (ISBI), pp. 506–509 (2009)

[10] Park, H., Bland, P.H., Hero III, A.O., Meyer, C.R.: Least Biased Target Selection in Probabilistic Atlas Construction. In: Duncan, J.S., Gerig, G. (eds.) MICCAI 2005. LNCS, vol. 3750, pp. 419–426. Springer, Heidelberg (2005)

[11] Klein, S., Staring, M., Murphy, K., Viergever, M.A., Pluim, J.P.W.: Elastix: A Toolbox for Intensity Based Medical Image Registration. IEEE Transactions on Medical Imaging 29(1), 196–205 (2010)

[12] Van der Lijn, F., De Bruijne, M., Hoogendam, Y.Y., Klein, S., Hameeteman, R., Breteler, M.M.B., Niessen, W.J.: Cerebellum Segmentation in MRI using Atlas Registration and Local Multi-Scale Image Descriptors. In: ISBI 2009, pp. 221–224 (2009)

[13] Udupa, J.K., Odhner, D., Falcão, A.X., Ciesielski, K.C., Miranda, P.A.V., Matsumoto, M., Grevera, G., Saboury, B., Torigian, D.: Automatic Anatomy Recognition via Fuzzy Object Models. In: SPIE on Medical Imaging: Image-Guided Procedures, Robotic Interventions, and Modeling, vol. 8316 (2012)

[14] Lötjönen, J., Koikkalainen, J., Thurfiell, L., Lundqvist, R., Waldemar, G., Soininen, H., Rueckert, D.: Improved Generation of Probabilistic Atlases for the Expectation Maximization Classification. In: The Eighth IEEE Intl. Symp. on Biomedical Imaging: From Nano to Macro (ISBI), pp. 1839–1842 (2011)

[15] Rusu, M., Bloch, N., Jaffe, C.C., Rofsky, N.M., Genega, E.M., Feleppa, E., Lenkinski, R.E., Madabhushi, A.: Statistical 3D Prostate Imaging Atlas Construction via Anatomically Constrained Registration. In: SPIE on Medical Imaging: Image-Guided Procedures, Robotic Interventions, and Modeling, vol. 8669 (2013)

[16] Tamez-Peña, J., González, P., Farber, J., Baum, K., Schreyer, E., Totterman, S.: Atlas Based Method for the Automated Segmentation and Quantification of Knee Features: Data from the Osteoarthritis Initiative. In: The Eighth IEEE Intl. Symp. on Biomedical Imaging: From Nano to Macro (ISBI), pp. 1484–1487 (2011)

[17] Acosta, O., Simon, A., Monge, F., Commandeur, F., Bassirou, C., Cazoulat, G., de Crevoisier, R., Haigron, P.: Evaluation of Multi-atlas-based Segmentation of CT Scans in Prostate Cancer Radiotherapy. In: The Eighth IEEE Intl. Symp. on Biomedical Imaging: From Nano to Macro (ISBI), pp. 1966–1969 (2011)

[18] Chen, A., Niermann, K.J., Deeley, M.A., Dawant, B.M.: Evaluation of Multi Atlasbased Approaches for the Segmentation of the Thyroid Gland in IMRT Head and Neck CT Images. In: SPIE on Medical Imaging: Image-Guided Procedures, Robotic Interventions, and Modeling, vol. 7962, pp. 1–8 (2011)

Extended Edge-Weighted Centroidal Voronoi Tessellation for Image Segmentation

Kangkang Hu and Yongjie Jessica Zhang*

Department of Mechanical Engineering, Carnegie Mellon University,
Pittsburgh, PA, USA
{kangkanh,jessicaz}@andrew.cmu.edu

Abstract. In this paper, we extend the basic edge-weighted centroidal Voronoi tessellation model (EWCVT) for image segmentation to a new advanced model, namely fuzzy and harmonic EWCVT model. This extended model introduces a fuzzy and harmonic form of clustering energy by combining the image intensity with cluster boundary information. Compared with the classic CVT and EWCVT methods, the fuzzy and harmonic EWCVT algorithm can not only overcome the sensitivity to the initialization and noise, but also improve the accuracy of clustering results, as verified in several biomedical images.

Keywords: centroidal Voronoi tessellation, fuzzy and harmonic model, image segmentation.

1 Introduction

Image segmentation has been one of the core topics in computer vision and image processing for decades. Its central task is to partition an image into subsets which share similar characteristics, such as color, brightness and texture. Pixels in one region are similar to each other with respect to some characteristics and adjacent regions are significantly different from it. There have been many methods proposed for image segmentation in the literature [4, 13]. Thresholding [1, 16] is a very common approach used for segmentation where an image is represented as groups of pixels with values greater than or equal to the threshold and values less than the threshold. Clustering [3, 8, 11] is also an approach for region segmentation where an image is partitioned into the sets or clusters of pixels having similarity in feature space. The edge detection method [12, 15] partitions an image by finding the pixels on the region boundary. However, these methods usually do not consider the spatial details and may cause leakage of the boundary for images with low contrast and large variation of intensity. The level set method [10, 14, 17] is typically a partial differential equation based variational method, which represents the evolving contour using a signed function. Then, according to the motion equation of the contour, one can easily derive a similar flow for the implicit surface that when applied to the zero-level will reflect the propagation of the contour. Level-set models are topologically flexible,

---

* Corresponding author.

Y.J. Zhang and J.M.R.S. Tavares (Eds.): CompIMAGE 2014, LNCS 8641, pp. 164–175, 2014.

but quite expensive in both computational time and memory. The graph-based method [2, 7] is a highly efficient and effective approach for image segmentation by partitioning the image into a small number of homogeneous regions, but it is still difficult to accurately segment an image.

Centroidal Voronoi tessellation (CVT) has been introduced to many fields such as image processing, data analysis, computational geometry, sensor network, and numerical partial differential equations [5]. The CVT is a special Voronoi tessellation whose generators are also the centroids (mass centers) of the corresponding Vornoi regions. In its simplest form, CVT-based algorithms reduce to the k-means clustering method [9]. The edge-weighted centroidal Voronoi tessellation (EWCVT) [18–20] greatly improves the classic CVT model by adding an edge energy term in the energy functional, and has been proven to be very effective and efficient for image segmentation. However, both the classic CVT and EWCVT are sensitive to initializations and noise, which makes the segmentation results inaccurate and unstable.

In this paper, we develop a new advanced model by combining the harmonic and fuzzy algorithms with the EWCVT. Compared with the classic CVT and EWCVT methods, our new method has two main advantages: 1) our algorithm is more stable and less sensitive to the initialization by imposing a soft membership on the data points; and 2) it improves the segmentation accuracy since the spatial information of local image features is integrated into both the similarity measure and the membership function to compensate for the effect of noise.

The remainder of this paper is organized as follows: Section 2 reviews the classic CVT and the EWCVT models. Section 3 discusses the new Fuzzy and Harmonic EWCVT model. Section 4 shows some results, and Section 5 presents conclusions and future work.

2   Review of CVT and EWCVT for Segmentation

Given an image $I(h, w)$ of size $M \times N$, where (h, w) are integer pairs that range over the image domain, $h = 1, \ldots, M$ and $w = 1, \ldots, N$. Let the dataset $X = \left\{x_{P(i)}\right\}_{i=1}^{n}$ denote all the pixel values $x_{P(i)} = I(h, w)$ of the image, where $n = M \times N$ is the total number of pixels and $i = 1, \ldots, n$. $P(i)$ represents the i-th pixel in the physical space. Let $C = \{c_l\}_{l=1}^{L}$ denote a set of typical intensity values for a greyscale image. The Voronoi region V_k in X corresponding to the level c_k $(k = 1, \ldots, L)$ can be defined as

$$V_k = \left\{x_{P(i)} \in X : dist\left(x_{P(i)}, c_k\right) \leq dist\left(x_{P(i)}, c_l\right), for\ l = 1, \ldots, L\right\}, \quad (1)$$

where $dist\left(x_{P(i)}, c_k\right)$ is a predefined measure of distance between $x_{P(i)}$ and c_k. Note that here the differences between intensity values are compared instead of the physical distances between pixels. The set $V = \{V_l\}_{l=1}^{L}$ is called a *Voronoi tessellation* or *Voronoi clustering* of the data set X. The set of chosen values $C = \{c_l\}_{l=1}^{L}$ are referred as the *Voronoi generators*.

For the classic CVT [6], $dist\left(x_{P(i)}, c_k\right) = \left|x_{P(i)} - c_k\right|$ is the Euclidean distance in the color space. Given any set of values $C = \{c_l\}_{l=1}^{L}$ and any partition

$U = \{U_l\}_{l=1}^L$ of X, the classical *clustering energy* of $(C;U)$ can be defined as follows:

$$E(C;U) = \sum_{l=1}^L \sum_{x_{P(i)} \in U_l} \left|x_{P(i)} - c_l\right|^2. \tag{2}$$

Note that $U = \{U_l\}_{l=1}^L$ are not necessarily the Voronoi regions corresponding to the set of generators $C = \{c_l\}_{l=1}^L$ in the definition. The construction of CVTs often can be viewed as an energy minimization process. Given a partition of X, denoted by $U = \{U_l\}_{l=1}^L$, the *centroid* of each cluster U_l is defined to be the intensity $c^* \in U_l$ which minimizes an objective function:

$$\min_{c \in U_l} \sum_{x_{P(i)} \in U_l} \left|x_{P(i)} - c\right|^2. \tag{3}$$

The classical clustering energy $E(C;U)$ is minimized only if $(C;U)$ form a CVT of X, i.e., U are Voronoi regions of X associated with the generators C and simultaneously C are the corresponding centroids of the region U.

As a follow-up, EWCVT [18] was developed by adding an edge related energy term to the CVT energy function. The domain of an image $I(h,w)$ is an index set $D = \{P(i) : i = 1, \ldots, n\}$, where $P(i)$ represents the i-th pixel in the physical space. Suppose that we have determined the clusters $\{U_l\}_{l=1}^L$ for a given image represented in the color space by $x_{P(i)}$ for $P(i) \in D$, there is a natural segmentation of the image which has L segments $D = \{D_l\}_{l=1}^L$ in the physical space defined by

$$D_l = \left\{P(i) : x_{P(i)} \in U_l\right\}. \tag{4}$$

For each pixel $P(i) \in D$, denote a local neighborhood as $N_\omega(P(i))$, which can be a $\omega \times \omega$ square centered at pixel $P(i)$ or a disk centered at pixel $P(i)$ with radius ω. For EWCVT, $dist\left(x_{P(i)}, c_k\right) = \sqrt{\left|x_{P(i)} - c_k\right|^2 + 2\lambda\tilde{n}_k(P(i))}$, where $\tilde{n}_k(P(i)) = |N_\omega(P(i))| - n_k(P(i)) - 1$ is the number of pixels within $N_\omega(P(i)) \setminus (D_k \cup P(i))$. $|N_\omega(P(i))|$ represents the number of pixels within the set $N_\omega(P(i))$. $n_k(P(i))$ denotes the number of pixels within $D_k \cap N_\omega(P(i)) \setminus P(i)$. Note that this distance combines the color information together with the physical information of the pixel $P(i)$. Here we can view $dist\left(x_{P(i)}, c_k\right)$ as the edge-weighted distance in the color space between $x_{P(i)}$ and c_k.

For any set of values $C = \{c_l\}_{l=1}^L$ and any partition $U = \{U_l\}_{l=1}^L$ (corresponding partition $D = \{D_l\}_{l=1}^L$ in the physical space) of X, we can define the edge-weighted CVT energy as

$$E_{EWCVT}(C;U) = \sum_{l=1}^L \sum_{x_{P(i)} \in U_l} \left(\left|x_{P(i)} - c_l\right|^2 + 2\lambda\tilde{n}_l(P(i))\right). \tag{5}$$

For the EWCVT, the *centroid* of each cluster U_l is defined as the intensity $c^* \in U_l$ which minimizes the objective function (5). The edge-weighted clustering energy $E(C;U)$ is minimized only if $(C;U)$ form an edge-weighted CVT of X, i.e., U are edge-weighted Voronoi regions of X associated with the generators C and simultaneously C are the corresponding centroids of the region U. In its simplest form, CVT and EWCVT algorithms reduce to the k-means clustering technique. It is also clear that the EWCVT algorithm will reduce to the classic CVT-based algorithm when the weight $\lambda = 0$.

3   Fuzzy and Harmonic EWCVT

The classic CVT and EWCVT have one drawback: they are sensitive to the initializations and noise. To overcome these limitations, in this section we propose a new extended model by combining the harmonic and fuzzy algorithms with the EWCVT. First, the harmonic edge-weighted CVT (HEWCVT) model is discussed by introducing the harmonic average idea. The fuzzy and harmonic edge-weighted CVT (FHEWCVT) algorithm is then proposed by combining the fuzzy idea together with HEWCVT.

3.1   Harmonic EWCVT

For HEWCVT, the definition of Voronoi region and edge-weighted distance $dist\left(x_{P(i)}, c_k\right)$ is the same as EWCVT. The EWCVT energy function defined in Section 2 is slightly different from the algorithm proposed in [18]. Here, we define the edge-weighted distance first and use the edge-weighted distance to define the EWCVT energy function. For any set of intensity values $C = \{c_l\}_{l=1}^{L}$ and any partition $U = \{U_l\}_{l=1}^{L}$ of X, we define the harmonic edge-weighted CVT energy by introducing the harmonic idea into the EWCVT method:

$$E_H\left(C; U\right) = \sum_{i=1}^{n}\left(L \bigg/ \sum_{l=1}^{L}\frac{1}{\left|x_{P(i)} - c_l\right|^2 + 2\lambda\tilde{n}_l(P(i))}\right). \qquad (6)$$

To calculate the centroids $\{c_k^*\}_{k=1}^{L}$, we minimize the HEWCVT energy function with respect to the centroid c_k $(k = 1,\ldots, L)$. Since $\tilde{n}(P(i))$ at each pixel $P(i)$ is fixed, we can obtain an iterative formula as follows:

$$c_k^* = \frac{\displaystyle\sum_{i=1}^{n} u_{ik}^{H} x_{P(i)}}{\displaystyle\sum_{i=1}^{n} u_{ik}^{H}}, \qquad (7)$$

where $u_{ik}^{H} = \left(\sum_{l=1}^{L}\frac{dist^2\left(x_{P(i)}, c_k\right)}{dist^2\left(x_{P(i)}, c_l\right)}\right)^{-2}$. Similarly, we can calculate all centroids $\{c_l^*\}_{l=1}^{L}$. For an arbitrary Voronoi tessellation $\left(\{c_l\}_{l=1}^{L}; \{V_l\}_{l=1}^{L}\right)$ of X where $V = \{V_l\}_{l=1}^{L}$ are the corresponding Voronoi regions associated with $C = \{c_l\}_{l=1}^{L}$, we often have $c_l \neq c_l^*$, for $l = 1,\ldots, L$, where $\{c_l^*\}_{l=1}^{L}$ are the corresponding centroids of $\{V_l\}_{l=1}^{L}$.

3.2 Fuzzy and Harmonic EWCVT

The fuzzy Voronoi region V_k in X corresponding to the level c_k $(k = 1, \ldots, L)$ can be defined as

$$V_k = \{x_{P(i)} \in X : prob\left(x_{P(i)}, c_k\right) \geq prob\left(x_{P(i)}, c_l\right), for \ l = 1, \ldots, L\}, \quad (8)$$

where $prob\left(x_{P(i)}, c_k\right)$ is a predefined measure which represents the degree of possibility of $P(i)$ to the kth cluster. The set $V = \{V_l\}_{l=1}^{L}$ is called a *fuzzy Voronoi tessellation* or *fuzzy Voronoi clustering* of the data set X. The set of chosen values $C = \{c_l\}_{l=1}^{L}$ are referred as the *fuzzy Voronoi generators*. The fuzzy edge-weighted distance D_{il} between $x_{P(i)}$ and c_l can be defined as

$$D_{il} = \mu_{il}^{\alpha}\left|x_{P(i)} - c_l\right|^2 + \lambda\mu_{il} \sum_{j \in N_w(P(i))} (1 - \mu_{jl}) + \lambda\left(1 - \mu_{il}\right) \sum_{j \in N_w(P(i))\backslash P(i)} \mu_{jl}, \quad (9)$$

where μ_{il} is the membership function which represents the degree of possibility of $P(i)$ to the lth cluster, and α is the fuzziness exponent. There are mainly two constraints for the membership matrix,

$$\begin{cases} \sum_{l=1}^{L} \mu_{il} = 1, \ \forall P(i) \in D, \\ 0 < \mu_{il} < 1, \ l = 1, \ldots, L. \end{cases} \quad (10)$$

For any set of intensity values $C = \{c_l\}_{l=1}^{L}$ and any partition $U = \{U_l\}_{l=1}^{L}$ of X, we define the fuzzy harmonic edge-weighted CVT energy as follows:

$$E_{FH}(C; U) = \sum_{i=1}^{n} L \bigg/ \sum_{l=1}^{L} \frac{1}{D_{il}}. \quad (11)$$

Here, we introduce a Lagrange multiplier ξ and define a new energy function named the Lagrange function,

$$\Lambda(\mu_{i1}, \ldots, \mu_{i1}, \xi) = \sum_{i=1}^{n} L \bigg/ \sum_{l=1}^{L} \frac{1}{D_{il}} + \xi(\sum_{l=1}^{L} \mu_{il} - 1). \quad (12)$$

We minimize the Lagrange function with respect to $\{\mu_{ik}^*\}_{k=1}^{L}$ and ξ, and then obtain a system of $L + 1$ equations for pixel $P(i)$ as

$$\begin{cases} \dfrac{L\left(\frac{1}{D_{ik}^2}\right)}{\left(\sum_{l=1}^{L} \frac{1}{D_{il}}\right)^2} \left(\alpha\mu_{ik}^{\alpha-1}\left|x_{P(i)} - c_k\right|^2 + \lambda \sum_{j \in N_w(P(i))} (1 - 2\mu_{jk})\right) + \xi = 0, \\ \sum_{k=1}^{L} \mu_{ik} = 1. \end{cases} \quad (13)$$

When $\alpha = 2$, the above system is linear, otherwise it becomes nonlinear. The Newton-Raphson method can be adopted to solve the above system to find its roots $\{\mu_{ik}^*\}_{k=1}^{L}$ and ξ.

To calculate the centroids $\{c_k^*\}_{k=1}^{L}$, we minimize the FHEWCVT energy function with respect to the centroid c_k $(k = 1, \ldots, L)$. We can get an iterative formula as follows:

$$c_k^* = \frac{\sum_{i=1}^{n} u_{ik}^{FH} \mu_{ik}^{\alpha} x_{P(i)}}{\sum_{i=1}^{n} u_{ik}^{FH} \mu_{ik}^{\alpha}}, \tag{14}$$

where $u_{ik}^{FH} = \left(\sum_{l=1}^{L} \frac{D_{ik}}{D_{il}}\right)^{-2}$. Similarly, we can calculate all centroids $\{c_l^*\}_{l=1}^{L}$. For an arbitrary fuzzy edge-weighted Voronoi tessellation $\left(\{c_l\}_{l=1}^{L}; \{V_l\}_{l=1}^{L}\right)$ of X where $V = \{V_l\}_{l=1}^{L}$ are the corresponding fuzzy edge-weighted Voronoi regions associated with $C = \{c_l\}_{l=1}^{L}$, we often have $c_l \neq c_l^*$, for $l = 1, \ldots, L$, where $\{c_l^*\}_{l=1}^{L}$ are the corresponding centroids of $\{V_l\}_{l=1}^{L}$. If $c_l = c_l^*$, for $l = 1, \ldots, L$, then we call the Voronoi tessellation $\{V_l\}_{l=1}^{L}$ a *fuzzy harmonic edge-weighted centroidal Voronoi Tessellation* of X. Similar to [18], we have the following theorem.

Theorem 1. *For an arbitrary Voronoi tessellation $\left(\{c_l\}_{l=1}^{L}; \{U_l\}_{l=1}^{L}\right)$ of X where $U = \{U_l\}_{l=1}^{L}$ are not necessarily the corresponding Voronoi regions associated with $C = \{c_l\}_{l=1}^{L}$. The fuzzy harmonic edge-weighted clustering energy $E(C; U)$ is minimized only if $(C; U)$ form a fuzzy harmonic edge-weighted CVT of X, i.e., U are fuzzy Voronoi regions of X associated with the generators C and simultaneously C are the corresponding fuzzy centroids of the region U.*

The construction of HEWCVT and FHEWCVT is an energy minimization process, where generators are updated by minimizing the corresponding objective functions. The detailed implementation is explained as follows.

Algorithms of HEWCVT and FHEWCVT (Implementation)

Given a positive integer L and digital image $X = \left\{x_{P(i)}\right\}_{i=1}^{n}$, choose arbitrary L intensity values $\{c_l\}_{l=1}^{L}$. The initialization of $\{c_l\}_{l=1}^{L}$ is completed by randomly picking L pixels in the images and using the corresponding intensity values as $\{c_l\}_{l=1}^{L}$. Then perform the following:

1. Determine the fuzzy edge-weighted Voronoi clusters $\{V_l\}_{l=1}^{L}$ of X associated with $\{c_l\}_{l=1}^{L}$;
2. If HEWCVT,

   For each cluster V_l $(l = 1, \ldots, L)$, determine the cluster means c_l^* by (7);

   Else if FHEWCVT,

   For all pixels, solve (13) to determine $\{\mu_{il}\}_{l=1}^{L}$ and take them as the new membership functions, and calculate $\{c_l^*\}_{l=1}^{L}$ using (14) and take them as the new generators;
3. If c_l^* and c_l are the same, return $(\{c_l\}_{l=1}^{L}; \{V_l\}_{l=1}^{L})$ and exit; otherwise, set $w_l = c_l^*$ for $l = 1, \ldots, L$ and return to Step 1.

4   Results and Discussion

To evaluate the performance of the proposed algorithm, we apply it to various synthetic and real images that are either clear of noise or corrupted by different types of noises. Table 1 shows the statistics information of all the testing examples. Fig. 1 shows segmentation results of a noisy two-class synthetic image with two clusters, here we choose two different density values (120 and 20) for initialization. Compared to CVT and EWCVT, it is obvious that HEWCVT and FHEWCVT are more accurate. The FHEWCVT method performs the best, it segments the image very accurately.

Table 1. Image segmentation statistics of the testing models

Image (Size)	Number of clusters	λ	α	Method	Time (s)			
Two-class (256 × 256)	2	0.5	1.2	Classic CVT	0.5			
				EWCVT	2.0			
				HEWCVT	4.0			
				FHEWCVT	7.0			
					Test 1	Test 2	Test 3	Test 4
Brain (192 × 192)	4	0.15	1.2	EWCVT	6.4	6.5	6.2	6.5
				HEWCVT	11.2	11.7	11.0	11.8
				FHEWCVT	26.1	27.4	26.4	27.2
Heart (453 × 451)	5	0.01	1.2	EWCVT	13.2	13.5	13.6	13.5
				HEWCVT	27.2	27.6	27.0	27.5
				FHEWCVT	46.2	47.1	46.6	47.0

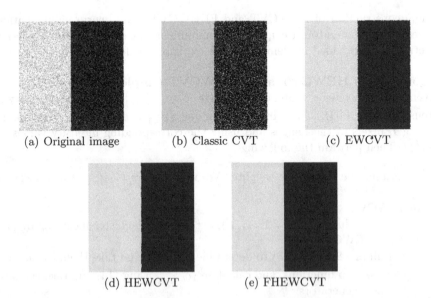

(a) Original image   (b) Classic CVT   (c) EWCVT

(d) HEWCVT   (e) FHEWCVT

Fig. 1. Segmentation results of a two-class synthetic image. (a) Original image; (b) classic CVT; (c) EWCVT; (d) HEWCVT; and (e) FHEWCVT.

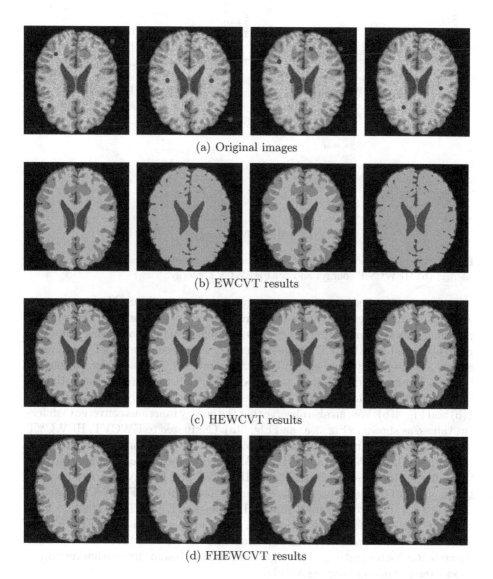

(a) Original images

(b) EWCVT results

(c) HEWCVT results

(d) FHEWCVT results

Fig. 2. Segmentation results of a noisy brain image. (a) Original images with 4 different initializations (each initialization has 4 input generators marked as red dots); four segmented results using EWCVT (b), HEWCVT (c) and FHEWCVT (d).

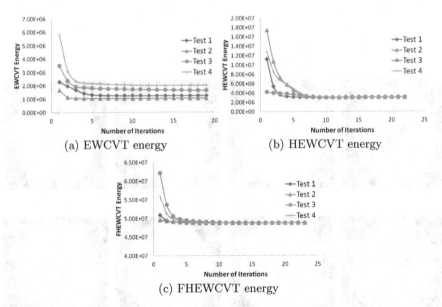

Fig. 3. Energy plots of the segmentation results for the noisy brain image. (a) EWCVT energy; (b) HEWCVT energy; and (c) FHEWCVT energy.

Figs. 2-3 and 4-5 show segmentation results of a noisy brain MRI image with four clusters and a heart CT image with five clusters respectively. For the same input image, we segment it four times with different initializations using EWCVT, HEWCVT and FHEWCVT. From the results, we can see that CVT based algorithms are essentially an energy minimization process. For each test, the energy function is minimized until it is converged. EWCVT is sensitive to the initialization. With different initializations, the results can be obviously different, see Fig. 2(b) and Fig. 4(b). We can also observe that the energy functions converge to different values, as shown in Fig. 3(a) and Fig. 5(a). Compared to EWCVT, HEWCVT and FHEWCVT are more stable and insensitive to initializations. For different initializations, the HEWCVT and FHEWCVT energy functions can always converge to similar optimal results. In addition, HEWCVT and FHEWCVT can improve the accuracy of the segmentation by capturing more features. FHEWCVT usually needs less iterations to converge to optimal results than EWCVT and HEWCVT, as shown in Fig. 3(c) and Fig. 5(c). However, it should be noted that the FHEWCVT algorithm usually consumes more time than other algorithms due to the expensive Newton-Raphson iterations. This algorithm also needs some human interaction to choose the parameters such as λ and α.

Discussion 1. Unlike EWCVT, HEWCVT uses a different form of the energy function to calculate the centroids. It uses information from all of the centers to calculate the harmonic average for each point. Due to the property of the harmonic mean, HEWCVT usually yields a better performance than EWCVT. EWCVT imposes hard membership on the data points: each data point is assigned to exactly one center. This means that each data point only has an influence over the center to

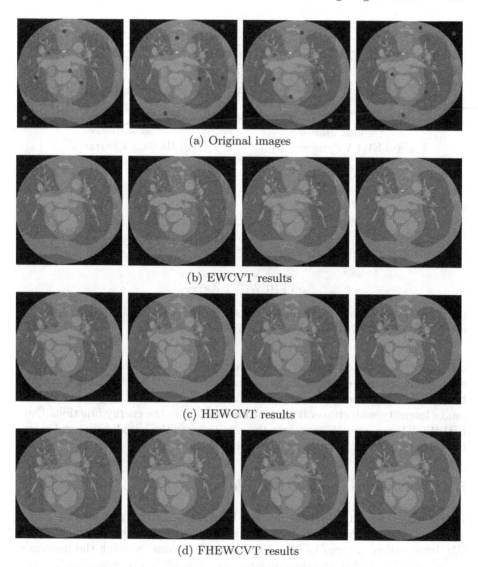

(a) Original images

(b) EWCVT results

(c) HEWCVT results

(d) FHEWCVT results

Fig. 4. Segmentation results of a heart image. (a) Original images with 4 different initializations (each initialization has 5 input generators marked as red dots); four segmented results using EWCVT (b), HEWCVT (c) and FHEWCVT (d).

which it is assigned. HEWCVT differs in that, for each data point, the objective function uses the distances to all centroids. This means that all centroids partially influence the harmonic average for each point. Thus HEWCVT is less sensitive to the initialization, especially when the number of clusters is large.

Discussion 2. FHEWCVT is a method of clustering which allows one piece of data belong to two or more clusters. It works by assigning membership to

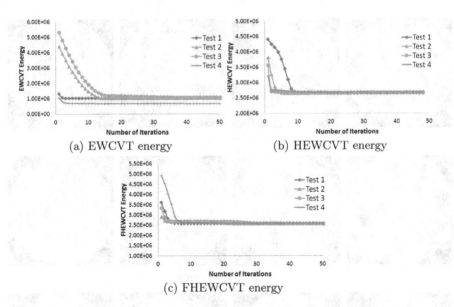

(a) EWCVT energy   (b) HEWCVT energy

(c) FHEWCVT energy

Fig. 5. Energy plots of the segmentation results for the heart image. (a) EWCVT energy; (b) HEWCVT energy; and (c) FHEWCVT energy.

each data point corresponding to each cluster. It is less affected by the presence of uncertainty or noise in the data since it has a soft membership function. FHEWCVT introduces the fuzzy and harmonic idea by combining the image intensity with cluster boundary information in the energy function. Thus FHEWCVT can not only overcome the sensitivity to the initialization and noise, but also improve the accuracy of clustering results.

5   Conclusions and Future Work

In this paper, we extend the traditional EWCVT algorithm and develop a new advanced model by combining the harmonic and fuzzy algorithms with EWCVT. We define different forms of objective energy functions by using the harmonic average and fuzzy idea, and then update generators of the corresponding Voronoi tessellations by minimizing the objective functions. Experiments indicate that the FHEWCVT algorithm can not only overcome the sensitivity to the initialization and noise but also improve the accuracy of clustering results. In the future we will apply our algorithm to more datasets and extend to 3D images.

References

1. Arifin, A.Z., Asano, A.: Image segmentation by histogram thresholding using hierarchical cluster analysis. Pattern Recognition Letters 27(13), 1515–1521 (2006)
2. Boykov, Y., Funka-Lea, G.: Graph cuts and efficient ND image segmentation. International Journal of Computer Vision 70(2), 109–131 (2006)

3. Cai, W., Chen, S., Zhang, D.: Fast and robust fuzzy c-means clustering algorithms incorporating local information for image segmentation. Pattern Recognition 40(3), 825–838 (2007)
4. Chan, T.F., Vese, L.A.: Active contour and segmentation models using geometric PDE's for medical imaging. In: Geometric Methods in Bio-medical Image Processing, pp. 63–75. Springer (2002)
5. Du, Q., Faber, V., Gunzburger, M.: Centroidal Voronoi tessellations: applications and algorithms. SIAM Review 41(4), 637–676 (1999)
6. Du, Q., Gunzburger, M., Ju, L., Wang, X.: Centroidal Voronoi tessellation algorithms for image compression, segmentation, and multichannel restoration. Journal of Mathematical Imaging and Vision 24(2), 177–194 (2006)
7. Felzenszwalb, P.F., Huttenlocher, D.P.: Efficient graph-based image segmentation. International Journal of Computer Vision 59(2), 167–181 (2004)
8. Hartigan, J.A., Wong, M.A.: Algorithm AS 136: a k-means clustering algorithm. Applied Statistics 28(1), 100–108 (1979)
9. Kanungo, T., Mount, D.M., Netanyahu, N.S., Piatko, C.D., Silverman, R., Wu, A.Y.: An efficient k-means clustering algorithm: analysis and implementation. IEEE Transactions on Pattern Analysis and Machine Intelligence 24(7), 881–892 (2002)
10. Li, C., Xu, C., Gui, C., Fox, M.D.: Distance regularized level set evolution and its application to image segmentation. IEEE Transactions on Image Processing 19(12), 3243–3254 (2010)
11. Li, Q., Mitianoudis, N., Stathaki, T.: Spatial kernel k-harmonic means clustering for multi-spectral image segmentation. IET Image Processing 1(2), 156–167 (2007)
12. Ma, W.Y., Manjunath, B.S.: Edgeflow: a technique for boundary detection and image segmentation. IEEE Transactions on Image Processing 9(8), 1375–1388 (2000)
13. Pal, N.R., Pal, S.K.: A review on image segmentation techniques. Pattern Recognition 26(9), 1277–1294 (1993)
14. Paragios, N., Deriche, R.: Geodesic active regions and level set methods for supervised texture segmentation. International Journal of Computer Vision 46(3), 223–247 (2002)
15. Senthilkumaran, N., Rajesh, R.: Edge detection techniques for image segmentation- a survey of soft computing approaches. International Journal of Recent Trends in Engineering 1(2), 250–254 (2009)
16. Tobias, O.J., Seara, R.: Image segmentation by histogram thresholding using fuzzy sets. IEEE Transactions on Image Processing 11(12), 1457–1465 (2002)
17. Vese, L.A., Chan, T.F.: A multiphase level set framework for image segmentation using the Mumford and Shah model. International Journal of Computer Vision 50(3), 271–293 (2002)
18. Wang, J., Ju, L., Wang, X.: An edge-weighted centroidal Voronoi tessellation model for image segmentation. IEEE Transactions on Image Processing 18(8), 1844–1858 (2009)
19. Wang, J., Ju, L., Wang, X.: Image segmentation using local variation and edge-weighted centroidal Voronoi tessellations. IEEE Transactions on Image Processing 20(11), 3242–3256 (2011)
20. Wang, J., Wang, X.: VCells: simple and efficient superpixels using edge-weighted centroidal Voronoi tessellations. IEEE Transactions on Pattern Analysis and Machine Intelligence 34(6), 1241–1247 (2012)

Knapsack Intersection Graphs and Efficient Computation of Their Maximal Cliques

Valentin E. Brimkov

Mathematics Department, SUNY Buffalo State College, Buffalo, NY 14222, USA
brimkove@buffalostate.edu

Abstract. As an image can easily be modeled by its adjacency graph, graph theory and algorithms on graphs are widely used in imaging sciences. In this paper we define a knapsack graph, which is an intersection graph of integer translates of knapsack polygons, and consider the maximal clique problem on such graphs. A major application of intersection graphs is found in visualization of relations among objects in a scene. Efficient algorithms for the maximal clique problem are applicable to problems of computer graphics and image analysis, while properties of the knapsack polygon have been used in obtaining theoretical results in discrete geometry for computer imagery. We first show that the maximal clique problem on knapsack graphs is equivalent to the maximal clique problem on intersection graphs of homothetic right triangles. The latter was shown to be equivalent to the maximal clique problem on max-tolerance graphs and solvable in optimal $O(n^3)$ time [28]. Thus, if the linear constraints defining the knapsack polygons are known, then the maximal clique problem on knapsack graphs can be solved using the algorithm from [28]. If the polygons are given by lists of their vertices and the defining constraints are unknown, we show how these can be found efficiently in computation time bounded by a low degree polynomial in the polygons size.

Keywords: Intersection graph, Max-tolerance graph, Knapsack graph, Maximal/maximum clique, Clique number.

1 Introduction

Graph theory and algorithms on graphs are widely used in image processing, as an image can easily be modeled by its adjacency graph [27]. The present paper is concerned with a class of intersection graphs. Given a family of sets S, its *intersection graph* is a graph with a vertex set labeled by the elements of S, in which $s_1, s_2 \in S$ are joined by an edge if and only if $s_1 \cap s_2 \neq \emptyset$. For pioneering contributions see the papers by Szpilrajn-Marczewski [40], Čulík [11], and Erdős, Goodman, and Pósa [14]. For various structural results the reader is referred to [32] and for related algorithmic issues to [19].

Intersection graphs appear applicable to numerous research domains, in particular computer imagery. A major application is found in representation and visualization of relations among objects in a scene. This includes data visualization for the purposes of software engineering [17], drawing Euler diagrams [38],

Y.J. Zhang and J.M.R.S. Tavares (Eds.): CompIMAGE 2014, LNCS 8641, pp. 176–187, 2014.
© Springer International Publishing Switzerland 2014

visualization of overlapping clusters on graphs [39], video database queries [43]; in graph-based recognition and visualization of grid patterns in street networks [21, 41], solid intersection [33, 34], and contingency tables [42]. Moreover, intersection graph-based discrete models of continuous n-dimensional spaces have been developed to solve problems of surface graphics [15].

Although any graph is an intersection graph of a certain family of sets [40], various classes of intersection graphs possess properties that are not featured by general graphs. For instance, some classical NP-hard problems, such as clique number, independence number, or chromatic number computation, are solvable in polynomial time on intersection graphs of specific families of sets. Algorithms for these kinds of problems are applicable to computer graphics and image analysis. Thus, maximal clique computation has been applied to image segmentation [24] and to deformable object model learning in image analysis [44]. For other applications in image processing see [36]. Maximal clique computation on certain intersection graphs is also relevant to problems of computer vision [3] and computer graphics [35], as well as to visualization in natural sciences [18].

Extensively studied are the cases of different classes of convex sets, in particular convex polygons (see, e.g., [2, 7–9, 16, 23, 25, 26, 28–31] for a number of samples). In the present paper we are concerned with the problem of finding the maximal cliques in an intersection graph of a set of convex polygons of a special type. For arbitrary convex polygons the maximal clique problem is known to be NP-hard [29]. Under certain essential restrictions (e.g., for the cases of rectilinear rectangles or homothetic triangles) the problem can be solved in polynomial time. Thus, it was recently shown that all maximal cliques in an intersection graph of a set of isosceles right triangles (called semi-squares) can be found in $O(n^3)$ time [28]. This is optimal, as the authors show that such an intersection graph can have $\Omega(n^3)$ maximal cliques.

Motivation for the results of [28] is seen in the equivalence of semi-square graphs with the well-known max-tolerance graphs [20]. The latter can be used to model certain biological problems related to comparison of DNA sequences. As we will see, the knapsack graphs studied in this paper are equivalent to the semi-square graphs and in turn to the max-tolerance graphs.

In the present paper we attempt to address the following questions:

- Are there other classes of intersection graphs that are equivalent to the semi-square and max-tolerance graphs?

- Are there any specific classes of convex polygons for whose intersection graphs the maximal cliques (and in turn, the chromatic number) can be found in polynomial time, provided that the polygons are non-homothetic and their sides are parallel to a non-constant number of directions?

To this end, we study intersection graphs of integer translates of knapsack polygons with parallel knapsack constraints, and show that on these graphs the maximal clique problem is equivalent to the one on semi-square (and thus on max-tolerance) graphs. Considering intersection graphs of integer polygons gives the paper a certain number-theoretic flavor that is uncommon for intersection graph theory. A specific motivation for studying knapsack graphs is seen in the fact that knapsack polytopes are lattice (or "digital") polytopes with special (in a sense, extreme) properties, which have been used for obtaining theoretical results in discrete geometry for computer imagery (see, for example, [6, 10, 12]).

Note that the polygons of the considered class may have an unbounded number of vertices [37] and are non-homothetic, in general (see Figure 1). Nevertheless, it follows that the max-clique problem on such graphs is equivalent to the one on semi-square graphs and thus can be solved in polynomial time.

The paper is organized as follows. In the rest of the present section we introduce some notions and notations to be used in the sequel. In Section 2 we first define knapsack graphs and then we demonstrate the equivalence of maximal clique problem on homothetic triangle graphs and knapsack graphs. In Section 3 we consider the non-trivial case where the polygons are given by their vertices and the knapsack constraints are not available. We conclude with some final remarks on future work and possible applications in Section 4.

1.1   Some Notions and Notations

A *clique* of an undirected simple graph G is a complete subgraph of G. A clique is *maximal* if it is not a proper subgraph of another clique, and *maximum* if no other clique of G has a greater number of vertices. The cardinality of a maximum clique is the graph *clique number*.

Given a set A, by $|A|$ we denote its cardinality and by $conv(A)$ its convex hull. $A \times B$ denotes their Cartesian product of sets A and B. Given two points x and y in the plane, by $\overline{xy}$ we denote the segment with endpoints x and y, by $|xy|$ the length of that segment, and by $\vec{xy}$ the vector with initial point x and terminal point y. By $\mathbf{u} + A$ we denote the translation of a set A by a vector $\mathbf{u} \in \mathbb{R}^2$.

A *supporting line* for a convex polygon P is a straight line l passing through a vertex of P so that the interior of P lies entirely on one side of l.

2   Knapsack Graphs

2.1   Defining Knapsack Graphs

In what follows we consider intersection graphs of families of sets that are integer translates of knapsack polygons. A knapsack polygon is defined as follows:

$$K(a,b,c) = conv(A), \quad A = \{(x,y) \in \mathbb{Z}^2 : ax + by \leq c, x, y \geq 0, a, b, c \in \mathbb{Z}_+\} \quad (1)$$

See Figure 1 for illustration.

In what follows, w.l.o.g. we will assume that $a \leq b \leq c$. Clearly, knapsack polygons are integer (i.e., their vertices have integer coordinates).

Now consider a family $\mathcal{F} = \{K_i := K(a, b, c_i), i = 1, 2, \ldots, n\}$ of n knapsack polygons having the same coefficients a and b and variable c's. (We will call the defining constraints $ax + by \leq c_i$ *parallel*, for short.) Consider a set $S(\mathcal{F}) = \{P_i, i = 1, 2, \ldots, n\}$ of arbitrary translates of these polygons by integer vectors,

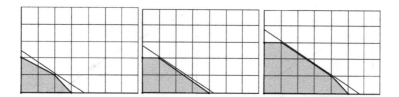

Fig. 1. Non-homothetic knapsack polygons determined by parallel linear constraints. The horizontal and vertical line segments depict the integer grid. In this and all the following figures a gray area represents a knapsack polygon and an uppermost slanted line segment represents a knapsack linear constraint defining the knapsack polygon.

i.e., $P_i = \mathbf{t_i} + K_i$ where $\mathbf{t_i} \in \mathbb{Z}^2$. Thus the polygons of $S(\mathcal{F})$ are integer. We are interested in the cliques of the intersection graph of $S(\mathcal{F})$, which will be referred to as a *knapsack graph*.

2.2 Equivalence of Maximal Clique Problem for Homothetic Triangle and Knapsack Graphs

Let $P \in S(\mathcal{F})$, i.e., $P = \mathbf{t} + K$ where $K = K(a, b, c) \in \mathcal{F}$. We define and denote the three extreme vertices of P as follows: $v^0 = \mathbf{t} + \mathbf{0}$, where $\mathbf{0} = (0, 0)$ is the zero-vector; $v^x = \mathbf{t} + (\lfloor c/a \rfloor, 0)$; $v^y = \mathbf{t} + (0, \lfloor c/b \rfloor)$.

The $\mathbf{t}$-translate of the triangle which determines $K(a, b, c)$ is $\triangle_P = \triangle v^0 q^x q^y$, where $q^x = \mathbf{t} + (c/a, 0)$ and $q^y = \mathbf{t} + (0, c/b)$.

We have the following fact.

Proposition 1. *For $P_1, P_2 \in S(\mathcal{F})$, $P_1 \cap P_2 \neq \emptyset$ if and only if $\triangle_{P_1} \cap \triangle_{P_2} \neq \emptyset$.*

Proof. Since $P_1 \subseteq \triangle_{P_1}$ and $P_2 \subseteq \triangle_{P_2}$, $P_1 \cap P_2 \neq \emptyset$ implies $\triangle_{P_1} \cap \triangle_{P_2} \neq \emptyset$.

Now let $\triangle_{P_1} \cap \triangle_{P_2} \neq \emptyset$. If $v_2^0 \in \triangle_{P_1}$, then by the definition of knapsack polygon, $v_2^0 \in P_1$ and $v_2^0 \in P_1 \cap P_2$. Otherwise, $P_2 \cap (\triangle_{P_1} \setminus P_1) \neq \emptyset$, which is possible only if the vertical leg L_1, or the horizontal leg L_2 of P_2, or both, intersect $\triangle_{P_1} \setminus P_1$. But the straight lines containing L_1 and L_2 are of the form $y = k_1$ and $x = k_2$, respectively, where k_1 and k_2 are integers. Hence, L_1 or L_2 intersect respectively the horizontal leg or the vertical leg of $\triangle_{P_1}$ at an integer point which is common for P_1 and P_2, and thus $P_1 \cap P_2 \neq \emptyset$. $\square$

Proposition 1 implies the equivalence of the maximal/maximum clique problem defined on the intersection graph of a set of homothetic right triangles and of a set of integer translates of knapsack polygons. As already mentioned, for the former the number of the maximal cliques does not exceed n^3 and these can be found in $O(n^3)$ time [28].[1] This is optimal since it matches a lower bound $\Omega(n^3)$ for the number of maximal cliques. Thus we have:

---

[1] Although in [28] the authors consider, for the sake of simplicity, isosceles right triangles (called semi-squares), their approach and results apply to arbitrary homothetic triangles.

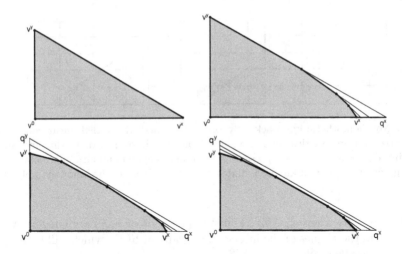

Fig. 2. Illustration to the different cases of supporting constraints

Corollary 1. *A knapsack graph can contain $\Theta(n^3)$ maximal cliques.*

If the knapsack polygons are given implicitly by the coefficients of the knapsack constraints, one can use the algorithm for triangles from [28] to find all maximal/maximum cliques in $O(n^3)$ time. In the next section we consider the less trivial case where the knapsack polygons are given by their vertices and the linear constraints defining them are unknown.

3   The Max Clique Problem for Knapsack Graphs When the Knapsack Constraints Are Unknown

Let the polygons $P_1, P_2, \ldots, P_n$ from $S(\mathcal{F})$ be given by lists of their vertices. Having the vertices of P_i $(1 \leq i \leq n)$, we also have the vertices of the corresponding knapsack polygon K_i. We want to find linear constraints $ax + by \leq c_i$, $i = 1, 2, \ldots, n$, which define the corresponding knapsack polygons from $\mathcal{F}$. The procedure for finding a, b and c_i relies on a series of observations and constructions. We start with a plain fact.

Fact 1. *The linear constraints $ax + by \leq c_i$ defining K_i for $i = 1, 2, \ldots, n$ can be chosen such that each line $ax + by = c_i$ is supporting to K_i.*

Thus we restrict ourselves to looking for constraints with that property. Given a knapsack polygon K, a supporting constraint can pass only through vertices with a special status. We distinguish between the following cases:

1. $K = \triangle_K$; then the polygon K has only three vertices: $v^0 = \mathbf{0}, v^x$, and v^y (Figure 2, top-left).

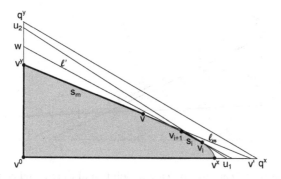

Fig. 3. Illustration to the proof of Fact 3

2. Let $s_1, s_2, \ldots, s_m$ be the sides of K different than $\overline{v^0 v^x}$ and $\overline{v^0 v^y}$. Side s_1 is incident with vertex v^x and side s_m is incident with vertex v^y. Let $l_1, l_2, \ldots, l_m$ be the respective straight lines containing these sides.

   2a. All these lines either intersect the segment $\overline{v^x q^x}$ or intersect the segment $\overline{v^y q^y}$ (Figure 2, top-right).

   2b. There is $k \in \mathbb{Z}_+$, such that the lines $l_1, \ldots, l_k$ intersect the segment $\overline{v^x q^x}$ and the lines $l_{k+1}, \ldots, l_m$ intersect the segment $\overline{v^y q^y}$ (Figure 2, bottom).

The following facts follow easily.

Fact 2. *In the framework of Case 1, a supporting line defining K can pass only through the points v^x or v^y.*

Fact 3. *In the framework of Case 2a, w.l.o.g. let all lines $l_1, l_2, \ldots, l_m$ intersect the segment $\overline{v^x q^x}$. Let $s_m = \overline{v v^y}$. Then all supporting lines defining K pass either through v or through v^y. See Figure 3.*

Proof. Clearly, l_m is a supporting line to K that defines K. Let $v' = l_m \cap \overline{v^x q^x}$. Assume that a supporting line l goes through a vertex v_i different from v and v^y. It intersects $\overline{v^x q^x}$ and $\overline{v^y q^y}$ at points u_1 and u_2, respectively, which are internal for these segments. Consider the side of K with endpoints s_i and s_{i+1} (as, possibly, $s_{i+1} = v$). Let l' be the line containing s_i. Since l intersects $\overline{v^y q^y}$, l' intersects it too, at a point w that is between v^y and u_2.

With these constructions, we obviously have $|wv_{i+1}| > |v^y v|$. We also have $|v^y v| > |vv'|$, otherwise v would not be a vertex of K. However, $|v_i v_{i+1}| < |vv'|$. Hence, $|v_i v_{i+1}| < |wv_{i+1}|$. Then v_{i+1} cannot be a vertex of K since the point $v_{i+1} + 2\overrightarrow{v_i v_{i+1}}$ would be a non-negative integer point under line l. Thus we are left with the possibility that all supporting lines that define K pass through v^x or v. □

Arguments analogous to those of the proof of Fact 3 imply Fact 4 below.

Fact 4. *In the framework of Case 2b, either none of the lines $l_1, \ldots, l_m$ intersect both $\overline{v^x q^x}$ and $\overline{v^y q^y}$ (Figure 2, bottom-left) or otherwise exactly one of the lines*

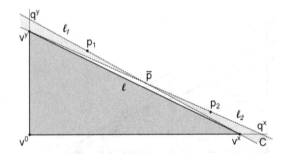

Fig. 4. Illustration to the concepts of leaning points and the related cone of supporting lines

l_k or l_{k+1} — say, l_k — *can intersect these two segments (Figure 2, bottom-right). In the former case, all supporting lines defining K pass through a vertex v which is the common endpoit of the segments s_k and s_{k+1}. In the latter case, all supporting lines defining K pass through one or both endpoints of segment s_k.*

Given a knapsack polygon K, we call *special* the vertex/vertices at which K admits a supporting defining line.

Next we are interested in determination of the set of all supporting lines that define a given knapsack polygon. All cases can be handled in an analogous manner, therefore we consider in more detail the simplest Case 1 with the help of Figure 4.

As we already discussed, all supporting lines defining K pass through the points v^x or v^y. Specifically, the lines through v^x form a doubly infinite cone with apex v^x. One of its border lines is line l through v^x and v^y. The other one is a line l_1 through v^x and an integer point p_1 in the first quadrant which is above the segment $\overline{v^x v^y}$ and is first met if one rotates l in clockwise direction about point v^x. Likewise, the lines through v^y form another cone with apex v^y and bordered by line l and a line l_2 defined by a closest integer point p_2 met by l upon counter-clockwise rotation about point p^y. We call p_1 and p_2 *leaning points* for polygon K. Clearly, all line directions contained in both cones are the lines of the cone C with apex $\bar{p} = l_1 \cap l_2$ and bounded by the lines l_1 and l_2.[2] See Figure 4.

Next we explain how the leaning points of a knapsack polygon can be found. First we formulate two subsidiary lemmas.

Lemma 1. *Let $\triangle ABC$ be a right triangle with rational vertices and with legs $\overline{AB}$ and $\overline{AC}$ parallel to the x- and y- axes, respectively. Let $l : ax + by = c$ be the straight line containing the hypotenuse $\overline{BC}$. W.l.o.g. assume that $A = \mathbf{0}$ and $a, b, c \in \mathbb{Z}_+$. Let p be an integer point that is met first when l is rotated clockwise*

---

[2] The lines l_1 and l_2 determine two supplementary cones; the one of interest does not contain K.

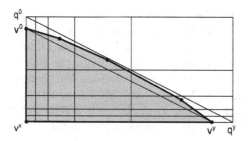

Fig. 5. Illustration to the construction used in the proof of Lemma 2

about point C. Then p is a vertex of the polygon $P = K(a, b, c - 1) = conv(M)$, where $M = \{(x, y) \in \mathbb{Z}^2 : ax + by < c,\ x, y \geq 0,\ a, b, c \in \mathbb{Z}_+\}$.

Proof. Let l' be a line supporting to P. Then l passes through a vertex q of P. Assuming that q does not possess the required property, there would be an integer point p which is strictly below l and strictly above l', which contradicts the definition of K as a convex hull of all integer points below l. $\square$

Lemma 2. *A point p defined as in Lemma 1 can be found in $O\left(\log \frac{c}{a} \log c\right)$ time.*

Remark 1. By Lemma 1, p is a vertex of the knapsack polygon $K(a, b, c - 1)$. Thus, to identify p it suffices to find the vertices of $K(a, b, c-1)$ and then to check which of them satisfies the required property. For this we will use a technique from [5] (initially presented in [4]) based on the approach from [22].

Proof of Lemma 2. We first briefly recall the construction from [5] restricted to two-dimensional knapsack polygons. Consider the sequences of rational numbers $\{x^1_j\}^\infty_{j=0}$ and $\{x^2_j\}^\infty_{j=0}$ where $x^1_0 = c/a$, $x^1_j = 2^{-j}c/a$ and $x^2_0 = c/b$, $x^2_j = 2^{-j}c/b$ for $j = 1, 2, \ldots$. For each of the two sequences determine integers P_1 with $0 < x^1_{P_1} \leq 1$, $x^1_{P_1-1} \geq 1$ and P_2 with $0 < x^2_{P_2} \leq 1$, $x^2_{P_2-1} \geq 1$. With the assumption $a \leq b$, we have $P_k \leq \log \frac{2c}{a}$.

Now consider the set of boxes $B_{k_1 k_2} = I_{k_1} \times I_{k_2}$, where $1 \leq k_1 \leq P_1$, $1 \leq k_2 \leq P_2$ and $I_{k_1} = [x_{k_1-1}, x_{k_1})$ and $I_{k_2} = [x_{k_2-1}, x_{k_2})$. See Figure 5. The overall number of boxes is bounded by $(\log \frac{2c}{a})^2$. Moreover, it was shown that each of them contains no more than one vertex of $K(a, b, c)$. In addition, all vertices satisfy the inequality $\bar{a}x + \bar{b}y \geq \bar{c}$ where $\bar{a} = \lfloor c/b \rfloor$, $\bar{b} = \lfloor c/a \rfloor$, and $\bar{c} = \bar{a}\bar{b}$. Then it follows that there are no more than $\log \frac{c}{a}$ boxes that can contain vertices of $K(a, b, c)$, and these boxes can easily be identified in $O\left(\log \frac{c}{a}\right)$ time. Moreover, if a box B contains a vertex, the latter is a solution to the integer linear program

$$\max ax + by, \quad \text{where} \quad ax + by \leq c,\ (x, y) \in B.$$

The above is a two-dimensional integer linear program with a fixed number of linear constraints. Such can be solved in linear time, that is, with $O(\log c)$ arithmetic operations [13]. Thus the computation of the $O\left(\log \frac{c}{a}\right)$ integer points that can be vertices of $K(a, b, c)$ takes $O\left(\log \frac{c}{a} \log c\right)$ time overall.

After having recalled the construction and the result from [5], it is easy to realize how the point p can be found. First we compute the set $\mathcal{P}$ of all integer points that are possible vertices of $K(a, b, c-1)$ in $O\left(\log \frac{c}{a} \log c\right)$ time. Then for each such point p_i we take the line through the points C and p_i. Having $O\left(\log \frac{c}{a}\right)$ points w, we have $O\left(\log \frac{c}{a}\right)$ such lines. We then choose the one which makes the largest angle with the x-axes. By construction, it is defined by the points C and $p \in \mathcal{P}$. By Lemma 1, the latter is a vertex of $K(a, b, c-1)$ and is the desired point satisfying the lemma's requirements. □

Using the algorithm of Lemma 2, we can find the leaning points of a knapsack polygon K. For example, in Case 1, the lemma is applied to the right triangle $\triangle v^x u v^y$ where $u = (v_1^x, v_2^y)$, and in Case 2a (ref. Figure 3) – to $\triangle v u v^y$ where $u = (v_1, v_2^y)$ (Case 2b being similar).

This completes the description of the computation of a cone of supporting lines associated with a knapsack polygon.

What remains to be explained is how to determine the coefficients a and b of the linear constraints defining $K_1, K_2, \ldots, K_n$ (and respectively, $P_1, P_2, \ldots, P_n$). Let $C_1, C_2, \ldots, C_n$ be the cones associated with the polygons $K_1, K_2, \ldots, K_n$ and $C_1^0, C_2^0, \ldots, C_n^0$ their translated copies so that the apex of each of them is at the origin. Clearly, all cones are contained in the 2nd and 4th quadrants. Every cone C_i^0 is defined by a pair of border lines g_i^1 and g_i^2 that intersect at the origin. Line g_i^1 is the one which is below line g_i^2 in the 4th quadrant. Next we sort the slopes of g_i^1 and then those of g_i^2 for $i = 1, 2, \ldots, n$, which takes $O(n \log n)$ time. Thus we find the two most internal lines g_1^* and g_2^* over the families g_i^1 and g_i^2. This gives us a cone C^* that is the intersection of all cones C_i^0, $i = 1, 2, \ldots, n$. It is easy to see that by construction the bit-size of g_1^* and g_2^* is polynomially bounded by the size of the problem input.

What we need last is a line from C^* that is internal for the cone and with coefficients that are polynomially bounded by the coefficients of g_1^* and g_2^*. Such can easily be found in different ways. For example, let $a_1 x + b_1 y = 0$ and $a_2 x + b_2 y = 0$ be the two border lines of C^*. Take points $r = (1, -a_1/b_1) \in g_1^*$ and $s = (1, -a_2/b_2) \in g_2^*$. The midpoint M of the segment $\overline{rs}$ belongs to the interior of C^*, so the line $h : ax + by = 0$ with $a = a_1 b_2 + a_2 b_1$, $b = 2a_1 a_2$ through the origin and M is internal for C^*.

By the construction of line h, it follows that every knapsack polygon K_i (and, respectively, the corresponding polygon P_i) admits a defining line $ax + by = c_i$ going through its special point(s), and the overall time complexity of finding these lines amounts to $O\left(n \log \bar{c} \log c + n \log n\right)$, where $\bar{c} = \max_{i=1}^n c_i/a_i$ and $c = \max_{i=1}^n c_i$. In sum, we can formulate the following theorem.

Theorem 1. *Let $P_1, P_2, \ldots, P_n$ be polygons that are integer translates of n knapsack polygons, as each polygon is given by a list of its vertices. One can compute linear constraints $ax + by \leq c_i$ defining knapsack polygons whose translates are $P_1, P_2, \ldots, P_n$. This can be accomplished with $O(n \log \bar{c} \log c + n \log n)$ arithmetic operations, where $\bar{c} = \max_{i=1}^n c_i/a_i$ and $c = \max_{i=1}^n c_i$. The maximal cliques of the intersection graph for the given polygons can be found in $O\left(n \log \bar{c} \log c + n^3\right)$ time.*

After finding all maximal cliques of a knapsack graph, one can easily identify the maximum ones as well as the clique number in $O(n^3)$ time.

4 Concluding Remarks

In this paper we defined knapsack graphs and considered the maximal clique problem on such graphs. We demonstrated its equivalence to the previously studied semi-square graphs and max-tolerance graphs, provided that the linear constraints defining the given polygons are known. For the case where they are unknown, we proposed an efficient algorithm for their computation. Improving its time-complexity is considered as a challenging future task. The presented results can be extended to more general polygons, possibly in higher dimensions. This can be another research direction. Work in progress is aimed at applying the presented results for identification of clusters of objects in a scene.

Proposition 1 demonstrated the equivalence of knapsack graphs and intersection graphs of homothetic triangles. As mentioned in the Introduction, the latter were proved to be equivalent to max-tolerance graphs [28]. In this last paper the authors explain in detail how the problem of finding the maximal cliques of a max-tolerance graph models the problem of identifying the maximal clusters of portions of DNA sequences obtained as a result of a query to a software tool like BLAST [1]. Thus the equivalence of knapsack and max-tolerance graphs makes the results of this paper potentially applicable to certain problems of computational biology, such as cluster analysis of biosequences.

Acknowledgements. The author thanks the two anonymous referees for their useful remarks and suggestions.

References

1. Altschul, W., Gish, W., Miller, W., Myers, E.W., Lipman, D.J.: Basic local alignment search tool. J. Mol. Biol. 215, 403–410 (1990),
   http://www.ncbi.nlm.nih.gov/BLAST/
2. Ambühl, C., Wagner, U.: The clique problem in intersection graphs of ellipses and triangles. Theory Comput. Syst. 38, 279–292 (2005)
3. Ballard, D.H., Brown, M.: Computer Vision. Prentice-Hall, Englewood Cliffs, N.J (1982)
4. Brimkov, V.E.: Vertices of the Knapsack Polytope. MS Thesis, University of Sofia (1984)
5. Brimkov, V.E.: A quasi-polynomial algorithm for the knapsack problem. Yugoslav J. Operations Research 4, 149–157 (1994)
6. Brimkov, V.E., Barneva, R.P.: On the polyhedral complexity of the integer points in a hyperball. Theoretical Computer Science 406, 24–30 (2008)
7. Brimkov, V.E., Kafer, S., Szczepankiewicz, M., Terhaar, J.: Maximal cliques in intersection graphs of quasi-homothetic trapezoids. In: Proc. MCURCSM 2013, Ohio, p. 10 (2013)

8. Brimkov, V.E., Kafer, S., Szczepankiewicz, M., Terhaar, J.: On intersection graphs of convex polygons. In: Barneva, R.P., Brimkov, V.E., Šlapal, J. (eds.) IWCIA 2014. LNCS, vol. 8466, pp. 25–36. Springer, Heidelberg (2014)
9. Cabello, S., Cardinal, J., Langerman, S.: The clique problem in ray intersection graphs. In: Epstein, L., Ferragina, P. (eds.) ESA 2012. LNCS, vol. 7501, pp. 241–252. Springer, Heidelberg (2012)
10. Coeurjolly, D., Brimkov, V.E.: Computational aspects of digital plane and hyperplane recognition. In: Reulke, R., Eckardt, U., Flach, B., Knauer, U., Polthier, K. (eds.) IWCIA 2006. LNCS, vol. 4040, pp. 291–306. Springer, Heidelberg (2006)
11. Čulík, K.: Applications of graph theory to mathematical logic and linguistics. In: Proc. Sympos. "Theory of Graphs and its Applications", Smolenice, 1963, pp. 13–20. Publ. House Czechoslovak Acad. Sci., Prague (1964)
12. de Vieilleville, F., Lachaud, J.-O., Feschet, F.: Maximal digital straight segments and convergence of discrete geometric estimators. In: Kalviainen, H., Parkkinen, J., Kaarna, A. (eds.) SCIA 2005. LNCS, vol. 3540, pp. 988–997. Springer, Heidelberg (2005)
13. Eisenbrand, F., Laue, S.: A faster algorithm for two-variable integer programming. In: Ibaraki, T., Katoh, N., Ono, H. (eds.) ISAAC 2003. LNCS, vol. 2906, pp. 290–299. Springer, Heidelberg (2003)
14. Erdős, P., Goodman, A.W., Pósa, L.: The representation of a graph by set intersections. Canad. J. Math. 18, 106–112 (1966)
15. Evako, A.V.: Topological properties of the intersection graph of covers of n-dimensional surfaces. Discrete Mathematics 147, 107–120 (1995)
16. Felsner, S., Müller, R., Wernisch, L.: Trapezoid graphs and generalizations, geometry and algorithms. Discrete Applied Mathematics 74, 13–32 (1993)
17. Fish, A., Stapleton, G.: Formal issues in languages based on closed curves. In: Proc. Distributed Multimedia Systems, pp. 161–167 (2006)
18. Gardiner, E.J.: Artymiuk, P.J., Willett, P.: Clique-detection algorithms for matching three-dimensional molecular structures. J. Molecular Graph Modelling 15(4), 245–253 (1997)
19. Golumbic, M.: Algorithmic Graph Theory and Perfect Graphs. Acad. Press (1980)
20. Golumbic, M., Trenk, A.: Tolerance graphs. Cambridge Studies in Advanced Mathematics, vol. 89. Cambidge University Press (2005)
21. Heinzle, F., Ander, K.H., Sester, M.: Graph based approaches for recognition of patterns and implicit information in road networks. In: Proc. 22nd International Cartographic Conference, A Coruna (2005)
22. Haies, A.C., Larman, D.S.: The vertices of the knapsack polytope. Discr. Appl. Math. 6, 135–138 (1983)
23. Imai, H., Asano, T.: Finding the connected components and a maximum clique of an intersection graph of rectangles in the plane. Journal of Algorithms 4, 300–323 (1983)
24. Ion, A., Carreira, J., Sminchisescu, C.: Image segmentation by figure-ground composition into maximal cliques. In: Proc. 13th International Conference on Computer Vision, Barcelona, pp. 2110–2117 (2011)
25. Jacobson, M.S., Morris, F.R., Scheinermann, E.R.: General results on tolerance intersection graphs. J. Graph Theory 15, 573–577 (1991)
26. Junosza-Szaniawski, K., Kratochvíl, J., Pergel, M., Rzążewski, P.: Beyond Homothetic Polygons: Recognition and Maximum Clique. In: Chao, K.-M., Hsu, T.-s., Lee, D.-T. (eds.) ISAAC 2012. LNCS, vol. 7676, pp. 619–628. Springer, Heidelberg (2012)

27. Klette, R., Rosenfeld, A.: Digital Geometry. Geometric Methods for Digital Picture Analysis. Morgan Kaufmann, San Francisco (2004)

28. Kaufmann, M., Kratochvíl, J., Lehmann, K., Subramanian, A.: Max-tolerance graphs as intersection graphs: cliques, cycles, and recognition. In: Proc. SODA 2006, pp. 832–841 (2006)

29. Kratochvíl, J.: Kuběna, A.: On intersection representations of co-planar graphs. Discrete Mathematics 178, 251–255 (1998)

30. Kratochvíl, J., Nešetřil, J.: Independent set and clique problems in intersection-defined classes of graphs. Comm. Math. Uni. Car. 31, 85–93 (1990)

31. Kratochvíl, J., Pergel, M.: Intersection graphs of homothetic polygons. Electronic Notes in Discr. Math. 31, 277–280 (2008)

32. McKee, T.A., McMorris, F.R.: Topics in Intersection Graph Theory. In: SIAM Monographs on Discrete Mathematics and Applications 2. SIAM, Philadelphia (1999)

33. Nakamura, H., Higashi, M., Hosaka, M.: Robust computation of intersection graph between two solids. Computer Graphics Forum 16, C79–C88 (1997)

34. Nakamura, H., Masatake, H., Mamoru, H.: Robust computation of intersection graph between two solids. Graphical Models 16(3), C79–C88 (1997)

35. Nandy, S.C., Bhattacharya, B.B.: A unified algorithm for finding maximum and minimum object enclosing rectangles and cuboids. Computers Math. Applic. 29(8), 45–61 (1995)

36. Paget, R., Longsta, D.: Extracting the cliques from a neighbourhood System. IEE Proc. Vision Image and Signal Processing 144(3), 168–170 (1997)

37. Rubin, D.S.: On the unlimited number of faces in integer hulls of linear programs with a single constraint. Operations Research 18, 940–946 (1970)

38. Simonetto, P., Auber, D.: An heuristic for the construction of intersection graphs. In: 13th International Conference on Information Visualisation, pp. 673–678 (2009)

39. Simonetto, P., Auber, D.: Visualise undrawable Euler diagrams. In: Proc. 12th IEEE International Conference on Information Visualisation, pp. 594–599 (2008)

40. Szpilrajn-Marczewski, E.: Sur deux proprisétés des classes d'ensembles. Fund. Math. 33, 303–307 (1945)

41. Tian, J., Tinghua, A., Xiaobin, J.: Graph based recognition of grid pattern in street networks. In: The International Archives of the Photogrammetry, Remote Sensing and Spatial Information Sciences, Advances in Spatial Data Handling and GIS. Lecture Notes in Geoinformation and Cartography, vol. 38, Part II, pp. 129–143 (2012)

42. Vairinhos, V.M., Lobo, V., Galindo, M.P.: Intersection graph-based representation of contingency tables, http://www.isegi.unl.pt/docentes/vlobo/ Publicacoes/3_17_lobo08_DAIG_conting_tables.pdf

43. Verroust, A., Viaud, M.-L.: Ensuring the drawability of extended euler diagrams for up to 8 sets. In: Blackwell, A.F., Marriott, K., Shimojima, A. (eds.) Diagrams 2004. LNCS (LNAI), vol. 2980, pp. 128–141. Springer, Heidelberg (2004)

44. Wang, X., Bai, X., Yang, X., Wenyu, L., Latecki, L.J.: Maximal cliques that satisfy hard constraints with application to deformable object model learning. Advances in Neural Information Processing Systems 24, 864–872 (2011)

Characterization of a Novel Imaging-Based Metric of Patellofemoral Separation Using Computational Modeling

Prahlad G. Menon[1,2,3,*] and Jacobus H. Muller[4,*]

[1] Sun Yat-Sen University - Carnegie Mellon University (SYSU-CMU)
Joint Institute of Engineering, Pittsburgh, PA, USA
[2] SYSU-CMU, Shunde International Joint Research Institute, Guangdong, China
[3] QuantMD, LLC, Pittsburgh, PA, USA
pgmenon@andrew.cmu.edu
[4] Biomedical Engineering Research Group,
Department of Mechanical and Mechatronic Engineering,
Stellenbosch University, Stellenbosch, South Africa
cobusmul@sun.ac.za

Abstract. We introduce patellofemoral separation (PFS) as a novel metric to quantify patella-trochlear proximity as a function of dynamic knee flexion. PFS is quantified in 4D (i.e. 3D+time) using accurate segmentation from pre-operative imaging data acquired in three discrete, quasi-static knee postures, up to the maximum bending limit (i.e. 40° of flexion), within the constraints of a standard computed tomography (CT) or magnetic resonance imaging (MRI) scanner. Additionally, in this study, in order to examine patient-specific patella postures over a full range from 0 to 90° of dynamic knee flexion and extension, we utilize a computational model to simulate dynamic patella kinematics beyond 40° of bending. The computational model was optimized to reproduce patella postures as determined from the imaging data. A method of shape-based interpolation of the acquired 3D components (i.e. bone and cartilage) of the knee was applied in order to recreate a continuous range of motion of the patella and femur during knee bending from 0° to 40° using imaging data and 0° to 90° from simulated data. Next, a regional Hausdorff distance mapping paradigm was applied to compare the separation of the 3D surfaces defined by the patella and femoral cartilage segmentations from the interpolated imaging-based and simulated knee postures, at 1°increments. This separation distance was termed as PFS and examined as a posture-varying color map on the patella cartilage surface. The mean PFS was computed as the mean HD of separation between patella and femoral cartilage, at each posture over the entire studied range of motion. Mean PFS was observed to decrease with increased knee flexion, evidencing increased proximity of the patella and femur and increased risk of contact. In order to automatically quantify signs of patellofemoral instability from pathological knee kinematics reconstructed using medical imaging, the limits of PFS defining the thresholds of pain will require to be determined by benchmarking the metric against patients with normal knee-function. The PFS metric may also find potential application as a biomarker for the identification of high localized patellofemoral pressure by predicting patellofemoral impingement.

---

[*] Joint first authors.

Y.J. Zhang and J.M.R.S. Tavares (Eds.): CompIMAGE 2014, LNCS 8641, pp. 188–203, 2014.
© Springer International Publishing Switzerland 2014

Keywords: Patellofemoral Separation, Biomarker, Computational Biomechanics of the Knee, Shape Interpolation, Procrustes Analysis, Iterative Closest Point based Registration and Interpolation.

1   Introduction

Efficient treatment strategies for injured knees rely on a fundamental understanding of the anatomy and biomechanical function of the knee [1]. To this end, there have been developments in the analysis of images of the knee to quantify anatomical shape and variability [2], derive kinematic relationships [3], and develop orthopedic solutions in terms of surgical tools and implants as well as surgical navigation [4]. These analyses is facilitated through segmentation and registration methods which are applied to scan data from a combination of imaging modalities, including Computed Tomography (CT), Magnetic Resonance Imaging (MRI), radiography and fluoroscopy.

It has been established that patellofemoral biomechanics is a function of the trochlea-patella shape, the active loading from the extensor mechanism, and the passive support from the peri-patellar ligamentous tissues [5]. Patellofemoral shape can potentially be quantified as a function of the anatomical geometry or patellofemoral pathology through image processing and analysis techniques which investigate the role of articular geometry in patellofemoral biomechanics.

Statistical shape modeling (SSM) has been used to visualize and classify the patellofemoral joint [2, 4, 6]. Zhu and Li [4] demonstrated the use of SSM to predict three dimensional (3D) patellofemoral shape from two dimensional (2D) images of a joint. Van Haver *et al.* [2] showed through an analysis on 20 normal and 20 dysplastic knees that SSM can potentially be used to classify patellofemoral dysplasia since it provides a method which factors in the full geometrical complexity of the trochlea. A distance map between a mean normal femur (mean of the 20 normal femurs) and a mean dysplastic femur (mean of the 20 abnormal femurs) illustrated the differences between the normal and abnormal femur and allowed for the identification of differences of specific geometrical features. Fitzpatrick *et al.* [6] utilized SSM to quantify variation between 15 femurs and patellae. A finite element model with which contact mechanics and articulation can be predicted was utilized with the SSM shape data to generate a statistical shape-function model with which the influence of changes in shape on patellofemoral mechanics could be quantified.

Investigations into patellofemoral shape have mainly focused on the trochlea, whereas few studies also include the patella. Fitzpatrick *et al.* [6] considered the patella in terms of contact and kinematics, whereas Borotikar *et al.* [3] considered the patella in terms of its *in*-vivo kinematics as depicted from MRI sequences. Baldwin *et al.* [7] utilized a verified computational model for tibiofemoral kinematics to predict patella kinematics and contact area. To our knowledge, there are no published results in which the spatial relationship between the patella and trochlea as a function of active knee flexion is quantified.

Further, *in-vivo* measurement and quantification of the intricate balance between the articular geometry, soft tissue stabilization and patellofemoral biomechanics remains challenging and to the author's knowledge, a robust methodology for the same has not yet been demonstrated. Baldwin *et al.* [7] showed that validated computational models are efficient tools for investigation into this problem. Some studies have illustrated the use of imaging techniques to quantify patellofemoral kinematics as a function of active knee flexion, but quantification of the accompanying soft tissue and contact kinetics are lacking [8]. The overarching goal of this study is to help in identifying a bridge between the patellofemoral kinematics and kinetics (i.e. patellofemoral biomechanics) and the articular geometry through a continuum shape analysis based on a novel shape-based patellofemoral distance-mapping paradigm.

This study presents a methodology with which the continuum patella-trochlea shape relationship can be quantified as a function of dynamic knee flexion through a novel patellofemoral separation (PFS) metric. As starting data to examine patient-specific patella postures over the full range from 0 to 90° of dynamic knee flexion and extension, we utilize a realistic computational model to simulate dynamic patella kinematics and then validate the results against the known quasi-static patella postures at discrete knee flexion angles reconstructed from *in-vivo* medical imaging data available for a range of 0 to 45° of knee bending (in extension and flexion). The computational model output then drives a novel shape-based distance mapping paradigm through which the patellofemoral joint can be characterized in terms of the separation between the patella and femoral cartilage structures through our PFS metric.

The methods followed in this study have been organized into sections which begin with a detailed delineation of our strategy to formulate a realistic computational model that simulates dynamic and active knee flexion. Next, we detail the strategy through which the predicted patellofemoral posture was validated against the known quasi-static patella postures at discrete knee flexion angles, and finally, our novel shape based distance mapping paradigm to express the patella kinematics in terms of the trochlear geometry and knee bending using the PFS metric is described.

2   Materials and Methods

2.1   Imaging

A CT scan (Siemens Emotion 16; 130 kV; Table 1) from the iliac spine down to the feet (knee in full extension), and a MRI scan (Siemens Symphony; 1.5 Tesla; Table 2) of the knee (at 16 degrees knee flexion), were obtained for one volunteer (male, 45 years old, 165 cm tall, 82 kg). An additional MRI scan was obtained while the volunteer maintained an isometric leg contraction at 40 degrees knee flexion. The femur, patella, tibia, and fibula were segmented from the CT scan.

The femoral, tibial and patella cartilage as well as the medial and lateral meniscus were segmented from the MRI scans. Registration techniques were used to co-register the osseous geometry segmented from CT images to the cartilage and menisci segmented from MRI data. This registration of the 3-D CT segmentations to the 3-D models in each MRI scan ensured point correspondence between the meshes of the 3D models in each of the three quasi-static knee bending postures. This paved the way to employ Procrustes analysis on this data (see section 2.3), since the registration of the 3-D CT segmentations to the 3-D models in each MRI scan inherently ensured point-correspondence between surface geometries at each posture. All processing (segmentation and registration) was performed in Mimics Innovation suite and 3-matic 6.0 (Materialise NV, Leuven, Belgium).

Table 1. CT scan settings

Parameter		Value
Acquisition		16 x 0.06 mm
Rotation time		1 sec
Pitch		1.5 mm
Slice		5 mm
Reconstruction Parameters	Slice	1 mm
	Recon increment	0.7 mm
	Field of view	250 mm
	Kernel/filter	B10s smooth

Table 2. MRI scan settings

Parameter		Value
Scan time		9.49 s
Contrast		TR 40, TE 24
Flip angle		8 degrees
Resolution	Field of view	200 mm
	Slice thickness	1.5 mm
	Base resolution	512
	Filter	Elliptical
Geometry	Single slab	
	Distance factor	50
	Slices per slab	72
Sequence	3-D	
	Bandwidth	132 Hz/Px

2.2   Computational Modeling

The computational model was formulated in a multibody simulation platform – ADAMS 2013.1 (MSC Software Corporation, Newport Beach, California, USA) which embodies an adapted formulation of the models in the Multibody Models of the Human Knee depository[1], from the Simtk database[2]. Similarities between the model presented in this study and the build in depository models are:

- The ligament model that is used.
- Soft tissue properties, including the stiffness and damping coefficients of the spring-damper units that represent the quadriceps and patella tendon, the medial and lateral collateral ligament, posterior and anterior cruciate ligament material and mechanical properties, and the meniscal-tibial ligaments stiffness profiles.
- The flexion force applied to the tibia to induce knee flexion.
- Ttibiofemoral compression force implemented through tibial mechanical axis.
- The tibiofemoral contact model and contact model parameters.
- The patellofemoral contact model and contact model parameters.

Modifications made to the build in models were:

- Our CT-segmented osseous models and MRI-segmented menisci (medial and lateral) replaced the osseous in the depository models.
- The Medial patellofemoral ligament and lateral patellofemoral ligament were included as peri-patellar stabilizers.

Osseous and Meniscal Model
The computational model included rigid 3D models of the distal femoral head, the proximal tibial and fibial head, the patella and medial and lateral menisci. The cartilage layers on the patella, femur and tibia were derived from the segmentation on the MRI obtained

---

[1]   https://simtk.org/home/mb_knee, 24/03/2014.
[2]   https://simtk.org/xml/index.xml, 24/03/2014.

at 16 degrees knee flexion. The medial and lateral menisci were each modeled as a subset of discrete elements which are connected by six-by-six stiffness matrices [9].

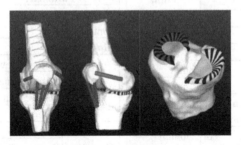

Fig. 1. Computational model with discretized menisci and medial and lateral patellofemoral ligaments. Red cylinders and blue spirals depict the quadriceps and patella tendon, respectively.

An in-house Matlab script (Matlab R2012a, Mathworks Inc., Natick, Massachusetts, USA) was developed to enable the division of the medial and lateral menisci into 34 equally-spaced discrete elements along the circumference (see Fig. 1). Parameters of the six-by-six stiffness matrices (see Equation 1) with which the discrete elements are connected were derived from [9] (see Table 3). Here, F_θ, F_r, F_z and T_θ, T_r, T_z represent the translational and torsional force components, and $K_\theta, K_r, K_z, Z_\theta, Z_r, Z_z$ represent the stiffness parameters in polar coordinates.

$$\begin{bmatrix} F_\theta \\ F_r \\ F_z \\ T_\theta \\ T_r \\ T_z \end{bmatrix} = \begin{bmatrix} K_\theta & K_{\theta r} & K_{\theta z} & 0 & 0 & 0 \\ K_{\theta r} & K_r & K_{rz} & 0 & 0 & 0 \\ K_{\theta z} & K_{\theta z} & K_z & 0 & 0 & 0 \\ 0 & 0 & 0 & Z_\theta & 0 & 0 \\ 0 & 0 & 0 & 0 & Z_r & 0 \\ 0 & 0 & 0 & 0 & 0 & Z_z \end{bmatrix} \begin{bmatrix} \theta \\ r \\ z \\ a \\ b \\ c \end{bmatrix} \quad (1)$$

Table 3. Meniscal stiffness matrix parameters

Parameter	Medial meniscus	Lateral meniscus
K_θ	320 [N/mm]	360 [N/mm]
$K_{\theta r}$	82.5 [N/mm]	22.5 [N/mm]
$K_{\theta z}$	82.5 [N/mm]	27.5 [N/mm]
K_r	270 [N/mm]	294 [N/mm]
K_{rz}	25 [N/mm]	75.5 [N/mm]
K_z	330 [N/mm]	330 [N/mm]
Z_θ	25 [N.mm/rad]	67.5 [N.mm/rad]
Z_r	25 [N.mm/rad]	27.5 [N.mm/rad]
Z_z	22.5 [N.mm/rad]	22.5 [N.mm/rad]

Soft Tissue Modeling

The quadriceps and patella tendons were modeled as idealized tension-only parallel spring-damper elements. The damping constant for the quadriceps was set to zero, whereas the patella tendon had a damping constant of 1 N.s/mm. The stiffness value for the quadriceps tendon was, $k_{QT} = 33$ N/mm, and the value for the patella tendon (three elements) was, $k_{PT} = 158$ N/mm [9, 10]. The meniscal ligaments were modeled as tension-only parallel spring-damper elements [9, 10], with the transverse ligament stiffness equal to 200 N/mm with a damping coefficient of 0.5 N.s/mm. The meniscal horn attachment ligament stiffness was set to 1000 N/mm and 0.5 N.s/mm damping.

The collateral ligaments (medial and lateral) and cruciate ligaments (anterior and posterior) were modeled on principles presented in the literature [11, 12]. The implementation was based on a script from the Multibody Models of the Human Knee depository[3] [9, 10]. The ligament tension (F_{lig}) was a function of the ligament stiffness (k), the current ligament length (l_{curr}), the zero-load length (l_0) and a non-linear strain level parameter ($\varepsilon_l = 0.03$; [11]). Blankevoort et al. [11] described the force-length relationship as shown in Equation 2:

$$F_{lig} = \begin{cases} \frac{1k\varepsilon^2}{4\varepsilon_l}; & 0 \leq \varepsilon \leq 2\varepsilon_l \\ k(\varepsilon - \varepsilon_l); & \varepsilon < 2\varepsilon_l \\ 0; & \varepsilon < 0 \end{cases} \tag{2}$$

where, $\varepsilon = \frac{l_{curr} - l_0}{l_0}$ is the ligament strain parameter. This was modified (Equation 3) by adding an error catch term associated with a damping coefficient ($c_r = 0.5$) [9, 10]:

$$F_{lig} = \begin{cases} \frac{1k\varepsilon^2}{4\varepsilon_l} - c_r v_{curr}; & 0 \leq \varepsilon \leq 2\varepsilon_l \\ k(\varepsilon - \varepsilon_l) - c_r v_{curr}; & \varepsilon < 2\varepsilon_l \\ -c_r v_{curr}; & \varepsilon < 0 \end{cases} \tag{3}$$

where, $v_{curr} = \frac{d}{dt} l_{curr}$ is the velocity of ligament lengthening.

The medial and lateral patellofemoral ligaments were simulated by discrete flexible links (with 15 elements) which were enabled to conform to the imaging-based osseous geometry, allowing for better simulation of the physiological loading directions of the patellofemoral ligaments. Material properties of Young's modulus, ($E = 19.1$ MPa), Density ($\rho = 1300$ kg/m^3) and Poisson ratio ($\upsilon = 0.4$) were based on models in the CES EduPack (CES EduPack 2013 V12.2.13, Granta Design Ltd). Attachment sites of ligaments and tendons were adjudged based on prior literature [13-15].

Contact Modeling
The tibiofemoral, tibio-meniscal, femoral-meniscal and patellofemoral interfaces were defined through a compliant contact (F_{cont}) algorithm [9, 16], in Equation 4:

$$F_{cont} = k_c \delta_{int}{}^{exp} + C_c \dot{\delta}_{int} \tag{4}$$

In Equation 4, k_c, C_c, and exp are contact parameters, and δ_{int} and $\dot{\delta}_{int}$ are respectively the amount of overlap and the speed of overlap between the interfacing bodies. Contact parameters for cartilage on cartilage were: contact stiffness $k_c = 500\,N/mm$, damping coefficient $C_c = 5\,N.s/mm$, and the elasticity exponent $exp = 1.5$;

---

[3] https://simtk.org/home/mb_knee, 24/03/2014.

and contact parameters for cartilage to meniscus contact were: contact stiffness $k_c = 19\,N/mm$, damping coefficient $C_c = 0.1\,N.s/mm$, and the elasticity exponent $exp = 3.37$. These values have been validated through a FEA solution set [9, 16].

Patella Posture Optimization

Three landmarks were defined on the patella with which its posture (position and orientation) could be quantified. These were located at the centroid of the patella (P_1), on the medial pole (P_2) and the distal pole (P_3). The points P_i are not collinear, and therefore enable patella rotation and translation to be accounted for by the optimization metric. Global linear traction paths (position vs. flexion angle) were derived for each landmark (D_1, D_2 and D_3) using the three imaging based postures at 2^0, 16^0 and 40^0 knee flexion. The traction paths were calculated as a displacement from the reference point (position at 2^0 knee flexion) in a Cartesian frame of reference (Equation 5):

$$
\begin{aligned}
D_1 &= f\left(P_{1,16°} - P_{1,2°}, P_{1,40°} - P_{1,2°}\right)_{XYZ} \\
D_2 &= f\left(P_{2,16°} - P_{2,2°}, P_{2,40°} - P_{2,2°}\right)_{XYZ} \\
D_3 &= f\left(P_{3,16°} - P_{3,2°}, P_{3,40°} - P_{3,2°}\right)_{XYZ}
\end{aligned}
\tag{5}
$$

The design variables for the optimization procedure were the soft tissue elements' initial strain. This included the medial and lateral patellofemoral ligaments, the patella tendon and quadriceps tendon. The objective was to minimize the difference between the computed patella traction and the traction paths defined in Equation 5. The following objective function was formulated (Equation 6):

$$
\min_{OBJ} = OBJ = \frac{\sum_i^n \sqrt{(D_{1,comp}-D_1)^2{}_i+(D_{2,comp}-D_2)^2{}_i+(D_{3,comp}-D_3)^2{}_i}}{n}
\tag{6}
$$

where, $D_{\#,comp}$ signifies the calculated position of the patella using the computational model, i is the current time step and n is the total number of time steps. The optimization distance metric is defined as:

$$
Opt_{metric} = \sum_i^n (D_{1,comp} - D_1)^2{}_i + (D_{2,comp} - D_2)^2{}_i + (D_{3,comp} - D_3)^2{}_i
\tag{7}
$$

The optimization procedure was implemented using the design evaluation toolbox of ADAMS and the built in generalized reduced gradient optimization algorithm [17].

2.3   Distance-Shape Mapping

A continuous distance-shape map depicting the regional shape-difference between the patella and the femoral cartilage segmentations was computed over the range of 0° to 90° of flexion and extension, respectively, using: a) the CT & MRI based quasi-static knee postures; as well as b) the results of dynamic computational modeling in flexion and extension, respectively. The description of our patellofemoral separation (PFS) metric and its method of computation are described in the following sub-sections.

Procrustes Analysis Based Shape Interpolation
The input data for this step included segmentations of the femur, patella, and their respective cartilage structures, at every available knee posture available from either image reconstruction or computational simulation, as described earlier. Each segmentation was sub-divided into a fine surface mesh and exported as STLs files for this phase of the analysis pipeline. It was ensured that each segmented structure had similar numbers of mesh vertices at each available knee posture, based on the registration step described in section 2.1. Procrustes analysis was applied in order to identify rigid transformations to co-register and then interpolate the point clouds defined by the vertices of 3D knee component shapes, between successive pairs of angular knee postures (say, a total of M postures), thereby defining a series of transformations (i.e. (M-1) transformation functions) which facilitated the creation of a continuous set of positions for each knee component over the angular range defined by the minimum to maximum knee bending for the given dataset viz. 0 to 40° for the imaging based data and 0 to 90° for the computational simulation results.

Each rigid transformation was established with the objective of minimizing the sum of square errors with the closest source vertices and target vertices, for a given pair of consecutive knee postures. Procrustes superimposition was performed to determine a linear transformation (translation, orthogonal rotation and scaling) for optimal conformance of each pair of point-clouds. For a collection of 3D mesh vertex coordinates, Y, the goal is to determine the optimal shape-preserving Euclidian transformation including, rotation and translation only, to be applied in order to bring them into alignment with a second set of vertex coordinates, X. The alignment error, shown in Equation 8 was minized:

$$\min_{b,T,c}\{\|Z - X\|: Z = bYT + c\} \qquad (8)$$

where, b is a scaling factor that stretches (b > 1) or shrinks (b < 1) the points, which was set to unity for this study; T is the orthogonal and rotation matrix; and c is a matrix with constant values in each column, used to shift or translate the points.

In result, the femur, patella and their respective cartilage segmentations were interpolated in terms of their spatial position in order to recreate an expected set of postures of the knee in 1° intervals over the angular range of flexion or extension de-fined by the input data. Each surface was prepared with a similar number and spacing of vertices.

Hausdorff Distance – Examining Patellofemoral Separation
An in-house plugin was developed in Paraview (Kitware, Inc., Clifton Park, NY) to compute a signed Hausdorff Distance (HD) defining the closest distance between points defining the patella and surface of the femur cartilage structures, at each interpolated knee posture. HD was encoded at the vertices of each of the compared segmented cartilage surfaces. This distance metric has been previously applied by our group to cardiac segmentations in order to analyze regional deformation [18-20]. The HD analysis inherently established point-correspondences between pairs of cartilage surfaces separated by 1^0 of bending.

The PFS metric represents a signature of regional patellofemoral separation over time and was computed as the HD averaged across the vertices on the patella surface facing the femur, at each knee posture. Further, in order to specifically establish a risk index for patellofemoral pain syndrome (PFPS) using our shape-derived PFS metric, the number of patella surfaces vertices, proximal to the femur, which were separated from the femur cartilage by under 1.5 mm was examined over the range of studied knee postures. Variation of the mean PFS below our 1.5 mm threshold for proximity was analyzed as a function of knee bending angle.

3   Results

3.1   Patella Posture Optimization

The computational knee posture optimization results are shown in Fig. 2A, as the optimization objective function was minimized.

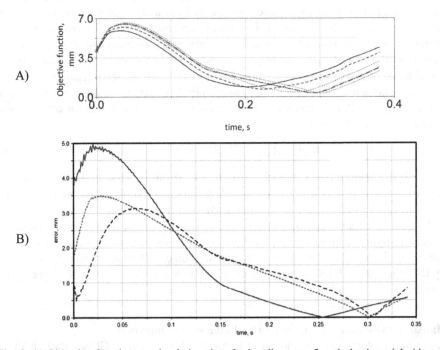

Fig. 2. A) Objective function vs. simulation time for bending over 5 optimization trials / iterations (Black: It 0, Blue: It 1, Gray: It 2, Red: It 3, Black dashed: It 4; Magenta: It 5); B) Error contributions from the three linear traction paths (Blue: D_1, Magenta: D_2, Red: D_3) over time

As a validation of the computational model's simulated knee flexion from 2 degrees to $40°$ knee flexion, the patella tracking was monitored as a function of knee flexion. Fig. 2 shows that the difference between simulated movement and in-vivo movement varied between 0.35 and 6.63 mm. The RMS value of the optimization distance metric (viz. the objective function) decreased from 2.91 to 2.64 by the 5th optimization iteration. The major contributor to the variance between the simulated and in-vivo movement was distance parameter D3 (maximum error = 5mm; see Fig. 2B). Patella kinematics as a function of bending in flexion and extension.

The mediolateral movement of the patella with reference to the transepicondylar axis center is expressed in Fig. 3. The reference axis was defined in such a way that movement from the reference point in a medial direction will increase positively whereas movement in a lateral direction will decrease negatively. It is evident that the patella displaced medially as the knee flexes up to 33°. From 33 to 90° the patella translated laterally again. The medial and lateral patellofemoral ligament tension as a function of active knee flexion is depicted in Fig. 4. As the knee flexes, both the medial and lateral ligament tensions decrease until 27 and 60° flexion respectively. The lateral ligament tension increases from 60° onwards.

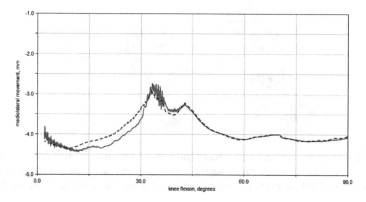

Fig. 3. Mediolateral translation of the patella as a function of active knee flexion (+ve: Medial and -ve: Lateral. Red line: flexion from 0° to 90°; Blue dashed: Extension from 90° to 0°.

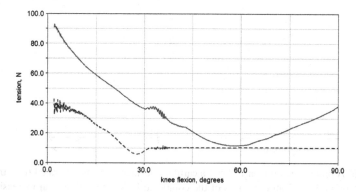

Fig. 4. Patellofemoral ligament tension. (Red: LPFL tension; Blue dashed: MPFL tension).

3.2   Distance Shape Mapping

The continuous PFS distance color map depicting the regional shape-difference between the patella and the femoral cartilage segmentations was computed over the
range of available quasi-static imaging-based segmentations are shown in Fig. 5.

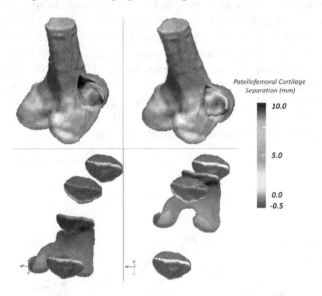

Fig. 5. The continuous distance-shape map depicting the regional HD separation between the
patella and the femoral cartilage image segmentations, colored on the patella cartilage at the 0^0
and 40^0 postures (Top Left and Right respectively), and at two intermediate positions (Bottom)

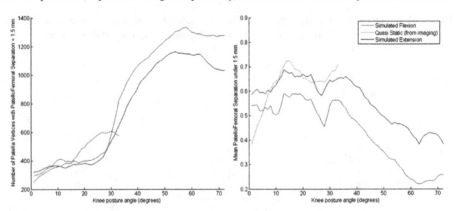

Fig. 6. Left: A plot of the number of patella cartilage surface vertices separated from the femoral cartilage by under 1.5 mm in terms of the computed PFS metric shows an increasing trend,
indicating that the patella gets closer to the femur with an increasing knee angle. Right: Variation of the mean PFS under 1.5 mm (i.e. our threshold for close proximity) over a range of knee
posture angles computed from: a) the interpolated image-segmentations (Green); b) the simulated flexion results (Red); and c) the simulated extension results (Blue). Our metric for high-
risk PFS (i.e. PFS < 1.5 mm) showed similar trends in each case.

A plot of the number of patella surface vertices separated from the femur cartilage by under 1.5 mm (our set threshold for high risk of impingement) showed a generally increasing trend (see Fig. 4, Left) indicating that impingement between the patella and femur is more likely with increasing knee flexion. This increasing trend was consistent between the analyses prepared using the different datasets examined in this study (viz. imaging-based segmentations and simulated knee postures) as the increasing area of the patella surface entering into the high-risk PFS threshold was confirmed by the results from the simulated flexion and extension data (red and blue curves in Fig. 6). Variation of the mean PFS in the high-risk (i.e. low PFS) regions computed from the image-segmentations and the simulated data was found to be very similar when examined as a function of knee angle (see Fig. 6B) under 40°. The PFS colored patella surfaces for 0, 10, 20, 30 and 40° knee flexion angles, in both flexion and extension are compared against the imaging-based actual reconstructions in Fig 7A.

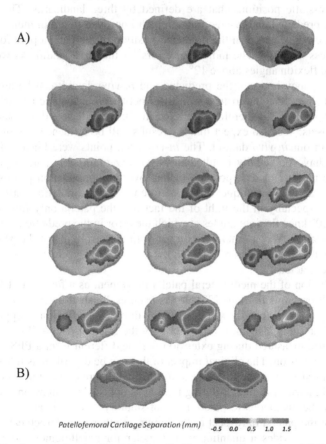

Patellofemoral Cartilage Separation (mm)   -0.5   0.0   0.5   1.0   1.5

Fig. 7. A) PFS colormaps for simulated flexion (Left); simulated extension (Middle); and image-segmentation based (Right) interpolated patella positions, for a range of knee postures i.e. 0, 10, 20, 30 and 40° from top to down, respectively. B) PFS colormaps at ~90° of knee flexion (Left) and extension (Right) based on the simulated knee postures.

Fig. 7B presents the expected PFS at 90° of flexion (Left) and extension (Right), based on the results of the patient-specific simulated knee postures, which were originally optimized to resemble the imaging segmentations at the acquired knee-postures. Note that these knee postures were impossible to obtain from imaging directly owing to space-constraints in the scanners but our optimized simulation results were sufficient to make a prediction of PFS.

4   Discussion

Patellofemoral posture prediction, i.e. patella position relative to the trochlea, by means of a computational model simulation has been compared to three quasi-static *in-vivo* measured postures. An optimization technique was used in an attempt to match the corresponding instances in the simulated dynamic patella movement to the *in-vivo* quasi-static positions that are defined by three landmarks. The RMS error between the predicted and *in-vivo* traction path improved to a minimum of 2.63 mm. The biggest error occurred in the predicted position of the patella pole for knee flexion angles less than 10°. The individual errors for the three landmarks were below 2 mm for knee flexion angles above 12°.

The discrepancy between the predicted and *in-vivo* dataset can be attributed to a number of factors. Patella posture will differ between quasi-static and dynamic knee flexion angles [21]. It is therefore expected that there will be a discrepancy between the two datasets. We also expect that the results will be influenced by the number of data points in our *in-vivo* dataset. The *in-vivo* data points were linearly interpolated, which may have potentially resulted in physically impossible patella positions. Increasing the number of data points will improve the optimization process. Notwithstanding, the applied technique with the aforementioned limitations still produced a good result, especially in the light of the fact that the patella only fully engages the trochlea at 20° knee flexion; angles at which the error in the prediction is below 2 mm for each landmark. We are therefore on par with the resolution of the MRI scan data from which the control parameters for the optimization technique for this flexion range were extracted.

The prediction of the mediolateral patella movement as a function of knee flexion concurs with previous findings [22]. It has been established by Amis *et al.* [22] that the traction path of the patella will be different during knee flexion as opposed to knee extension. Our study also shows that not only the traction path will be different, but the PFS metric measured during extension will be different form a PFS metric measured during extension. The clinical impact of this can be described as follows:

The results show that the PFS metric for this case increased as the knee flexes, and that the PFS metric was greater during flexion as opposed to extension. Theoretically, the PFS will be analogous to patellofemoral stability since it is an indication of the proximity of the patella in respect to the femur, in other words trochlear engagement. PFS therefore provides a quantitative parameter for patellofemoral stability. Additionally, the PFS metric also serves as an indication of patellofemoral "impingement", i.e. area of close proximity between the patella and trochlea. High patellofemoral contact pressure at the osseo-chondro interface has been described as one of the possible mechanical etiological factors for patellofemoral pain [23]. The PFS metric is equivalent to the patellofemoral contact area, since it indicates the proximity of the patella to the trochlea. Since patellofemoral contact pressure is a normalization of the contact force:contact area ratio, it follows that patellofemoral impingement (expressed by the PFS metric) may potentially indicate the risk of higher contact pressure, without the need to perform timeous finite element analysis.

The key contributions of this study in terms of analysis of patellofemoral separation in the context of patellofemoral contact, are three-fold:

First, we demonstrate a methodology to optimize a computational model for knee biomechanics to match medical imaging based knee postures. Further, we interpolate the postures of knee surface segmentations available at a few discrete knee bending positions from medical imaging data in order to create a set of segmentations for full, continuous range of motion of the knee. Second, we establish that the range of motion of the patella can be characterized for its time-varying regional distance with respect to the femur in terms of the regional shape difference between the patella and femoral cartilage structures. This was established using a novel shape-based patellofemoral distance-mapping paradigm to characterize patellofemoral separation. Finally, we establish mean patellofemoral separation as a heat map computed on the patella cartilage surface, over the entire studied range of motion and further formulate an a novel patellofemoral proximity metric, PFS, which represents a patient-specific fingerprint of the regional function of the knee. PFS was observed to decrease with increased knee flexion, evidencing increased proximity of the patella and femur. Quantification of patellofemoral distance characteristics may have application in tailoring personalized diagnostics and treatment strategy for patients with PFPS.

There are limitations to this study. Only three *in-vivo* data points for computational model optimization was available to spatial and imaging constraints. Using fluoroscopy and 2D to 3D registration techniques, it may be possible to establish a more complete dataset of patient-specific knee postures. We did not correlate PFS to FEA pressure predictions. The latter is a subject of our ongoing studies.

5   Conclusion

In summary, this paper describes a methodology to predict a novel metric of regional patellofemoral separation (PFS) in knee postures which are difficult to acquire in closed CT and MR imaging systems due to space constraints. This metric can potentially be utilized in for different purposes: It has potential to be used as quantification of patellofemoral stability since it graphically shows how "well" the patella is seated in the trochlear groove. It may be used to elucidate differences between patients, e.g. characterize patient-specific PFS between anterior knee pain and pain free controls. The outcome from such an analysis can lead to a better understanding of the threshold for high-risk of pain in terms of PFS. In future studies, we will aim to characterize a library of normal and abnormal knee joints using the proximity distance metric, using an image data from a series of retrospectively studied patients and normal controls. A larger cohort study would help establish a mean healthy patellofemoral proximity distance metric as well as a mean abnormal proximity distance metric, for a healthy and abnormal dataset, respectively. This would take us one step closer to establishing our PFS metric as a biomarker for abnormal knee function.

Acknowledgements. The authors acknowledge the Department of Mechanical and Mechatronic Engineering at Stellenbosch University for their financial assistance and facilities, and Dr. van Wagening & Partners at Stellenbosch Medi-Clinic's Radiology department for the CT and MRI scans. We also thank Mr. Johan van der Merwe at BERG, Stellenbosch, for his inputs on the script used to discretize the menisci for our computational models.

References

[1] Goldblatt, J.P., Richmond, J.C.: Anatomy and biomechanics of the knee. Operative Techniques in Sports Medicine 11, 172–186 (2003)

[2] Van Haver, A., Mahieu, P., Claessens, T., Li, H., Pattyn, C., Verdonk, P., et al.: A statistical shape model of trochlear dysplasia of the knee. The Knee

[3] Borotikar, B.S., Sipprell III, W.H., Wible, E.E., Sheehan, F.T.: A methodology to accurately quantify patellofemoral cartilage contact kinematics by combining 3D image shape registration and cine-PC MRI velocity data. Journal of Biomechanics 45, 1117–1122 (2012)

[4] Zhu, Z., Li, G.: Construction of 3D human distal femoral surface models using a 3D statistical deformable model. Journal of Biomechanics 44, 2362–2368 (2011)

[5] Senavongse, W., Farahmand, F., Jones, J., Andersen, H., Bull, A.M.J., Amis, A.A.: Quantitative measurement of patellofemoral joint stability: Force–displacement behavior of the human patella in vitro. Journal of Orthopaedic Research 21, 780–786 (2003)

[6] Fitzpatrick, C.K., Baldwin, M.A., Laz, P.J., FitzPatrick, D.P., Lerner, A.L., Rullkoetter, P.J.: Development of a statistical shape model of the patellofemoral joint for investigating relationships between shape and function. Journal of Biomechanics 44, 2446–2452 (2011)

[7] Baldwin, M.A., Clary, C., Maletsky, L.P., Rullkoetter, P.J.: Verification of predicted specimen-specific natural and implanted patellofemoral kinematics during simulated deep knee bend. Journal of Biomechanics 42, 2341–2348 (2009)

[8] Draper, C.E., Besier, T.F., Santos, J.M., Jennings, F., Fredericson, M., Gold, G.E., et al.: Using real-time MRI to quantify altered joint kinematics in subjects with patellofemoral pain and to evaluate the effects of a patellar brace or sleeve on joint motion. Journal of Orthopaedic Research 27, 571–577 (2009)

[9] Guess, T.M., Thiagarajan, G., Kia, M., Mishra, M.: A subject specific multibody model of the knee with menisci. Medical Engineering & Physics 32, 505–515 (2010)

[10] Bloemker, K.H., Guess, T.M., Maletsky, L., Dodd, K.: Computational knee ligament modeling using experimentally determined zero-load lengths. Open Biomed. Eng. J. 6, 33–41 (2012)

[11] Blankevoort, L., Kuiper, J.H., Huiskes, R., Grootenboer, H.J.: Articular contact in a three-dimensional model of the knee. Journal of Biomechanics 24, 1019–1031 (1991)

[12] Wismans, J., Veldpaus, F., Janssen, J., Huson, A., Struben, P.: A three-dimensional mathematical model of the knee-joint. Journal of Biomechanics 13, 677–685 (1980)

[13] LaPrade, R.F., Engebretsen, A.H., Ly, T.V., Johansen, S., Wentorf, F.A., Engebretsen, L.: The Anatomy of the Medial Part of the Knee. The Journal of Bone & Joint Surgery 89, 2000–2010 (2007)

[14] Terry, G.C., LaPrade, R.F.: The posterolateral aspect of the knee. Anatomy and surgical approach. Am. J. Sports Med. 24, 732–739 (1996)

[15] Victor, J., Wong, P., Witvrouw, E., Sloten, J.V., Bellemans, J.: How isometric are the medial patellofemoral, superficial medial collateral, and lateral collateral ligaments of the knee? Am. J. Sports Med. 37, 2028–2036 (2009)

[16] Guess, T.M., Liu, H., Bhashyam, S., Thiagarajan, G.: A multibody knee model with discrete cartilage prediction of tibio-femoral contact mechanics. Computer Methods in Biomechanics and Biomedical Engineering 16, 256–270 (2011, 2013)

[17] Gabriele, G.A., Ragsdell, K.M.: The Generalized Reduced Gradient Method: A Reliable Tool for Optimal Design. Journal of Manufacturing Science and Engineering 99, 394 (1977)

[18] Adhyapak, S., Menon, P., Mehra, A., Tully, S., Rao Parachuri, V.: Rapid Quantification of Mean Myocardial Wall Velocity in Ischemic Cardiomyopathy by Cardiac Magnetic Resonance: An Index of Cardiac Functional Abnormalities during the Cardiac Cycle. J. Clin. Exp. Cardiolog. 5, 2 (2014)

[19] Adhyapak, S.M., Menon, P.G., Rao Parachuri, V.: Restoration of optimal ellipsoid left ventricular geometry: lessons learnt from in silico surgical modeling. Interact. Cardiovasc. Thorac. Surg. 18, 153–158 (2014)

[20] Menon, P.G., Morris, L., Staines, M., Lima, J., Lee, D.C., Gopalakrishnan, V.: Novel MRI-derived quantitative biomarker for cardiac function applied to classifying ischemic cardiomyopathy within a Bayesian rule learning framework, pp. 90341L-90341L-6 (2014)

[21] Müller, J.H., Scheffer, C., Elvin, A., Erasmus, P.J., Dillon, E.M.: Patella tracking with peripatellar soft tissue stabilizers as a function of dynamic subject-specific knee flexion. Journal of Mechanics in Medicine and Biology 11, 18 (2011)

[22] Amis, A.A., Senavongse, W., Bull, A.M.J.: Patellofemoral kinematics during knee flexion-extension: An in vitro study. Journal of Orthopaedic Research 24, 2201–2211 (2006)

[23] Sanchis-Alfonso, V., Besier, T., Draper, C., Pal, S., Fredericson, M., Gold, G., et al.: Imaging and Musculoskeletal Modeling to Investigate the Mechanical Etiology of Patellofemoral Pain. In: Anterior Knee Pain and Patellar Instability, pp. 269–286. Springer, London (2011)

Feature-Sensitive and Adaptive Mesh Generation of Grayscale Images

Ming Xu[1], Zhanheng Gao[2], and Zeyun Yu[1,*]

[1] Department of Computer Science, University of Wisconsin,
Milwaukee, WI 53211, USA
yuz@uwm.edu
[2] College of Computer Science and Technology, Jilin University, Changchun, China

Abstract. In the current paper, we present a series of algorithms to generate high quality, feature-sensitive, and adaptive meshes from a given grayscale image. The Canny's edge detector is employed to guarantee that important image features are preserved in the meshes. A halftoning-based sampling strategy is adopted to provide feature-sensitive and adaptive point distributions in the image domain. A Delaunay-triangulation is used to generate initial triangulation of the image, followed by iterative mesh smoothing for mesh quality improvement. Experimental results on several medical images have shown that the proposed method is effective in producing adaptive meshes with high-quality and well-preserved features.

Keywords: Mesh generation, Feature sensitivity, Adaptivity, Delaunay triangulation, Medical images.

1 Introduction

Imaging technologies have been widely used in many aspects of science and engineering. Some popular examples in biomedical applications are computerized tomography (CT), magnetic resonance imaging (MRI), ultrasound (US), single photon emission computed tomography (SPECT), positron emission tomography (PET), and light/electron microscopy (LM/EM) [1, 2]. With new developments in hardware and software, many imaging modalities often provide image resolutions in the order of thousands of pixels in each x- or y-dimension. Additionally, with the increasing use of three-dimensional (3D) imaging technologies, it is now not uncommon to see a single image volume exceeding the size of one Gigabyte or more. The growing availability of high-resolution and volumetric images has posed challenges on data storage and transmission and thus triggered the need for algorithms to represent images more efficiently. The goal of the current study is to explore an image representation method by decomposing a 2D image into a set of non-overlapping triangles that cover the entire image domain. The mesh is adaptive such that important image features or regions of interest are captured by small mesh elements and regions of little interest are represented by large (sparse) elements.

---

* Corresponding author.

Y.J. Zhang and J.M.R.S. Tavares (Eds.): CompIMAGE 2014, LNCS 8641, pp. 204–215, 2014.

Mesh representation of images is typically performed in two steps in previous work: node generation and Delaunay triangulation of the nodes. Different mesh generation methods often differ from each other in node generation and can be classified into three categories: (1) content-adaptive node generation with various types of local feature measurements [5, 6, 7, 8, 9], (2) greedy (iterative) node insertion starting from a coarse mesh of an image [10, 11, 12, 13, 14], and (3) greedy (iterative) node removal starting from a dense mesh containing all pixels of an image [11, 15, 16, 17]. Besides the ability of representing faithfully the original images, a good mesh generator is expected to be fast and able to generate high-quality meshes with as few nodes as possible. The mesh quality is important for restoring images from meshes because of the interpolation required in the image re-sampling step. It is also critical when the meshes are used for subsequent applications such as finite element simulations. Most of the approaches mentioned above, however, do not take mesh quality into serious consideration except the method described in [8], where some mesh post-processing strategies are carried out by adding new mesh nodes. It is known that mesh quality can be efficiently improved by moving mesh nodes without adding additional ones [18, 19, 20, 21]. This strategy had been recently used in [22] for image triangulation by optimizing an objective function that incorporates both image intensities and mesh quality. There are two major drawbacks of this approach: low speed due to a numerical scheme adopted to minimize the energy function, and high approximation errors because of the assumption of a constant intensity in each triangle. Therefore, a good mesh generator from images is still in great need.

In the current paper, we present a series of algorithms to generate high quality, feature-sensitive, and adaptive meshes from a given grayscale image. The Canny's edge detector is employed to guarantee that important image features are preserved in the meshes. A halftoning-based sampling strategy [6] is adopted to provide feature-sensitive and adaptive point distributions in the image domain. A Delaunay-triangulation is used to generate initial triangulation of the image, followed by iterative mesh smoothing for mesh quality improvement. The rest of this paper is organized as follows. In Section 2, the detail of each step of the proposed image-based mesh generation is given. Some experimental results on selected medical images are presented in Section 3, followed by our conclusions in Section 4.

2   Method

The proposed method includes three main steps. In the first step, we generate three kinds of mesh nodes: (1) Canny's points, (2) halftoning points, and (3) uniform points. In the second step, an initial triangular mesh is generated from these points by using a popular open source mesh generator. Finally, the initial mesh is smoothed to increase the shape of the triangles and align the mesh to image features, where the modified versions of the conventional centroid Voronoi diagram (CVT) and optimal Delaunay triangulation (ODT) smoothing methods are adopted.

2.1   Node Generation

In order to have adaptive and feature-sensitive meshes for a given image, we need to generate initial mesh nodes that possess these properties. To this end, we would like to generate dense mesh node distributions on or near curved-boundary or tiny features of the image, and sparse mesh node distributions on straight-boundary features or background of the image.

Canny Sample Points. Image edges are important features in an image and need to be preserved in the obtained meshes. Canny edge detector is a well-known method to deal with boundary extraction. Initial Canny edge points are strictly attached to the boundary of the features of the image. Figure 1(b) displays the result of the Canny edge detector running on an image of 192*256 pixels shown in Figure 1(a). While the Canny edge detector can represent the image edges quite faithfully, the edge points are too dense to yield quality meshes if all these edges are used as mesh nodes. Our strategy is to implement an adaptive sampling on the Canny edge points. We note that an image usually contains features with high curvature and features with relatively straight edges. An example of curved-boundary and tiny features is displayed in red in Figure 1(b). The blue rectangle in the Figure 1(b) shows an example of straight-boundary features. Our interest is to generate dense sample points on curved-boundary features and sparse sample points for straight-boundary features.

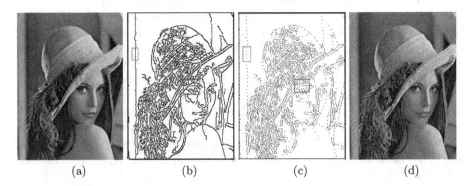

(a)   (b)   (c)   (d)

Fig. 1. (a) The original image of 192*256 pixels. (b) The result image of the canny edge detector, where $\sigma = 0.7$, lower threshold $= 0.1$, and higher threshold $= 0.6$. The region in red shows an example of curved-boundary or tiny features. The region in blue is an example of straight-boundary features. (c) The adaptively sampled points from (b). The red and blue rectangles show the results of curved-boundary and straight-boundary features respectively. (d) The final result of adaptive node generation. The green points are the canny edge points and the red points are the halftoning and uniform sample points.

In our method, we take the curvature information of every Canny's edge point into account and use the principal component analysis (PCA) to determine the sampling density. The PCA method can detect the overall attribute of the neighbors of a certain size by a statistical way, and this method can be easily extended to three dimensional images. We traverses every edge point, denoted as $\overline{P}$. Let all the edge points within $\overline{P}$'s $K \times K$ neighborhood be $P_1, P_2, ..., P_n$, where n is the number of neighboring edge points of $\overline{P}$ in its neighborhood. K is a parameter based on the density of the features in the original image, and is locally calculated for each edge point in the method described below. The covariance matrix is first calculated in the following expression:

$$\sum_{j=1}^{n} \left(P_j - \overline{P}\right) \left(P_j - \overline{P}\right)^T \in \mathbb{R}^{2 \times 2}. \tag{1}$$

Then we calculate the two eigenvalues of this covariance matrix, denoted by λ_1, λ_2 (assuming $\lambda_1 \geqslant \lambda_2$). We decide the sample radius which we call as $R(\overline{P})$ using the following equation:

$$R(\overline{P}) = \begin{cases} 1 & (\lambda_1 - \lambda_2)/(\lambda_1 + \lambda_2) \leq 0.3 \\ 3 & 0.3 < (\lambda_1 - \lambda_2)/(\lambda_1 + \lambda_2) \leq 0.5 \\ 5 & else \end{cases} \tag{2}$$

The current Canny's edge point $\overline{P}$ survives (i.e., being a valid sampling point) if and only if there is no other existing sampling point found within the neighborhood of size $K \times K$, where $K = 2 \times R(\overline{P}) + 1$. Figure 1(c) shows the sampled points with the PCA strategy. As we have discussed, tiny features and features with high curvature have dense sample points (see the red rectangle for example). On the other hand, big features or features with straight lines have sparsely sampled points (see the blue rectangle for example).

Halftoning Sample Points. The edge points described above only capture the pixels on or near the image edges. In order to have a decent initial mesh, one has to scatter some more points in the non-edge regions of the image. To this end, we adopt the halftoning sample points based on the approach described in [6]. This method generates the sample points based on the second derivatives of an image, where most of the sample points found are placed near the image features (edges). Below we give a brief summary of this approach. The interested reader is referred to [6] for more details.

The first step of this method is to extract the image feature map by calculating the Hessian matrix described in the following equation:

$$H(x, y) = \begin{pmatrix} f_{xx}''(x, y) & f_{xy}''(x, y) \\ f_{xy}''(x, y) & f_{yy}''(x, y) \end{pmatrix}. \tag{3}$$

We then calculate the two eigenvalues of the above Hessian matrix:

$$\lambda_{1,2}(x, y) = \frac{1}{2} \left(f_{xx}''(x, y) + f_{yy}''(x, y)\right) \pm \sqrt{\frac{1}{4} \left(f_{xx}''(x, y) - f_{yy}''(x, y)\right)^2 + \left(f_{xy}''(x, y)\right)^2} \tag{4}$$

The image feature map is generated in the following equation (where $G(x, y) = max(|\lambda_1(x, y)|, |\lambda_2(x, y)|)$):

$$\sigma(x, y) = \left(\frac{G(x, y)}{A}\right)^\gamma,\tag{5}$$

where A is the largest value of $G(x,y)$, and γ is a parameter and in this paper $\gamma = 1.0$.

The Floyd-Steinberg diffusion algorithm [3] is then used to scan the whole image pixel by pixel and compare each pixel's feature map value with a threshold q as follows:

$$b(x, y) = \begin{cases} 1 & if \sigma(x, y) \geq q \\ 0 & otherwise \end{cases}\tag{6}$$

A point (x,y) is chosen as a sample point if $b(x, y) = 1$. The parameter q determines the number of mesh nodes that can be generated using this method. In our method, $q = 0.3$. To dynamically update the feature map $\sigma(x, y)$, this method computes the quantization error $e(x, y)$ by:

$$e(x, y) = \sigma(x, y) - (2q) b(x, y)\tag{7}$$

And the the feature map is updated by the diffusion procedure towards the right and down directions:

$$\begin{aligned}
\sigma(x, y + 1) &= \sigma(x, y + 1) + \omega_1 e(x, y) \\
\sigma(x + 1, y - 1) &= \sigma(x + 1, y - 1) + \omega_2 e(x, y) \\
\sigma(x + 1, y) &= \sigma(x + 1, y) + \omega_3 e(x, y) \\
\sigma(x + 1, y + 1) &= \sigma(x + 1, y + 1) + \omega_4 e(x, y)
\end{aligned}\tag{8}$$

where $\omega_1 = 7/16$, $\omega_2 = 3/16$, $\omega_3 = 5/16$, $\omega_4 = 1/16$.

The above updating scheme is applied to every pixel until the bottom of the image is reached. A point (x, y) is said to be a halftoning sample point if the final $b(x, y)$ is non-zero and no Canny's points are found in its 7×7 neighborhood.

Uniform Sample Points. Although the halftoning sample points can cover most non-edge regions of the image, it is possible the no point (either Canny or halftoning) is found in regions of almost constant intensities. We therefore generate some points uniformly to cover the rest of the images where the first two types of sample points are not located. Again, a point (x, y) is said to be a valid uniform sample point if no Canny's or halftoning points are found in its 7×7 neighborhood.

Figure 1(d) shows the final result of the sample point generation, where green points are Canny's sample points and red points correspond to the other two types.

2.2 Mesh Generation via Delaunay Triangulation

The sample points found above are used to generate our initial mesh for a given image by using the Delaunay triangulation. We employed a popular open source software [4] in this paper. Figure 2(a) shows the initial triangle mesh generated by the Delaunay triangulation. As can be seen in Figure 2(a), the quality of the initial triangular mesh is not good. Hence a mesh smoothing scheme performing on this initial mesh is necessary, as described below. The smoothed mesh is expected to be not only well shaped and sized but also strictly attached to the features (edges) of the image.

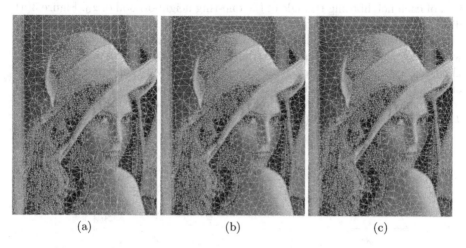

(a)   (b)   (c)

Fig. 2. (a) Initial triangle mesh generated by Delaunay triangulation. (b) The smoothed mesh by the CVT method based on the image features after five iterations. (c) The smoothed mesh by the ODT method based on the image features after five iterations.

2.3 Mesh Smoothing

We extend several traditional mesh smoothing methods, including Optimal Delaunay Triangulations (ODT) and Centroid Voronoi Tessellations (CVT) [18, 19], to the image domain, in order to enhance the quality of the mesh. While the traditional mesh smoothing techniques only take the mesh quality into account, we will develop two new methods based on the ODT and CVT schemes to incorporate image feature information into mesh quality improvement. Both ODT and CVT are ropology-preserving, meaning that they only move mesh nodes without modifying the mesh topology. In the context of image triangulation, we restrict ourselves to moving only halftoning and uniform sample points but keeping Canny's points unchanged because of the feature-preservation purpose.

Image-Based CVT Scheme. The traditional CVT method traverses every vertex of the triangle mesh, denoted by x_0, and finds its new position x^* as follows:

$$x^* = \frac{1}{|\Omega_0|} \sum_{T_j \in \Omega_0} |T_j| \cdot C_j, \tag{9}$$

where $|\Omega_0|$ is the area of the one-ring neighborhood of x_0, $|T_j|$ is the area of a triangle T_j in the one-ring neighborhood of x_0, and C_j is the centroid of the triangle T_j.

In order to take the image features into account, we add the gradient information of each neighboring triangle of the one-ring neighborhood of x_0. Figure 3(a) displays how to calculate the gradient information of T_j. First we calculate the centroid of this triangle, called C_j, and its gradient magnitude $g(C_j)$. Secondly, we connect the three vertices of this triangle with C_j yielding three sub-triangles: ΔabC_j, Δbx_0C_j, and ΔC_jx_0a. Thirdly, we calculate every sub-triangles centroid and their gradient magnitudes. Then the average of these four gradient values (a red points and three green points in Figure 3(a)) is calculated to get the triangle T_j's gradient information $g(T_j)$.

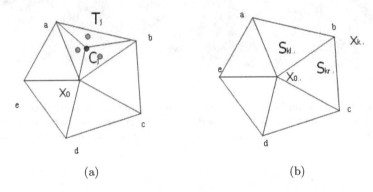

(a)   (b)

Fig. 3. (a) The one-ring neighborhood of x_0. T_j is one of the adjacent triangles in the neighborhood. C_j is the centroid of the T_j. (b) The one-ring neighborhood of x_0. x_k is one of the neighboring vertices of x_0. S_{kl} and S_{kr} are the left and right triangles of edge x_0x_k respectively.

The proposed image-based CVT scheme is as follows:

$$x^* = \frac{\sum_{T_j \in \Omega_0} |T_j| \cdot C_j \cdot g(T_j)}{\sum_{T_j \in \Omega_0} |T_j| \cdot g(T_j)} \tag{10}$$

Image-Based ODT Scheme. Similar to the CVT scheme, the traditional ODT method is defined based on the one-ring neighborhood of a vertex in the mesh as follows:

$$x^* = x_0 - \frac{1}{2\,|\Omega_0|} \sum_{\substack{x_k \in \Omega_0 \\ x_k \neq x_0}} (S_{kl} + S_{kr})\,(x_0 - x_k), \tag{11}$$

where S_{kl} is the left triangle of edge $x_0 x_k$ and S_{kr} is the right triangle of edge $x_0 x_k$ (see Figure 3(b)).

In the proposed work, we modify the original ODT method by taking the gradient information into account as below:

$$x^* = x_0 - \frac{\sum_{\substack{x_k \in \Omega_0 \\ x_k \neq x_0}} (S_{kl} \cdot g\,(S_{kl}) + S_{kr} \cdot g\,(S_{kr})) \cdot (x_0 - x_k)}{\sum_{\substack{x_k \in \Omega_0 \\ x_k \neq x_0}} (S_{kl} \cdot g\,(S_{kl}) + S_{kr} \cdot g\,(S_{kr}))}, \tag{12}$$

where $g\,(S_{kl})$ is the averaged gradient magnitude of left triangle of edge $x_0 x_k$ and $g\,(S_{kr})$ is the averaged gradient magnitude of right triangle of edge $x_0 x_k$.

Edge Flipping Strategy. Although the traditional and our modified CVT/ODT methods are intended to move vertices without changing the mesh topology, it is often beneficial to change the mesh topology by using the widely-used edge-flipping technique. In our implementation, we traverse every vertex of the mesh one by one using either image-based CVT or image-based ODT method. The CVT or ODT method and the edge-flipping scheme are applied to the mesh alternatively. Typically five iterations of applying ODT/CVT and edge-flipping to the meshes would be sufficient, as demonstrated below in the results.

The final result of the image-based CVT and ODT methods are shown in Figure 2 (b) and (c) respectively, for the initial mesh in Figure 2(a). In both cases, the smoothed meshes have good quality mesh. Moreover, the mesh nodes are better attached along the feature boundary in the image. Also, dense sample points are placed near the image features and sparse sample points are placed in the background or the regions of low-curvature features. From the point of view of the image segmentation, the results retain the fidelity of the boundaries of the objects in Figure 2 (b) and (c).

3   Experimental Results

In this section, we will provide the results of our methods running on some biomedical images. The number of iterations in the mesh smoothing step is set as 5. The code was written in c++ and compiled in Windows Visual Studio 2010. The total running time for a 2D image of size 256×256 is less than one second on a Pentium IV PC with a 2.0 GHz CPU and 2 GB memory.

Figure 4 displays the result of our method running on a 128×128 heart image (courtesy of Dr. Andrew McCulloch, UCSD). In (a) we can see that the most important feature in this image is the ventricle in the middle of this image.

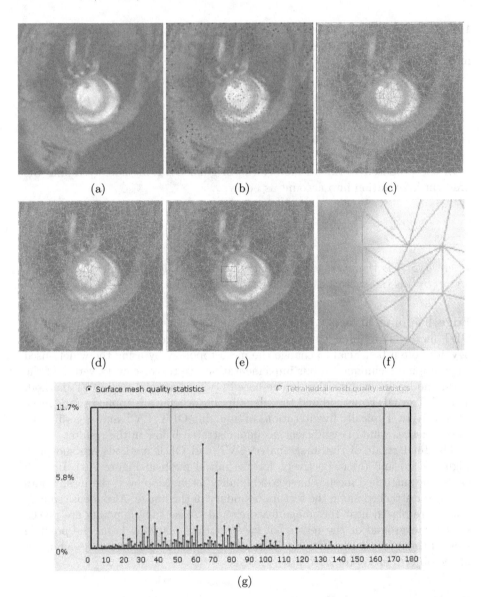

(a)   (b)   (c)

(d)   (e)   (f)

(g)

Fig. 4. Result of our method running on a 128×128 heart image. (a) The original image. (b) The result of the sample point generation. Green points are Canny's sample points. Red points are halftoning and uniform sample points. (c) The result of initial mesh generated by Delaunay triangulation. (d) The result of the image-based ODT method. (e) The result of the image-based CVT method. (f) A closeup look at the rectangular region in (e). (g) A quantitative measure of the quality of the final triangulations. The minimum angle is 4.57 degree. The maximum angle is 165.96 degree. The minimum size of the triangles is 0.499. The maximum size of the triangles is 32.99.

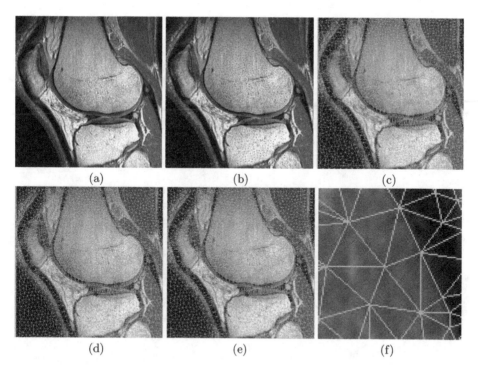

Fig. 5. Result of our method running on a 256 × 256 knee image. (a) The original image. (b) The result of the sample point generation. Green points are Canny's sample points. Red points are halftoning and uniform sample points. (c) The result of initial mesh generated by Delaunay triangulation. (d) The result of the image-based ODT method. (e) The result of the image-based CVT method. (f) A closeup look at the rectangular region in (e).

(b) shows the result of the sample points found. The Canny's sample points (in green) occupy the most area of the left-top of this image. (c) is the result of initial mesh generated by Delaunay triangulation. The mesh smoothing, as shown in (d) and (e), provide better quality of the meshes. Also, the closeup view shows that the triangles are well aligned along the boundary of the ventricle.

Secondly, we test the proposed method on a 256 × 256 knee MRI image taken from GE-Healthcare. In Figure 5(c), the initial mesh has the same shortcoming as in the initial mesh of the heart image. But this mesh quality is improved by the mesh smoothing, as seen in (d) and (e). A closeup view of the mesh is shown in (f), from which one can see the alignment of the mesh with image features.

Finally in Figure 6(a), we show a 256 × 256 noisy image of partial cardiac cells (courtesy of Dr. Masahiko Hoshijima, UCSD). (b) and (c) show the sample points found and the initial mesh by Delaunay triangulation. The smoothed meshes in (d) and (e) show that the proposed method can generate high quality meshes even for very noisy images.

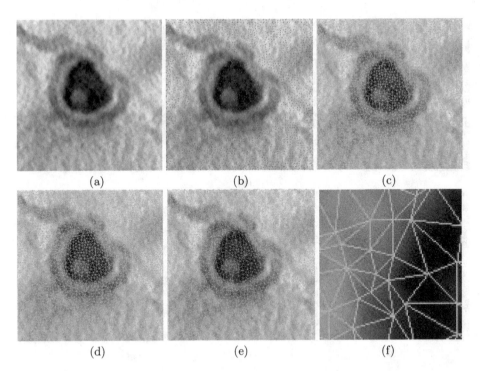

(a)   (b)   (c)

(d)   (e)   (f)

Fig. 6. Result of our method running on a 256×256 cardiac cell image. (a) The original image. (b) The result of the sample point generation. Green points are Canny's sample points. Red points are halftoning and uniform sample points. (c) The result of initial mesh generated by Delaunay triangulation. (d) The result of the image-based ODT method. (e) The result of the image-based CVT method. (f) A closeup look at the rectangular region in (e).

4   Conclusion

In the present paper, a method was descried to generate meshes from 2D grayscale images. Numerous experimental results have shown that the meshes obtained by the proposed method are adaptive, feature sensitive, and have high mesh quality. All these properties are critical in subsequent image-based applications such as image segmentation and finite element simulations. Part of our ongoing work is to utilize the generated meshes to segment the original images into distinctive feature regions and background. As the number of triangles obtained is typically much smaller than the number of pixels in the original images, it is expected that the triangulated images would provide a tremendous speedup in image segmentation.

References

1. Haidekker, M.A.: Medical Imaging Technology, Springer Briefs in Physics (2013)
2. Chandler, D., Roberson, R.W.: Bioimaging: Current Concept in Light & Electron Microscopy. Jones & Bartlett Learning (2008)

3. Floyd, R., Steinberg, L.: An adaptive algorithm for spatial gray scale. In: SID Int. Symp. Digest of Tech. Papers, pp. 36–37 (1975)
4. Shewchuk, J.: Triangle: A Two-Dimensional Quality Mesh Generator and Delaunay Triangulator, http://www.cs.cmu.edu/~quake/triangle.html
5. Ramponi, G., Carrato, S.: An adaptive irregular sampling algorithm and its application to image coding. Image and Vision Computing 19(7), 451–460 (2001)
6. Yang, Y., Wernick, M.N., Brankov, J.G.: A fast approach for accurate content-adaptive mesh generation. IEEE Transactions on Image Processing 12(8), 866–881 (2003)
7. Kim, T.-S., Lee, W.H.: 3-D MRI and DT-MRI Content-adaptive Finite Element Head Model Generation for Bioelectromagnetic Imaging. In: Recent Advances in Biomedical Engineering (2009)
8. Cuadros-Vargas, A.J., Nonato, L.G., Minghim, R., Etiene, T.: Imesh: An Image Based Quality Mesh Generation Technique. In: Proceedings of the XVIII Brazilian Symposium on Computer Graphics and Image Processing (2005)
9. Tu, X., Adams, M.D.: Improved Mesh Models of Images Through the Explicit Representation of Discontinuities. Canadian Journal of Electrical and Computer Engineering 36(2), 78–86 (2013)
10. Garland, M., Heckbert, P.S.: Fast Polygonal Approximation of Terrains and Height Fields. CMU-CS-95-181 (1995)
11. Adams, M.D.: A Highly-Effective Incremental/Decremental Delaunay Mesh-Generation Strategy for Image Representation. Signal Processing 93(4), 749–764 (2013)
12. Sarkis, M., Diepold, K.: Content Adaptive Mesh Representation of Images Using Binary Space Partitions. IEEE Trans. Image Process. 18(5), 1069–1079 (2009)
13. Bougleux, S., Peyré, G., Cohen, L.D.: Image Compression with Anisotropic Geodesic Triangulations. In: IEEE 12th International Conference Computer Vision, pp. 2343–2348 (2009)
14. Li, P., Adams, M.D.: A Tuned Mesh-Generation Strategy for Image Representation Based on Data-Dependent Triangulation. IEEE Trans. Image Process. 22(5), 2004–2018 (2013)
15. Demaret, L., Dyn, N., Iske, A.: Image Compression by Linear Splines over Adaptive Triangulations. Signal Processing 86(7), 1604–1616 (2006)
16. Demaret, L., Iske, A.: Anisotropic Triangulation Methods in Adaptive Image Approximation. In: Approximation Algorithms for Complex Systems. Springer Proceedings in Mathematics, vol. 3, pp. 47–68 (2011)
17. Adams, M.D.: A Flexible Content-Adaptive Mesh-Generation Strategy for Image Representation. IEEE Transactions on Image Processing 20(9), 2414–2427 (2011)
18. Chen, L.: Mesh smoothing schemes based on optimal Delaunay triangulations. In: Proceedings of the 13th International Meshing Roundtable, pp. 109–120 (2004)
19. Chen, L., Xu, J.: Optimal Delaunay triangulation. Journal of Computational Mathematics 22(2), 299–308 (2004)
20. Gao, Z., Yu, Z., Holst, M.: Quality Tetrahedral Mesh Smoothing via Boundary-Optimized Delaunay Triangulation. Computer Aided Geometric Design 29(9), 707–721 (2012)
21. Gao, Z., Yu, Z., Holst, M.: Feature-Preserving Surface Mesh Smoothing via Suboptimal Delaunay Triangulation. Graphical Models 75(1), 23–38 (2013)
22. Goksel, O., Salcudean, S.E.: Image-Based Variational Meshing. IEEE Transactions on Medical Imaging 30(1), 11–21 (2011)

Subdividing Prismatic Meshes by Cutting Flow

Xiaotian Yin[1], Wei Han[1], Xianfeng Gu[2], and Shing-Tung Yau[1]

[1] Mathematics Department, Harvard University, Cambridge, MA, USA
{xyin,weihan,yau}@math.harvard.edu
[2] Computer Science Department, Stony Brook University, Stony Book, NY, USA
gu@cs.sunysb.edu

Abstract. This paper is motivated by the problem of subdividing a prismatic mesh to a tetrahedral mesh with prescribed boundary conditions and without inserting Steiner points. We show that this 3D subdivision problem can be modeled as a 2D cutting flow problem. Then we propose a complete solution to the cutting flow problem, covering all possible combinations of base domain topology and boundary condition. We not only provide provable sufficient and necessary conditions for existence of solutions, but also provide linear algorithms to compute a solution whenever there is one.

Keywords: Cutting Flow Problem, Graph Algorithm, Tetrahedral Mesh, Prismatic Mesh.

1 Introductions

A prismatic mesh consists of a set of triangular prisms, where each prism is a volumetric element bounded by two triangular faces and three quadrilateral faces, and different prisms are glued together along same type of faces (i.e. triangle to triangle, quadrangle to quadrangle). It in general comes in layers, where each layer is an extrusion of a triangular mesh (i.e. base mesh) along a line interval (i.e. fiber).

1.1 Motivations

Prismatic meshes have attracted significant interest in various areas, including computer-aided-design, computational fluid dynamics, biomedical computing, etc. They are especially useful for modeling geometries that are layered inherently. One of such applications, to name a few, is for the wall of heart, which is a laminated muscle consisting of three separate layers, each with a separate family of fiber and myocyte orientations. The boundary-layer mesh is also used to model the boundary of viscous flows, where the prismatic layers have the advantages of less computational errors [13,8]. Another targeted application is the face offsetting mesh over a Lagrangian surface mesh or level-set iso-surface, which is used to model the dynamic moving interface for crystal growth, multi-phase flows, etc [6]. In addition, it is also used to model three-dimensional space-time

Y.J. Zhang and J.M.R.S. Tavares (Eds.): CompIMAGE 2014, LNCS 8641, pp. 216–227, 2014.

finite elements (called *space-time slabs*) by extruding a two-dimensional space triangular mesh into prisms by a height of $\triangle t$ in the time direction [10].

In spite of their modeling power and wide usage, prismatic meshes are often required to be converted to tetrahedral meshes, especially for the purpose of computation and simulation. In finite element methods, many solvers are designed for tetrahedral meshes and do not support prismatic elements [7,12]. In computer graphics, many efficient algorithms for volume rendering, iso-contouring and particle advection only work for meshes of tetrahedra [1,9]. Therefore how to triangulate a prismatic mesh becomes a desirable task.

1.2   Related Work

Splitting a single prism into three tetrahedra is an easy task, but cutting a set of prisms consistently is much more challenging. Here we only consider conversions without inserting additional points (i.e. Steiner points). Under certain circumstances user may wish to have control on the boundary triangulation, i.e. the subdivision of the quadrilateral faces on the boundary of the prismatic mesh, and the internal subdivision must conform to such boundary conditions. In addition, the underlying base mesh may have various topologies, which could bring another level of difficulty to the problem of extending the boundary triangulation into the inside.

There has been a rich literature on triangulating non-tetrahedral elements, such as [7,9,11,3,12,1,4,14]. They are either using iterative methods or direct methods, allowing or not allowing Steiner points, topologically or geometrically. However, for the problem of triangulating prismatic meshes without inserting Steiner points, none of the above work provided a complete solution considering both boundary conditions and base mesh topologies.

For example, [4] proposes an algorithm to subdivide a volumetric mesh consisting of mixed elements (pyramids, prisms, and hexahedra) into tetrahedra by comparing and ordering vertex indices. However, it assigns boundary conditions on their own (i.e. free boundary) instead of following the user specified boundary conditions, while the latter makes a completely different problem.

Another work that is most similar to this work is [14], which considers prescribed boundary conditions for prismatic mesh subdivision. However, it only works on topological disks but not on other types of topologies. Moreover, in their most basic case (i.e. restricted boundary condition), they only provide the sufficient condition for non-existence of solutions while no necessary condition is considered.

In comparison, in this work we consider both boundary conditions and base topologies. Under this general framework, we provide complete solutions to all possible combinations of these two factors, which are summarized in Table 1. In the remaining part of this paper, we first formulate the 3D prismatic mesh subdivision problem as a 2D graph problem: the cutting flow problem (section 2). Then we present our solutions to the cutting flow problem in the most basic setting (section 3) as well as other extended settings (section 4). Finally we discuss the complexity and limitations of our algorithms (section 5).

Table 1. Out solution covers all possible base topologies and boundary conditions

Bnd / Topo	Fixed	Free
Simply-Connected & Planar	**Conditionally Solvable** Section 3, Theorem 1	
Multiply-Connected & Planar	**Always Solvable** Section 4.1, Theorem 2	**Always Solvable** Section 4.4, Theorem 5
Multiply-Connected & Non-Planar	**Always Solvable** Section 4.2, Theorem 3	
Simply-Connected & Non-Planar	**Always Solvable** Section 4.3, Theorem 4	

2   Problem Formulation

2.1   Intuition

We subdivide each layer in a prismatic mesh separately, and formulate this problem as an equivalent 2D graph flow problem in the underlying base mesh. The work is based on the following intuition. For every individual prism in the mesh, as shown in Figure 1, each quadrilateral face should be split into two triangles, either through the *diagonal* (lower-left to upper-right) or *anti-diagonal* (lower-right to upper-left). We model such a splitting process by assigning directed flows across edges of the base triangular face. If a quadrilateral face is split along diagonal, we put a flow into the base triangle across the corresponding base edge; otherwise, put a flow out of the base triangle.

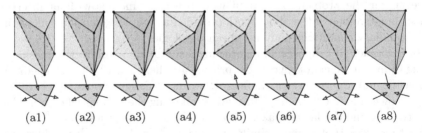

(a1)   (a2)   (a3)   (a4)   (a5)   (a6)   (a7)   (a8)

Fig. 1. The intuition: subdividing each individual prism by cutting flow. (a1) to (a6) are valid cuttings, (a7) and (a8) are invalid.

The above idea suggests that subdividing a prismatic mesh is equivalent to finding a flow on the base mesh satisfying the following requirements:

1. Each base triangle should have both inflow and outflow (Figure 1).
2. The flow must get out of one triangle and into an adjacent triangle.
3. If the flow across boundary edges is specified, it should remain fixed.

2.2   Cutting Flow Problem

A triangular mesh $M = (V, E, F)$ is either *planar* if it can be embedded in the plane by one-to-one correspondence, or *non-planar* otherwise. A mesh is either *simply-connected* if any loop on the surface can smoothly contract to a single point without leaving the surface, or *multiply-connected* otherwise.

Given M, we define its *dual graph* (Figure 2) as $G^* = (V^*, E^*)$. Due to the fact that M has only triangular faces, vertices in G^* has degree no more than 3. In a dual graph G^*, we define *edge cut* as a group of edges whose removal makes the graph disconnected. The *edge-connectivity* $\lambda(G^*)$ is the size of a smallest edge cut. If G^* has edge-connectivity 2, we call it a *cluster*. If it has edge-connectivity 1, we call it a *tree*. If G^* only consists of a single vertex, we define its edge-connectivity as 0 and treat it as a degenerated tree.

We define the *augmented dual graph* (Figure 2) as $\widetilde{G^*} = (V^* \cup \widetilde{V}, E^* \cup \widetilde{E})$, which incudes a set of virtual edges $\widetilde{E}$ that corresponds to the boundary edges in M, plus a set of virtual vertices $\widetilde{V}$ placed off the boundary of M to bound the virtual edges in $\widetilde{E}$. In the rest of the paper we will use G^* to denote the dual graph or the augmented dual graph interchangeably unless otherwise noted.

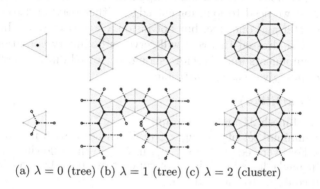

(a) $\lambda = 0$ (tree) (b) $\lambda = 1$ (tree) (c) $\lambda = 2$ (cluster)

Fig. 2. Dual graph G^* (solid dark in upper row) and its augmentation $\widetilde{G^*}$ (dotted dark in lower row) overlayed on primal mesh M (shaded as green)

Now we can transform the 3D subdivision problem to a 2D flow problem:

Problem 1 (The Cutting Flow Problem). Given a triangular mesh M with augmented dual graph $\widetilde{G^*} = (V^* \cup \widetilde{V}, E^* \cup \widetilde{E})$, find a flow (called cutting flow) on the edge set of $\widetilde{G^*}$, such that:

– Fixed Boundary: *The flow on $\widetilde{E}$ is given as input and cannot be changed.*
– No Source/Sink: *Every vertex in V^* must have both inflow and outflow.*

3   Solution: Basic Setting

This section shows how to solve the cutting flow problem for simply-connected and planar meshes (i.e. topological disks), by first partitioning the input mesh into simpler sub-components (Section 3.1), then solving each special case (Section 3.2, 3.3), and finally solving the general case (Section 3.4).

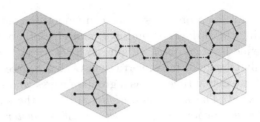

Fig. 3. Partition a dual graph G^* into a minimal set of sub-components of trees (pink) and clusters (other colors) by removing a set of cut edges (dotted)

3.1 Partition

Given a simply-connected planar triangular mesh M, its dual graph G^* can be partitioned into a set of sub-components: clusters (with edge-connectivity 2) and trees (with edge-connectivity 1 or 0). Here we require the set to be *minimal*, meaning that the union of any two sub-components is neither a tree nor a cluster. This implies that we need to look for cut edges either between two clusters or between one cluster and one tree, but not inside a tree (Figure 3). In addition, all the cut edges addressed this way will serve as boundary conditions for the resulting sub-components and therefore should be solved during partition. The following procedure gives such a partition:

Procedure 1 (*Partition*)

- *Input*: Primal mesh M and dual graph G^*.
- *Output*: A minimal set of cut edges $\mathfrak{E}$ in G^* assigned with flow directions.
- *Procedure*: For every edge $e^* = (v_1^*, v_2^*)$ in G^*, do the following:
  1. If the primal edge e in M does not connect two boundary vertices, ignore e^* and continue to the next one;
  2. If $deg(v_1^*) < 3$ and $deg(v_2^*) < 3$, ignore e^* and continue to the next one;
  3. Otherwise, add e^* to $\mathfrak{E}$ and solve it by cases:
     (a) Both v_1^* and v_2^* have degree 3 in G^*: assign e^* with flow $v_1^* \to v_2^*$;
     (b) One vertex (say v_1^*) has degree less than 3 (i.e. e^* connects a tree and a cluster, and $deg(v_1^*) = 2$):
        - If none of v_1^*'s incident edges has been solved: assign e^* with an arbitrary direction, say $v_1^* \to v_2^*$;
        - Otherwise, at least one of v_1^*'s incident edges has been solved :
           * If v_1^* already has an inflow: assign e^* with $v_1^* \to v_2^*$;
           * If v_1^* already has an outflow: assign e^* with $v_1^* \leftarrow v_2^*$.

Lemma 1. If a tree sub-component is generated from Procedure 1, it always has a mixed boundary condition.

3.2 Solving Trees

Given a simply-connected planar triangular mesh M, if the dual graph G^* is a tree, the solvability depends on the boundary condition. There are only three possible cases (A, B and C), some are solvable (A and B) while others are not solvable (C).

Case A: If G^* is a tree with mixed boundary condition and every leaf vertex has mixed boundary condition, we can use the following Procedure 2 to solve it (Figure 4).

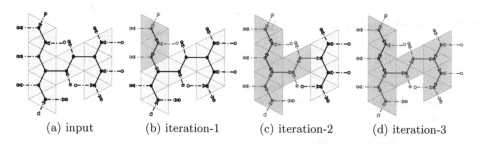

| (a) input | (b) iteration-1 | (c) iteration-2 | (d) iteration-3 |

Fig. 4. Tree of Case A: all the leaves have mixed boundary. It can be completely solved by Procedure 2.

Procedure 2 (*Solving Mixed Tree with Mixed Leaves*)

- *Input*: A mixed-boundary tree G^* that all its leaves are mixed-boundary.
- *Output*: A cutting flow for G^*.
- *Procedure*: Repeat the following steps to iteratively solve and remove branches until G^* is empty:
  1. Pick a leaf vertex v_0^* (always with a mixed boundary), trace a branch of degree-2 vertices ($m > 0$): $(v_0^*)v_1^* \cdots v_{m-1}^*(v_m^*)$, until reaching a vertex v_m^* of one of the following two cases:
     (a) A junction of multiple branches (i.e. degree 3); or
     (b) Another leaf (i.e. degree 1).
  2. Solve this branch as: $v_0^* \to v_1^* \to \cdots \to v_m^*$
  3. If v_m^* is a junction (i.e. there are other branches left), then replace this branch (excluding v_m^*) with a virtual edge carrying the same flow direction as that between v_{m-1}^* and v_m^*.
  4. Otherwise, this is the only branch left in G^* and is already solved. Exit.

Procedure 2 only terminates at step 4, where the whole tree is solved. In fact, when a branch is solved in step 3 and removed from G^*, the remaining G^* is still a tree and all the leaves still have mixed boundary.

Case B: If G^* is a tree with mixed boundary condition but some of its leaf vertices has uniform boundary condition, we use Procedure 3 in below to solve the branches bounded by these uniform-boundary leaves (Figure 5), and then the remaining part of G^* is a smaller tree with all mixed-boundary leaves, which is of Case A.

Procedure 3 (*Solving Mixed Tree with Uniform Leaves*)

- *Input*: A mixed-boundary tree G^* that at least one leaf has uniform boundary.

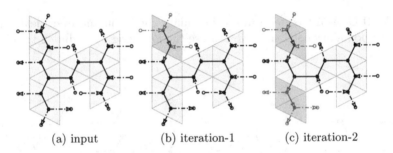

(a) input   (b) iteration-1   (c) iteration-2

Fig. 5. Tree of Case B: the whole tree has mixed boundary but at least one leaf has uniform boundary. It can be converted to Case A (shaded by light green in c) by Procedure 3.

- *Output*: A cutting flow for G^*.
- *Procedure*: Repeat the following steps to iteratively solve and remove branches with uniform leaves:
    1. Pick a leaf vertex v_0^* with uniform boundary condition (supposing inflow without loss of generality). If there is no such leaf, exit the procedure; Otherwise, go to the next step.
    2. Starting from this leaf trace a branch of degree-2 vertices ($m > 0$): $(v_0^*)v_1^* \cdots v_{m-1}^*(v_m^*)$, such that all the vertices before (but not including) v_m^* have the same boundary flow (i.e. inflow) and v_m^* is in one of the following conditions:
        (a) v_m^* is degree 3; or
        (b) v_m^* is degree 2 but with a different boundary flow (i.e. outflow);
    3. Assign edge directions along this branch conforming to the boundary flow at v_0^* (i.e. inflow): $v_0^* \to v_1^* \to \cdots \to v_m^*$
    4. Replace the branch (excluding v_m^*) with a virtual edge carrying the same flow direction (i.e. inflow to v_m^*).

In this case, G^* has leaves with uniform boundary condition. After each iteration, a branch with uniform-boundary leaf will be either completely solved and removed (following step 2a), or trimmed to a shorter branch with mixed-boundary leaf (following step 2a). Therefore every iteration removes a uniform-boundary leaf and possibly introduces a new mixed-boundary leaf. In addition, if there are any original mixed-boundary leaves in the input graph G^*, they remain untouched. Therefore after this procedure, G^* will be a tree with only mixed-boundary leaves and can thus be further solved by Procedure 2.

Case C: If G^* is a tree with uniform boundary condition, it is easy to prove that there is no solution to the cutting flow problem, as shown in Lemma 2 and illustrated in Figure 6.

Lemma 2. A tree G^* with uniform boundary condition has no cutting flow solution.

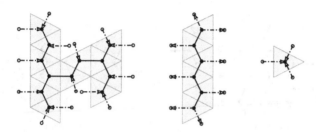

Fig. 6. Tree of Case C: all the boundary flows are uniformly inflow (or uniformly outflow). There is no cutting flow solution by Lemma 2. Here are three examples.

Overall: Based on the above discussions of case A, B and C, we have the following obvious conclusion for trees:

Lemma 3. A tree G^* is solvable if and only if the boundary condition is mixed.

3.3 Solving Clusters

If the dual graph G^* is a cluster, the solvability does not depend on the boundary condition. Let $O(G^*)$ be the subgraph (a cycle) spanned by the most outside layer of vertices in G^*, $I(G^*)$ be the subgraph spanned by the remaining vertices, and $B(G^*)$ be the set of edges bridging vertices in $O(G^*)$ and vertices in $O(I(G^*))$.

Actually a cluster G^* can always be solved using Procedure 4 iteratively by *front-advancing* and *divide-and-conquer*. We first solve the frontier $O(G^*)$ and edges in $B(G^*)$ (illustrated in Figure 7), then partition the remaining part $I(G^*)$ into smaller clusters and trees with appropriate boundary conditions, and solve them iteratively.

Procedure 4 (*Solving Cluster*)

- *Input*: A cluster G^* with arbitrary boundary condition.
- *Output*: A cutting flow for G^*.
- *Procedure*:
    1. Trace the frontier cycle $O(G^*) = v_0^* v_1^* \cdots v_m^*$ and solve it as: $v_0^* \to v_1^* \to \cdots \to v_m^* \to v_0^*$. If $I(G^*)$ (and thus $B(G^*)$) is empty, then everything is solved and exit. Otherwise, go to the next step.
    2. Solve edges in $B(G^*)$: for each $v^* \in O(I(G^*))$ that is incident to some edges in $B(G^*)$:
        (a) If v^* is incident to at least 2 edges in $B(G^*)$, then assign one edge with inflow and the others with outflow (both with respect to v^*);
        (b) If v^* is incident to only 1 edge in $B(G^*)$, then assign this edge with an arbitrary direction.
    3. Remove $O(G^*)$ from G^*, and let $G^* := I(G^*)$ where $B(G^*)$ will serve as the new boundary.

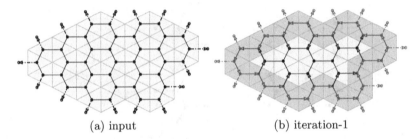

(a) input   (b) iteration-1

Fig. 7. Solving Clusters. A cluster (a) can be completely solved by Procedure 4. (b) shows the first iteration of front-advancing, where edges in $O(G^*)$ (red) and edges in $B(G^*)$ (blue) are solved in step 1 and step 2; Thereafter, edges in $I(G^*)$ (black) will be solved in step 4 using divide-and-conquer.

    4. Partition the updated G^* into trees and clusters by Procedure 1, then solve each of them by cases:
      (a) For each tree sub-component, solve it using Procedure 2;
      (b) For each cluster sub-component, call Procedure 4 recursively.

Procedure 4 always terminates with a valid cutting flow solution and will not get stuck anywhere else, which leads to the following Lemma 4:

Lemma 4. A cluster G^* is always solvable regardless of the boundary condition.

3.4   Solving General Meshes

For an arbitrary simply-connected planar triangular mesh M, the dual graph G^* is in general a union of trees and clusters. We do "divide-and-conquer" again, similar to the way we handle the inner part of a cluster (Section 3.3). But the difference is that, here the boundary condition for a general G^* is specified by user and could be arbitrary. Even worse, if G^* itself is a tree and the given boundary condition is uniform, it has been shown unsolvable. Fortunately, we can prove that this is the only case that does not admit any solution. In any other case, i.e. G^* has a mixed boundary condition or has at least one cluster sub-component, we can always find a solution. Algorithm 1 shows the procedures to process a general G^*, Theorem 1 justifies the solvability.

Algorithm 1 (Solving Simply-Connected Domain)

  – *Input*: A simply-connected planar G^* with arbitrary boundary condition.
  – *Output*: A cutting flow for G^*.
  – *Procedure*:
    1. If G^* is a tree with uniform boundary, report unsolvable and exit.
    2. Partition G^* into sub-components $\{G_1^*, \cdots, G_n^*\}$ (by Procedure 1).
    3. For each tree sub-component G_i^*:
      (a) If it has leaves with uniform boundary, call Procedure 3 to preprocess it and then call Procedure 2 to solve it;
      (b) Otherwise, call Procedure 2 directly to solve it.
    4. For each cluster sub-component G_j^*, call Procedure 4 to solve it directly.

Theorem 1. *A simply-connected planar triangular mesh M (with dual graph G^*) has cutting flow solutions unless and only unless G^* is a tree and the boundary condition is uniform.*

Corollary 1. *A simply-connected planar triangular mesh M (with dual graph G^*) is solvable if boundary condition is mixed.*

4   Solutions: Extended Settings

Here we show how to solve more complicated cases.

4.1   Multiply-Connected Planar Domain

If a planar mesh M has more than one boundary (i.e. a topological disk with one or more holes), it can be cut into to a simply-connected planar domain. This can be easily done on the dual graph G^* by a Breadth-First-Search (BFS), finding and removing a set of edges $\mathfrak{E}$, turning G^* into a tree $\overline{G^*} := G^*/\mathfrak{E}$ (Figure 8). Whenever we remove an e^*, assign it with an arbitrary flow direction. Obviously, the resulting $\overline{G^*}$ has a mixed boundary because every edge in $\mathfrak{E}$ will introduce an inflow and an outflow on the boundary of $\overline{G^*}$. By Corollary 1, $\overline{G^*}$ can always be solved by Algorithm 1.

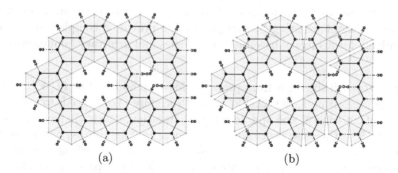

(a)   (b)

Fig. 8. Multiply-connected planar domain (a) can be converted to simply-connected planar domain (b) with mixed boundary condition by removing a set of edges $\mathfrak{E}$ (dotted red) from G^*

Theorem 2. *A multiply-connected planar domain is always solvable.*

4.2   Multiply-Connected Non-planar Domain

If the input mesh M is multiply-connected but not planar, it must be a surface with handles (i.e. genus greater than 0), with or without boundary. This can be solved in exactly the same way as in Section 4.1. Therefore we have:

Theorem 3. *A multiply-connected non-planar domain is always solvable.*

4.3 Simply-Connected Non-planar Domain

If a planar mesh M is both simply-connected and non-planar, it must be a closed surface of genus zero (i.e. topological sphere). Such a mesh can be partitioned to two simply-connected pieces, each with a boundary. To make things simple, we partition G^* into: $G^* = G_1^* \cup G_2^*$ by removing a set of edges $\mathfrak{E}$, where G_1^* consists of a single vertex v_0^* and $\mathfrak{E}$ consists of three edges in G^* that are incident to v_0^*. Then we assign one edge in $\mathfrak{E}$ with inflow and the other two with outflow (all with respect to v_0^*). Now both G_1^* and G_2^* are simply-connected planar domains with mixed boundary condition. By Corollary 1 we have:

Theorem 4. A simply-connected non-planar domain is always solvable.

4.4 Free Boundary

For an input mesh M with boundary but without specified boundary flow directions, regardless it is simply-connected or multiply-connected, planar or non-planar, we can simply assign the boundary of G^* with both inflow and outflow, therefore turning a free boundary graph into a mixed boundary graph that is always solvable according to Corollary 1.

Theorem 5. A free boundary mesh is always solvable.

5   Conclusions and Remarks

In this paper we study the problem of converting a prismatic mesh to a tetrahedral mesh without inserting Steiner points. We provide a complete solution to this problem for arbitrary base mesh topologies and arbitrary boundary conditions.

Complexity: All the algorithms proposed here are bounded by $O\left(|V^*| + |E^*|\right)$ in time. In Algorithm 1, the "divide" part (Procedure 1) only needs to keep track of the set of cut edges $\mathfrak{E}$ and update it in each iteration, which will have an overall cost of $O\left(|E^*|\right)$ (because every edge will appear in $\mathfrak{E}$ in at most one iteration). For the "conquer" part (Procedure 2, 3 and 4), it is easy to verify that every edge in the original input will only be solved once in the whole process, therefore the overall cost is bounded by $O\left(|V^*| + |E^*|\right)$. For any other combination presented in Section 4, it will take an extra pre-processing step in linear time (i.e. either a BFS on G^* or a traverse of the boundary of G^*). Therefore the time complexity is still $O\left(|V^*| + |E^*|\right)$.

Limitations: The algorithms proposed in this paper only work on an input prismatic mesh with given qualities but are not designed to improve the quality of the elements. This work only considers topological (or combinatorial) information but not the geometric aspect, plus that Steiner points are not allowed. Therefore it may result in skewed tetrahedra if the given prismatic mesh has some bad elements. However, the mesh quality can be improved, either using pre-processing (e.g. [6]) or post-processing (e.g. [2,5]), which are beyond the scope of this paper but would be an interesting direction for further exploration.

References

1. Albertelli, G., Crawfis, R.A.: Efficient subdivision of finite-element datasets into consistent tetrahedra. In: Proceedings of the 8th Conference on Visualization, VIS 1997, pp. 213–219. IEEE Computer Society Press, Los Alamitos (1997)
2. Au, P., Dompierre, J., Labbé, P., Guibault, F., Camarero, R.: Proposal of benchmarks for 3D unstructured tetrahedral mesh optimization. In: Proceedings of the 7th International Meshing, pp. 459–478 (1998)
3. Connell, S.D., Braaten, M.E.: Semi-structured mesh generation for 3d Navier-Stokes calculations. In: AIAA 12th Computational Fluid Dynamics Conference, pp. 369–380 (1995)
4. Dompierre, J., Labbé, P., Vallet, M.-G., Camarero, R.: How to subdivide pyramids, prisms, and hexahedra into tetrahedra. In: 8th International Meshing Roundtable, pp. 195–204 (1999)
5. Freitag, L.A., Ollivier-Gooch, C.: Tetrahedral mesh improvement using swapping and smoothing. International Journal for Numerical Methods in Engineering 40(21), 3979–4002 (1998)
6. Jiao, X.: Face offsetting: A unified approach for explicit moving interfaces. J. Comput. Phys. 220, 612–625 (2006)
7. Loehner, R.: Matching semi-structured and unstructured grids for Navier-Stokes calculations. In: AIAA 11th Computational Fluid Dynamics Conference, pp. 555–564 (1993)
8. Longest, W., Kleinstreuer, C.: Comparison of blood particle deposition models for non-parallel flow domains. Journal of Biomechanics 36(3), 421–430 (2003)
9. Max, N., Becker, B., Crawfis, R.: Flow volumes for interactive vector field visualization. In: Proceedings of the 4th Conference on Visualization, VIS 1993, pp. 19–24. IEEE Computer Society, Washington, DC (1993)
10. N'dri, D., Garon, A., Fortin, A.: A new stable space-time formulation for two-dimensional and three-dimensional incompressible viscous flow. International Journal for Numerical Methods in Fluids 37(8), 865–884 (2001)
11. Pirzadeh, S.: Unstructured viscous grid generation by advancing layers method. In: AIAA 12th Computational Fluid Dynamics Conference (1993)
12. Pirzadeh, S.: Three-dimensional unstructured viscous grids by the advancing-layers method. AIAA Journal 34(1), 43–49 (1996)
13. Taylor, C.A., Hughes, T.J.R., Zarins, C.K.: Finite element modeling of blood flow in arteries. Computer Methods in Applied Mechanics and Engineering 158(1-2), 155–196 (1998)
14. Yin, X., Han, W., Gu, X., Yau, S.-T.: The cutting pattern problem for tetrahedral mesh generation. In: Quadros, W.R. (ed.) Proceedings of the 20th International Meshing Roundtable, vol. 90, pp. 217–236. Springer, Heidelberg (2011)

Segmentation of Skin Lesions Using Level Set Method

Zhen Ma and João Manuel R.S. Tavares

Instituto de Engenharia Mecânica e Gestão Industrial,
Faculdade de Engenharia, Universidade do Porto
Rua Dr. Roberto Frias, s/n, 4200-465 Porto, Portugal

Abstract. Diagnosis of skin cancers with dermoscopy has been widely accepted
as a clinical routine. However, the diagnostic accuracy using dermoscopy relies
on the subjective judgment of the dermatologist. To solve this problem, a computer-aided diagnosis system is demanded. Here, we propose a level set method
to fulfill the segmentation of skin lesions presented in dermoscopic images. The
differences between normal skin and skin lesions in the color channels are
combined to define the speed function, with which the evolving curve can be
guided to reach the boundary of skin lesions. The proposed algorithm is robust
against the influences of noise, hair, and skin textures, and provides a flexible
way for segmentation. Numerical experiments demonstrated the effectiveness
of the novel algorithm.

keywords: medical imaging, melanoma, image segmentation, level set method.

1   Introduction

Nowadays, skin cancer has become one of the most frequent forms of cancer [1, 2].
An early diagnosis of skin cancer is critical for improving the prognosis, because
patients with certain conditions, for example, the melanoma, can have a very high
survival rate if the cancers are detected at the early stages and treated properly [3].
Dermoscopy is a non-invasive imaging technique developed to assist this diagnostic
process, and has been reported to considerably improve the detection rate of skin
cancers [4]. Nonetheless, it was also pointed out that the diagnostic accuracy using
dermoscopy largely depends on dermatologists' experience [5]. In order to eliminate
this subjectivity, a computer-aided diagnosis (CAD) system is demanded.

The first step of a CAD system is to segment skin lesions in the images; the accuracy of segmentation has a deterministic influence on the later analysis. The appearance of skin lesions varies considerably among different skin conditions; meanwhile,
the influences of noise, hairs, skin texture, and air bubbles may appear simultaneously
in the image and make the segmentation even harder. Many algorithms have been
proposed to solve the segmentation problem, and the majority of them are based on
thresholding and clustering. For example, a double thresholding process was used in
[6] to segment the boundaries of skin lesions based on the intensity of the converted
images. A dermatologist-like tumor extraction algorithm and its improved version
were developed in [7, 8] that combined the thresholding with the iterative region
growing for segmentation. A 2D color clustering algorithm was proposed in [9];

Y.J. Zhang and J.M.R.S. Tavares (Eds.): CompIMAGE 2014, LNCS 8641, pp. 228–233, 2014.

a supervised algorithm based on a neural network and an unsupervised algorithm based on modified JSEG algorithm were proposed in [10] and [11], respectively.

The level set method was initially developed to track curve evolution in computational physics; however, it has been successfully applied to many areas of image processing [12]. For the segmentation of dermoscopic images, the level set method is less sensitive to the influence of noise; and the implicit tracking provides an efficient way to obtain the boundary and the regions of skin lesions simultaneously. Here, a new algorithm based on the level set method was proposed to fulfil the segmentation task. Following the statistical features of dermoscopic images in different color spaces, the contrasts of the lightness and saturation between the skin lesions and the surrounding normal skin were used as the clues for segmentation and were combined to define a region-based external force, following which the evolving curve can contract to the boundary of the skin lesion in a robust way.

In the next section, the level set method is reviewed; then, the proposed algorithm is introduced, including the equation of motion and the evolution process; afterwards, numerical experiments are presented, and according to the segmentation results, implementation issues of the algorithm are discussed. In the last section, the conclusions and perspectives of future work are indicated.

2   Methodology

The level set method was proposed to solve the topological changes during the curve evolution [13]. In this method, the evolving curve is embedded into a higher-dimensional level set function $\phi(x, y, t)$ as its zero level set, and the evolution is tracked by finding the zero level set of the function $\phi(x, y, t)$ at the time t. The equation of motion of a level set method is normally written as:

$$\frac{\partial \phi}{\partial t} + F|\nabla \phi| = 0, \tag{1}$$

where $\phi(x, y, t)$ is the level set function and F is the speed function. The main idea of using the level set method for segmentation is to model the segmentation as a process of curve evolution. Hence, a proper speed function needs to be defined, with which the curve can reach the object boundary and achieve a stable status there.

2.1   Equation of Motion

The color distribution of skin lesions is normally inhomogeneous. If the curve evolves inside the region of skin lesions, it can be easily attracted to the inner boundaries and cause wrong segmentation. Therefore, in the proposed algorithm, the curve evolution is constrained to contraction in the region of normal skin. By this way, the initial curves are required to cover the entire regions of the skin lesions. The values of the level set function $\phi(x, y, 0)$ are then defined as the signed distance function to the initial curves with positive (negative) sign inside (outside) the curves.

The lightness difference between normal skin and skin lesions provides an important clue for segmentation. Nevertheless, the appearance of skin lesions has large variations among different conditions, and in many cases, its main dissimilarity to the normal skin is the chromaticity which is often perceptually affected by lightness variations. Thus, in order to use the color information efficiently, the RGB color space in the images are converted to the *CIE L*a*b** and *CIE L*u*v** color spaces. Although the lightness is separated from the color representation in the two *CIE* color spaces, the chromaticity channels a^*, b^*, u^* and v^* are coordinates in the color diagram and are unsuitable to be used directly to define the speed function. Instead, the color saturation was adopted to combine the lightness and chromaticity for segmentation. Saturation is a measure that describes the colorfulness of a color relative to its lightness, but is not officially defined in the *CIE* color system. The definition of saturation in computer vision was adopted here with its value calculated as:

$$S = \begin{cases} 0 & \text{if } R + G + B = 0 \\ 1 - \frac{min(R,G,B)}{(R+G+B)/3} & \text{otherwise} \end{cases} . \tag{2}$$

Then, the equation of motion of the proposed level set model is defined as:

$$\frac{\partial \phi}{\partial t} + P_L(x,y) * P_S(x,y) * (1 + \kappa)|\nabla \phi| = 0, \tag{3}$$

where κ is the curve curvature; $P_L(x,y)$ and $P_S(x,y)$ are the Gaussian probability density distribution function of the lightness and saturation channels of the normal skin, respectively. The curvature defined in the speed function acts as the internal force to smooth the curve during the evolution.

The speed function in Eq. (3) includes the statistical information of lightness and saturation values of normal skin. However, this information is unavailable before segmentation; hence, to obtain an approximation of these values, the Otsu's method [14] is applied to classify the image pixels based on the lightness values. Supposing Ω_0 is the set composed by pixels that represent the normal skin according to the classification of the Otsu's method, the following region is used to calculate the statistical values:

$$\Omega_S = \{(x,y)|-50 < \phi(x,y,0) < 0\} \cap \Omega_0. \tag{4}$$

The region Ω_S belongs to a neighboring external band of the initial curves; as the skin lesions are completely inside the initial curves, this region can provide an approximation of the statistical distributions of the lightness and saturation of the normal skin. These statistical values are then updated along with the curve evolution. With Eq. (3), the evolving curves will contract to the places where either the lightness or the saturation is appreciably different to normal skin.

2.2   Evolution

As referred before, the $a^*, b^* u^*, v^*$ channels in the *CIE L*a*b** and *L*u*v** color spaces are the positions of a color relative to the color bases and diagram. Their locations reflect the perceptual difference between the normal skin and skin lesions; pixels of the same group should have coordinates near each other, and pixels from the different group should have coordinates with a large distance. Accordingly, the image pixels can be classified into two groups based on their distances to the spatial color centers of normal skin and skin lesions. Nonetheless, the spatial centers of the two groups are unknown either. Yet, given that the skin lesions are inside the evolving curves, a neighboring external region Ω_S is used to calculate the spatial centers of normal skin in the color space as:

$$\Omega_S^{(t)} = \{(x, y) | -50 < \phi(x, y, t) < 0\}, \tag{5}$$

and the internal region of the curve is used to calculate the centers of the skin lesions. Along with the contraction of the curve, the spatial centers of the skin lesions and the surrounding normal skin will become more accurate. With the classification based on the Euclidean distance in the color spaces, the statistical distribution of the saturation values of normal skin can be better reflected. Hence, the statistical vales are updated during the evolution in the region $\Omega_0^{(t)} \cap \Omega_S^{(t)}$ where $\Omega_0^{(t)}$ is the set composed by pixels representing the normal skin at the time t. Additionally, in light with the color classification, the speed function in Eq. (3) is modified as:

$$F^*(x, y) = \begin{cases} 0.5 * F(x, y) & \text{if } (x, y) \text{ represents skin lesions at the time } t \\ F(x, y) & \text{otherwise} \end{cases}. \tag{6}$$

With the modified speed function, the evolving curve can be further attached to the boundary of skin lesions.

3   Experiments

An image database containing 68 dermoscopic images was used to test the performance of the proposed segmentation algorithm, in which 58 were diagnosed as nevus and 10 as melanomas. CUDA implementation of the proposed algorithm was adopted to enhance the computational efficiency. The obtained segmentation results were quite promising and, for their quantitative analysis, the exclusive-or measure defined below was used to evaluate the difference between the ground truth and the segmentation result:

$$D(C_0, C_1) = Area\big(inside(C_0) \oplus inside(C_1)\big)/Area\big(inside(C_0)\big), \tag{7}$$

where C_0 is the ground true boundary, C_1 is the contour obtained by the algorithm, and $\oplus$ is the exclusive-or operator. Fig. 1 illustrates four segmentation examples in the image database; one can verify the robustness of the proposed approach against the different imaging conditions. For the proposed algorithm, the mean and the standard deviation of the exclusive-or measure on this image database are 0.1036 and 0.0485, respectively.

There is no restrict on the shape of the initial curves in the proposed algorithm; however, the initial curves are required to cover the complete region of the skin lesions. If the neighboring region of the initial curves is affected appreciably by unwanted influences, the algorithm may not achieve satisfactory results; to avoid this situation, the initial curves are defined manually. Meanwhile, in the segmentation, the size of the neighboring region of the evolving curves affects the statistical information of normal skin around the skin lesions. A larger neighboring region around the initial curve can capture the variations of normal skin more accurately, but is more likely to introduce unwanted influences. The band size was chosen as 50 in the experiments and led to satisfactory results.

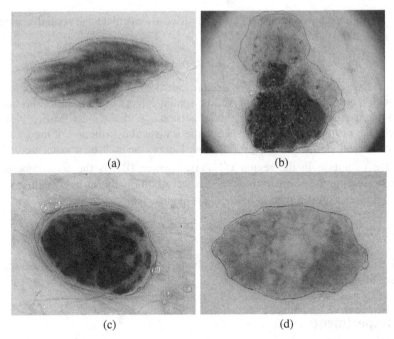

(a)   (b)

(c)   (d)

Fig. 1. Segmentation examples using the proposed algorithm, red contours – segmentation results of the proposed algorithm; blue contours – ground truths: (a) image with nevi, $D(C_0, C_1) = 0.0833$; (b) image with melonoma, $D(C_0, C_1) = 0.1590$; (c) image with nevi, $D(C_0, C_1) = 0.0868$; (d) image with melanoma, $D(C_0, C_1) = 0.0447$

4   Conclusion

A novel level set method was proposed to segment skin lesions. The proposed algorithm combines the various information contained in dermoscopic images, and defines the speed function based on the converted color channels. Numerical experiments illustrated the effectiveness and robustness of the algorithm, and the implementation issues were discussed based on the tests.

The differences between the skin lesions and normal skin were efficiently used in the proposed algorithm. With the region-based external forces, the proposed algorithm is not sensitive to the unwanted influences presented in the images. The future work will continue to improve its robustness and accuracy.

Acknowledgement. This work was done in the scope of the project "A novel framework for supervised mobile assessment and risk triage of skin lesions via non-invasive screening", with the reference PTDC/BBB-BMD/3088/2012, financially supported by Fundação para a Ciência e a Tecnologia (FCT), in Portugal.

References

1. Jemal, A., Siegel, R., Xu, J., Ward, E.: Cancer statistics. CA Cancer J. Clin. 60(5), 288–296 (2010)
2. American Cancer Society. Cancer facts & figures (2013),
   http://www.cancer.org/acs/groups/content/
   @epidemiologysurveilance/documents/document/acspc-036845.pdf
3. Balch, C.M., Buzaid, A.C., Soong, S.J., Atkins, M.B., Cascinelli, N., Coit, D.G., Fleming, I.D., Gershenwald, J.E., Houghton Jr., A., Kirkwood, J.M., McMasters, K.M., Mihm, M.F., Morton, D.L., Reintgen, D.S., Ross, M.I., Sober, A., Thompson, J.A., Thompson, J.: Final version of the American Joint Committee on Cancer staging system for cutaneous melanoma. J. Clin. Oncol. 19(16), 3635–3648 (2001)
4. Grin, C.M., Kopf, A.W., Welkovich, B., Bart, R.S., Levenstein, M.: Accuracy in the clinical diagnosis of malignant melanoma. Arch. Dermatol. 126(6), 763–766 (1990)
5. Kittler, H., Pehamberger, H., Wolff, K., Binder, M.: Diagnostic accuracy of dermoscopy. Lancet Oncol. 3(3), 159–165 (2002)
6. Xu, L., Jackowski, M., Goshtasby, A., Roseman, D., Bines, S., Yu, C., Dhawan, A., Huntley, A.: Segmentation of skin cancer images. Image Vision Comput. 17(1), 65–74 (1999)
7. Iyatomi, H., Oka, H., Saito, M., Miyake, A., Kimoto, M., Yamagami, J., Kobayashi, S., Tanikawa, A., Hagiwara, M., Ogawa, K., Argenziano, G., Soyer, H.P., Tanaka, M.: Quantitative assessment of tumor extraction from dermoscopy images and evaluation of computer-based extraction methods for automatic melanoma diagnostic system. Melanoma Res. 16(2), 183–190 (2006)
8. Iyatomi, H., Oka, H., Celebi, M.E., Hashimoto, M., Hagiwara, M., Tanaka, M., Ogawa, K.: An improved Internet-based melanoma screening system with dermatologist-like tumor area extraction algorithm. Comput. Med. Imaging Graph. 32(7), 566–579 (2008)
9. Schmid, P.: Segmentation of digitized dermatoscopic images by two-dimensional color clustering. IEEE T. Med. Imaging 18(2), 164–171 (1999)
10. Donadey, T., Serruys, C., Giron, A., Aitken, G., Vignali, J.-P., Triller, R., Fertil, B.: Boundary detection of black skin tumors using an adaptive radial-based approach. In: SPIE Med. Imaging, vol. 3379, pp. 810–816 (2000)
11. Celebi, M.E., Aslandogan, Y.A., Stoecker, W.V., Iyatomi, H., Oka, H., Chen, X.: Unsupervised border detection in dermoscopy images. Skin Res. Technol. 13(4), 454–462 (2007)
12. Ma, Z., Tavares, J.M.R.S., Jorge, R.N.M., Mascarenhas, T.: A review of algorithms for medical image segmentation and their applications to the female pelvic cavity. Comput Methods Biomech. Biomed. Engin. 13(2), 235–246 (2010)
13. Osher, S.J., Sethian, J.: Fronts propagating with curvature-dependent speed: algorithms based on Hamilton-Jacobi formulations. J. Comput. Phys. 79(1), 12–49 (1998)
14. Otsu, N.: A threshold selection method from gray-level histograms. IEEE T. Syst. Man Cyb. 9(1), 62–66 (1979)

Wavelet-Based Computer-Aided Detection of Bright Lesions in Retinal Fundus Images*

Isabel N. Figueiredo and Sunil Kumar

CMUC, Department of Mathematics, University of Coimbra, Portugal
{isabelf,skumar}@mat.uc.pt

Abstract. Computer-aided detection and diagnosis of diabetic retinopathy with retinal fundus images is the necessary step for the implementation of a large scale screening effort in regions where ophthalmologists are not available. In this paper we propose computer-aided binary detector of bright lesions in retinal fundus images. It is based on wavelets for multiresolution feature discrimination and support vector machine (SVM) for classification. After thresholding the sub-band images resulting from the Isotropic Undecimated Wavelet Transform (IUWT) decomposition of the input image, we employ an approach based on the image Hessian eigenvalues and multi-scale image analysis, for designing good feature descriptors of bright lesions. These are afterwards used in the SVM model classifier. Experimental results on our current data set show that the proposed method is efficient and achieves a very good success rate.

Keywords: Diabetic retinopathy, Bright lesions, Fundus images, Computer-aided diagnosis.

1 Introduction

Diabetic retinopathy (DR) is a condition occurring in persons with diabetes, which causes progressive damage to the retina, the light sensitive lining at the back of the eye. It is a serious sight-threatening complication of diabetes. Often there are no visual symptoms in the early stages of diabetic retinopathy. Early detection and treatment can limit the potential for significant vision loss from diabetic retinopathy. Therefore, it is vital, for a diabetic patient to have regular eye examinations. Fundus images are visual records which document the current ophthalmoscopic appearance of a patient's retina, the retinal vasculature, and the optic nerve head (optic disc) from which the retinal vessels enter the eye.

Diabetic retinopathy lesions may be classified as red lesions, such as microaneurysms and hemorrhages, and bright lesions, such as exudates, drusen and cotton-wool spots. In this paper, our aim is to develop a system for the detection of bright lesions in retinal fundus images. Some computer-aided systems for

---

* This work was partially supported by the project PTDC/MATNAN/0593/2012, and also by CMUC and FCT (Portugal), through European program COMPETE/ FEDER and project PEst-C/MAT/UI0324/2011).

Y.J. Zhang and J.M.R.S. Tavares (Eds.): CompIMAGE 2014, LNCS 8641, pp. 234–240, 2014.

bright lesions can be found in [1–3], and a survey of various methods related to diabetic retinopathy is available in [4].

In this work we develop a combined wavelet and support vector machine based system for automated detection of bright lesions. In a first step we derive efficient feature descriptors by thresholding different sub-band images resulting from the Isotropic Undecimated Wavelet Transform (IUWT) [5] decomposition of the original image, and employing an image analysis approach, relying on the image Hessian eigenvalues and multiscale analysis. In the second step we use these derived features as inputs to the SVM model, for binary classification. The experimental results on our current dataset show that the proposed method gives 95% accuracy. The motivation for using the wavelet-based approach proposed in this paper is related to the fact that the IUWT has been used, recently and with success, in image processing of retinal fundus images, for vessel detection and measurement [6]. Moreover, the success of the image Hessian eigenvalues and multiscale analysis, in designing shape filters for automatic detection of blood and bleeding in wireless capsule endoscopy images in [7–9], motivated the authors to use a similar, yet different approach in this paper. Finally, the good discriminative characteristic of the wavelet-based bright lesion detectors introduced in this work, has induced the authors to using a SVM binary classifier, for automated classification.

After this introduction the rest of this paper consists of Section 2, where the methodology is described, and Section 3, where the experimental results are reported as well as some conclusions and future research plans.

2 Methodology

In order to improve the quality of the original input RGB color fundus image, we use enhanced images obtained with the technique described in [10, 11]. We then process the green channel I_G of the enhanced RGB image (a channel which exhibits a good contrast between bright regions versus background and dark structures), using the methodology explained in this section. It includes the detection of the optic disc (OD), a bright structure that should be avoided in all the detection procedure, for not to being misunderstood, by the detectors, as a bright lesion.

2.1 Optic Disc Localization and Detection

We use a strategy based on the following four main steps, and that is illustrated in Figure 1 for a single image.

1. Firstly, the following curvature identification function (herein called $\mathcal{OD}_{loc}$) is applied for locating the OD

$$\mathcal{OD}_{loc} := -\mathcal{K}\min(\mathcal{H}, 0),$$

where $\mathcal{K}$ and $\mathcal{H}$ are, respectively, the Gaussian and mean curvatures of the image I_G, interpreted as the graph of a function defined over the pixel domain.

In fact, the OD appears as a concave region (protrusion) in the green channel I_G. Mathematically, this $\mathcal{OD}_{loc}$ function filters out the convex parts of the graph of I_G, and its value is closely related to the size of the protrusions in the image. Consequently, the OD location in the frame can be inferred by identifying the locations where $\mathcal{OD}_{loc}$ is higher. In [12, 13] the same curvature function was used (with success) for detecting colonic polyps (which are round-shaped protusion objects), in wireless capsule endoscopy images.

2. Secondly, to detect the OD boundary we extract 15% highest pixels in $\mathcal{OD}_{loc}$. The connected component, in the thresholded image, whose product between its area and its $\mathcal{OD}_{loc}$ mean intensity is maximum, is considered to be the location of the OD. Consequently, its centroid is the estimated OD center location.

3. Thirdly, based on the OD localization and an estimated general OD size, we define a small region of interest (ROI), containing the previous OD location. The edges of this ROI are also computed using Canny edge detector [14].

4. Finally, to the edges of this ROI, a circular Hough transform (CHT) [15, 16] is applied to segment the OD.

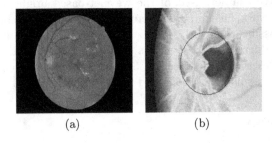

(a)   (b)

Fig. 1. (a) Enhanced image with OD localized. (b) The determined OD boundary.

2.2 Wavelet-Based Bright Lesion Detectors

The Isotropic Undecimated Wavelet Transform (IUWT) [5] is characterized by a a simple implementation of its direct and inverse transform. Denoting by $C_0 = I_G$ the enhanced green channel of the input image, then at each iteration j, the scaling coefficients C_j are computed by lowpass filtering (where filtering is applied by convolution and separably along each dimension), and the wavelet coefficients W_j (hereafter called wavelet levels) are defined just by scaling coefficient subtraction, i.e, $W_{j+1} = C_{j+1} - C_j$. Starting with the filter $h_0 = [1/16, 1/4, 3/8, 1/4, 1/16]$, which is derived from the cubic B-spline, at each scale $j \geq 2$ the filter h_j is augmented by inserting $2^j - 1$ zeros between each pair of adjacent coefficients of h_0. The scaling coefficient C_{j+1} is defined from the previous C_j using separable convolution with h_j in each dimension. The reproduction of the original image I_G is achieved just by adding all the wavelet coefficients and the final computed scaling coefficient, as follows: $I_G = C_m + \sum_{j=1}^{m} W_j$.

For each enhanced image we compute $I_n = \sum_{j=2}^{n} W_j$, for $n = 2, 3, 4, 5,$, with W_j the wavelet level at iteration j of the enhanced green channel I_G. Then, we extract the 20% highest pixels in I_n to identify the bright regions. We then take the product of this thresholded image with I_n and also with the optic disc mask (created from the OD location). The resulting image is denoted by F_n. The first and second rows of Figure 2 show the four images I_n and F_n, respectively, corresponding to the input image displayed in Figure 1. As expected, and as it can be observed in this Figure 2, due to the IUWT definition, larger details/features/objects are better perceived with higher wavelet levels. We also apply to F_n the adaptive Wiener filter, using neighborhoods of size $[15, 15]$, for smoothing and enhancing. As a result of these thresholding and smoothing operations, the bright lesions appear as isolated bright elongated patches or blobs outstanding to their surroundings (see the second row in Figure 2).

We then look for blob or elongated bright structures in each image F_n, using the eigenvalues of the image Hessian matrix and multiscale image analysis. For each scalar image $F_n : \Omega \subseteq \mathbb{R}^2 \to \mathbb{R}$, where Ω is the pixel domain, we first define the Hessian matrix of one point (x, y), and at a scale s, by

$$H_s(x, y) = \begin{pmatrix} (F_n)_{xx}^s(x, y) & (F_n)_{xy}^s(x, y) \\ (F_n)_{xy}^s(x, y) & (F_n)_{yy}^s(x, y) \end{pmatrix}.$$

Here $(F_n)_{xx}^s$, $(F_n)_{xy}^s$ and $(F_n)_{yy}^s$ are the second-order partial derivatives of F_n and the scale s is involved in the calculation of these derivatives. Suppose $\lambda_{s,1}$ and $\lambda_{s,2}$ are the two eigenvalues of the Hessian matrix H_s. Note that in a blob region, these two eigenvalues have the same sign and similar magnitudes, whereas if one eigenvalue's absolute value is large and the other one is small or close to zero, an elongated structure is locally predominant (see [17]). Without loss of generality we assume that $|\lambda_{s,1}| \leq |\lambda_{s,2}|$. Then, setting $G_s = \lambda_{s,1}^2 + \lambda_{s,2}^2$,

$$f_1 = \exp\left(-\beta G_s^2\right) \quad \text{and} \quad f_2 = 1 - \exp\left(-\alpha \left(\frac{\lambda_{s,1}}{\lambda_{s,2}}\right)^2\right),$$

and motivated by [17], we define the blob (B_s) and ridge (R_s) detectors (at each point of the domain) by

$$B_s = \begin{cases} 0, & \text{if } \lambda_{s,1}\lambda_{s,2} < 0 \text{ or } |\lambda_{s,2} - \lambda_{s,1}| > \delta \\ (1 - f_1)f_2, & \text{otherwise,} \end{cases}$$

and

$$R_s = \begin{cases} 0, & \text{if } \lambda_{s,2} > 0, \\ (1 - f_1)(1 - f_2), & \text{otherwise,} \end{cases}$$

with α and β parameters which control the sensitivity of the functions and δ a user chosen threshold. Therefore, B_s or R_s are close to 1 if a blob or a tubular structure, respectively, is present at the current location. In order to automatically detect bright lesions of different sizes, a multiscale approach is now necessary. The response of the detector functions B_s and R_s will be maximum at a scale that approximately matches the size of the bright lesion to be detected. Hence, at each point of the domain we define the functions

$$B_n = \max_{s_{min} \leq s \leq s_{max}} (B_s.F_n), \qquad R_n = \max_{s_{min} \leq s \leq s_{max}} (R_s.F_n),$$

where s_{min} and s_{max} are the minimum and maximum scales at which the bright lesions are expected to be found. The final detectors are the sums $S_n = B_n + R_n$, for $n = 2, 3, 4, 5$ (these are shown in the last row of Figure 1). Finally, we consider the maximum of each function S_n as inputs to the SVM model classifier, described in the next section.

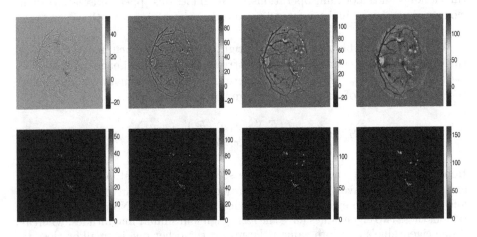

Fig. 2. First row: Images $I_n, n = 2, 3, 4, 5$. Second row: Detectors $S_n, n = 2, 3, 4, 5$.

3   Experimental Results and Conclusion

We now assess the effectiveness of the proposed bright lesion detection methodology. We performed experiments on our current data set, consisting of 112 representative bright lesion images and 222 representative images without bright lesions. Figure 3 shows the ROC (receiver operating characteristic) curves of the four different features (the maximum of S_n, $n = 2, 3, 4, 5$). Each ROC curve, is a graphical plot of the sensitivity, or true positive rate, versus false alarm rate (1-specificity), for a binary classifier system as its discrimination threshold is varied. One can observe from this Figure 3 that the maxima of functions S_n are very promising discriminative features.

For implementation the SVM binary classifier, we consider the library LIB-SVM [18]. The feature vector is built using the maximum value of each function S_n, $n = 2, 3, 4, 5$. In order to avoid over-fitting problem, we exploited 5-fold cross validation. The optimal values of the the regularization and kernel parameters for the SVM classifier were found by grid search [18]. Before training, all features were normalized to the range $[-1, 1]$ to avoid dominance of features with

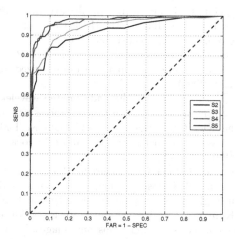

Fig. 3. ROC curve for features corresponding to $S_n, n = 2, 3, 4, 5$ (in the legend Sn represents S_n)

greater numeric ranges. To assess the classification of the current dataset by SVM, we use a standard performance measure, the accuracy (the number of correct predictions divided by the sum of number of positives and negatives). The experimental results show that the proposed methodology achieves 95% accuracy on our current data set.

We close this paper with some conclusions and future plans. We have described a computer-aided procedure for bright lesions detection in retinal fundus images. The method consists of the following main steps: the optic disc location (for avoiding interference in the detection), the determination of the several wavelet levels (that embody the different lesion sizes : small image details are visible in low levels while larger in higher levels), the computation of the sum of the blob and ridge detectors (to account for the different bright lesion shapes : blob-like or tubular-like) and finally the application of the SVM binary model classifier. The current experimental results demonstrate the efficacy of the proposed method. In the future we intend to test it in a much larger data set and analyse the feasibility of using the blob and ridge detectors separately, and combined with extra textural descriptors, with the aim of developing bright lesion shape classification.

References

1. Sánchez, C.I., Hornero, R., López, M.I., Aboy, M., Poza, J., Abásolo, D.: A novel automatic image processing algorithm for detection of hard exudates based on retinal image analysis. Medical Engineering & Physics 30, 350–357 (2008)
2. Phillips, R., Forrester, J., Sharp, P.: Automated detection and quantification of retinal exudates. Graefe's Archive for Clinical and Experimental Ophthalmology 231, 90–94 (1993)

3. Wang, H., Hsu, W., Goh, K.G., Lee, M.L.: An effective approach to detect lesions in color retinal images. In: Proceedings of the IEEE Conference on Computer Vision and Pattern Recognition, vol. 2, pp. 181–186 (2000)
4. Winder, R., Morrow, P., McRitchie, I., Bailie, J., Hart, P.: Algorithms for digital image processing in diabetic retinopathy. Computerized Medical Imaging and Graphics 33, 608–622 (2009)
5. Starck, J.L., Fadili, J., Murtagh, F.: The undecimated wavelet decomposition and its reconstruction. IEEE Transactions on Image Processing 16, 297–309 (2007)
6. Bankhead, P., Scholfield, C.N., McGeown, J.G., Curtis, T.M.: Fast retinal vessel detection and measurement using wavelets and edge location refinement. PloS One 7(3), e32435 (2012)
7. Figueiredo, I.N., Kumar, S., Leal, C., Figueiredo, P.N.: Computer-assisted bleeding detection in wireless capsule endoscopy images. Computer Methods in Biomechanics and Biomedical Engineering: Imaging & Visualization 1, 198–210 (2013)
8. Figueiredo, I.N., Kumar, S., Leal, C., Figueiredo, P.N.: An automatic blood detection algorithm for wireless capsule endoscopy images. In: Tavares, J., Jorge, N. (eds.) Computational Vision and Medical Image Processing, VIPIMAGE 2013, pp. 198–210. Taylor & Francis Group, London (2014) ISBN 978-1-138-00081-0 198–210
9. Kumar, S., Figueiredo, I.N., Graca, C., Falcao, G.: A gpu accelerated algorithm for blood detection in wireless capsule endoscopy images. In: Tavares, J.M., Renato, R.S.N.J. (eds.) Developments in Medical Image Processing and Computational Vision. Lecture Notes in Computational Vision and Biomechanics. Springer (2014)
10. Ferreira, J., Bernardes, R., Baptista, P., Cunha-Vaz, J.: Earmarking retinal changes in a sequence of digital color fundus photographs. In: IFMBE Proc., vol. 11, pp. 1727–1983 (2005)
11. Foracchia, M., Grisan, E., Ruggeri, A.: Luminosity and contrast normalization in retinal images. Medical Image Analysis 9(3), 179–190 (2005)
12. Figueiredo, I.N., Kumar, S., Figueiredo, P.N.: An intelligent system for polyp detection in wireless capsule endoscopy images. In: Tavares, J., Jorge, N. (eds.) Computational Vision and Medical Image Processing, VIPIMAGE 2013, pp. 229–235. Taylor & Francis Group, London (2014)
13. Figueiredo, P.N., Figueiredo, I.N., Prasath, S., Tsai, R.: Automatic polyp detection in pillcam colon 2 capsule images and videos: preliminary feasibility report. Diagnostic and Therapeutic Endoscopy, 1–7 (2011)
14. Canny, J.: A computational approach to edge detection. IEEE Transactions on Pattern Analysis and Machine Intelligence PAMI-8, 679–698 (1986)
15. Hough, P.V.C.: Methods and means for recognizing complex patterns. U.S. Patent 3 069 654 (December 1962)
16. Kimme, C., Ballard, D., Sklansky, J.: Finding circles by an array of accumulators. Commun. ACM 18, 120–122 (1975)
17. Frangi, A.F., Niessen, W.J., Vincken, K.L., Viergever, M.A.: Multiscale vessel enhancement filtering. In: Wells, W.M., Colchester, A.C.F., Delp, S.L. (eds.) MICCAI 1998. LNCS, vol. 1496, pp. 130–137. Springer, Heidelberg (1998)
18. Chang, C.C., Lin, C.J.: LIBSVM: A library for support vector machines. ACM Transactions on Intelligent Systems and Technology 2, 27:1–27:27 (2011)

Computing Probabilistic Optical Flow
Using Markov Random Fields*

Dongzhen Piao[1], Prahlad G. Menon[2,3], and Ole J. Mengshoel[1]

[1] Carnegie Mellon University Silicon Valley, Moffett Field, CA, USA
{dongzhen.piao,ole.mengshoel}@sv.cmu.edu
[2] SYSU-CMU Joint Institute of Engineering, Pittsburgh, PA, USA
[3] Shunde International Joint Research Institute, Shunde, China
pgmenon@andrew.cmu.edu

Abstract. Optical flow methods are often used in image processing, for example for object recognition and image segmentation. Traditional optical flow methods use numerical methods, assuming intensity constancy of pixels' movements. In this work we describe a probabilistic method of modeling the optical flow problem, and discuss the use of Gibbs sampling for optimization of the computed optical flow vector field. In experiments involving test images as well as medical image slices through the short-axis of the left ventricle of the heart, our probabilistic method is compared with the classic Horn-Schunck optical flow method. We demonstrate that our proposed approach probabilistic optical flow method is robust to changes in the shape and intensity of objects tracked. This is a useful property when identifying cardiac structures from time-resolved medical images of the heart, where the shape of the cardiac structures change between consecutive temporal frames of the cardiac cycle.

Keywords: Optical flow, Markov Random Fields, Gibbs Sampling.

1 Introduction

One fundamental problem when processing temporal image sequences is to compute optical flow, *i.e.*, the movement of objects and pixels between consecutive images. Once optical flow is found, it can be used in a wide range of tasks, including image segmentation, 3D shape acquisition, perceptual organization, and object recognition. Many optical flow methods have been investigated, such as differential methods (Horn-Schunck [1] and Lucas-Kanade [2]), region-based matching, frequency-based methods, and phase-based methods.

One key assumption in most existing optical flow methods is the *invariance of pixel intensity*, meaning that the intensity of each pixel in the original image should be the same as the intensity of the corresponding pixel in the moved image. While this assumption often works, it will not hold in many real-world situations due to changing illumination conditions or changing object surface

---

* This research is funded in part by CMU-SYSU Collaborative Innovation Research Center and the SYSU-CMU International Joint Research Institute.

Y.J. Zhang and J.M.R.S. Tavares (Eds.): CompIMAGE 2014, LNCS 8641, pp. 241–247, 2014.

direction. In these circumstances, algorithms that assume invariant pixel intensity often yield poor results. Another problem with most traditional optical flow methods is that they result in lack of smoothness on object boundaries, *i.e.*, they often produce abrupt optical flow changes. In order to get a smooth flow boundary, images usually need to go through a smoothing pre-processing step, before the optical flow method is applied. Alternatively, post-processing can be performed on an optical flow result to make it smoother.

In this paper, we present a new approach of modeling and solving optical flow problems, using probabilistic graphical models. We discuss the intuitions that guide the design of the model, a Markov random field. We show that this method is able to handle changing pixel intensities when an object moves and also performs smoothing of object boundaries, without separate pre- or post-processing operations on the image. Our probabilistic optical flow method has an essential robustness when it comes to variations in pixel brightness, compared to traditional brightness constancy assumptions often made when solving the optical flow problem. This makes our method conducive to application in identification of cardiac structures from time-resolved medical imaging data, wherein the shape and intensity of tracked objects (such as the left ventricle) change between consecutive temporal frames of the cardiac cycle.

2   Probabilistic Optical Flow

Traditional optical flow methods use numerical methods to compute optical flow [3]. In contrast, we assign a probability to each optical flow, thus obtaining the problem of finding the most probable optical flow in a Markov random field.

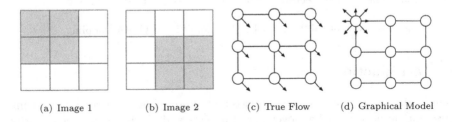

(a) Image 1   (b) Image 2   (c) True Flow   (d) Graphical Model

Fig. 1. Sample images that illustrate a probabilistic Markov random field formulation of optical flow

Imagine that we are trying to find the optical flow from Image 1 to Image 2 in Fig. 1. There is a black 2x2 square in the top left corner of Image 1, and it moved to the bottom right corner in Image 2. The true optical flow is shown in Fig. 1(c). If we didn't know the true flow, how many possible optical flow assignments are there? For simplicity, assume that each pixel in Image 1 can only move one pixel (to its 8 neighboring pixels) or not move at all (shown in Fig. 1(d)). Then each pixel's optical flow has 9 possible assignments. Since there are 9 pixels, there are 9^9 possible assignments. Finding the optimal optical flow involves finding the "best" assignment among these 9^9 possible assignments.

We denote all the pixels in Image 1 as $\boldsymbol{p} = \{p_i\}, i = 1, \ldots, 9$, and the corresponding optical flow as $\boldsymbol{F} = \{F_i\}$. We assign each optical flow instantiation a probability, with higher probability given to instantiations that satisfy the following three intuitions (intensity, distance, and neighbor) better. A Markov Random Field (MRF) [4] is constructed for the optical flow $\boldsymbol{F}$, as seen in Fig. 1(d). Here, each pixel's optical flow $F(p_i)$ is a random variable (the circles), and neighboring pixels' flows are connected by an edge. We define the following three different factors on the MRF.

1. Intensity Factor ϕ_I: $\phi_I(F_i) = \exp(-E_I(F_i))$, where $E_I(F_i)$ is the **Intensity Energy** of optical flow, is defined on each pixel p_i:

$$E_I(F_i) = (I(p_i) - I'(p_i + F_i))^2/\alpha^2. \tag{1}$$

Here, $I(p)$ and $I'(p)$ are the pixel intensities in the first and second images, respectively.[1] The α parameter controls the variance of intensity energy, specifically how much more likely same-intensity movement is compared to changing-intensity movement. In this way, we can deal with images whose object pixel intensities change, greatly broadening the applicability of optical flow methods.

2. Distance Factor ϕ_D: $\phi_D(F_i) = \exp(-E_D(F_i))$, where $E_D(F_i)$ is the **Distance Energy** of optical flow, is defined on each pixel p_i:

$$E_D(F_i) = |F_i|^2/\beta^2. \tag{2}$$

Here, $|F_i|$ is the length of flow vector F_i. The β parameter controls variance of distance energy. **Distance Energy** gives lower energy to shorter optical flow vectors, favoring short movements.

3. Neighbor Factor ϕ_N: $\phi_N(F_i, F_j) = \exp(-E_N(F_i, F_j))$, where $E_N(F_i, F_j)$ is **Neighbor Energy**, is defined on every pair of adjacent pixels $(p_i, p_j) \in \boldsymbol{E}$:

$$E_N(F_i, F_j) = |F_i - F_j|^2/\gamma^2. \tag{3}$$

Here, $|F_i - F_j|$ is the length of the vector difference between F_i and F_j, and γ is a variance parameter. **Neighbor Energy** gives lower energy when neighboring pixels' intensities are similar, thus attempting to let pixels of the same object move together, and smoothing flow transitions at object boundaries.

Adding (1), (2), and (3), the total energy $E(\boldsymbol{F})$ of the probabilistic optical flow model is:

$$E(\boldsymbol{F}) = \sum_i E_I(F_i) + \sum_i E_D(F_i) + \sum_{(i,j) \in \boldsymbol{E}} E_N(F_i, F_j)$$
$$= \sum_i \frac{(I(p_i) - I'(p_i + F_i))^2}{\alpha^2} + \sum_i |F_i|^2/\beta^2 + \sum_{(i,j) \in \boldsymbol{E}} |F_i - F_j|^2/\gamma^2. \tag{4}$$

---

[1] The **Intensity Energy** assigns high energy to flow values that greatly change pixel intensity, making them less likely to happen. On the other hand, if a pixel's intensity didn't change after the movement, i.e., $I(p_i) = I'(p_i + F_i)$, then the energy of that flow will be 0, which makes it more likely to have happened.

The probability distribution over optical flow is $P(\boldsymbol{F}) = \frac{1}{Z}\exp(-E(\boldsymbol{F}))$. We use Gibbs sampling [5] to find the optical flow with highest probability, and use simulated annealing [6] to speed up the sampling process.

3   Experiment

3.1   Methods

We conduct experiments on several images to validate our method. We also compare our results to results from a traditional optical flow method, the Horn-Schunck method [1]. We denote our probabilistic optical flow method as the **POF** method, and the Horn-Schunck method as the **HS** method.

To evaluate optical flow results, we compute the difference between calculated (using **POF** or **HS**) flow vectors and ground truth flow vectors. The magnitude of difference will be available for visual inspection. We also measure **RMSE** (Root Mean Squared Error) of calculated flow vectors. With ground truth flow vectors given as $\boldsymbol{F}^* = \{F_i^*\}, i = 1, \ldots, N$, where N is total number of pixels, the RMSE of any optical flow $\boldsymbol{F}$ is $RMSE(\boldsymbol{F}) = \sqrt{(\sum_i |F_i - F_i^*|^2)/N}$, where $|F_i - F_i^*|$ is the length of the difference between flow vectosr F_i and F_i^*.

3.2   Experiment on Synthetic Images

Fig. 2 contains synthetic images with multiple rectangles with changing intensity. The original and moved images are shown in Fig. 2(a) and Fig. 2(e) respectively. The ground truth of optical flow between these two images is shown in Fig. 2(b), using the color and vector palette in Fig. 2(f). The center of the palette in

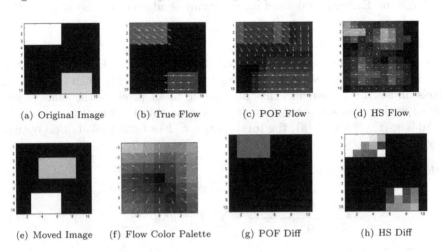

(a) Original Image   (b) True Flow   (c) POF Flow   (d) HS Flow

(e) Moved Image   (f) Flow Color Palette   (g) POF Diff   (h) HS Diff

Fig. 2. Performance comparison of optical flow computation using our POF method in (c) compared to the HS method in (d), using a simulated pair of images in (a) and (e), wherein two rectangular objects move while also changing their intensity

Fig. 2(f) (black area) represents no movement ($F_x = 0, F_y = 0$), and different flow directions are distinguished by different hues. We are only concerned about the movement of the objects (bright rectangles), thus the black background is not included in the comparison.

The optical flow results for the POF and HS methods are shown, respectively, in Fig. 2(c) and Fig. 2(d). The differences between computed flows and ground truth are shown in Fig. 2(g) and Fig. 2(h). A brighter pixel represents a larger magnitude of the difference vector. From Fig. 2(c) and Fig. 2(d), we can see that both methods identified two moving objects. However, the HS method's result has major differences between neighboring pixels, and the flow values are very inconsistent. In contrast, the POF method perfectly captured the true optical flow, see Fig. 2(g). The RMSE is also drastically better for POF: For POF, RMSE = 0.4, while for HS, RMSE = 2.6.

3.3   Experiment on Cardiac Images

In Fig. 3, we show two images of the left ventricle of the heart, seen in a short-axis slice, in consecutive time frames, extracted from York University's Cardiac MRI dataset[2] [7]. The original and moved images correspond to patient 1, slice 5, at time frames 1 and 5 respectively. The left ventricle is identified in both images, by inner boundary and outer boundary. Since ground truth of the true optical flow solution for the entire image was not available, as a substitute ground truth we calculated the movement of the boundaries of the left ventricle, *i.e.*, the endo- and epicardial walls. This was done by segmenting their contours maunually at the first and

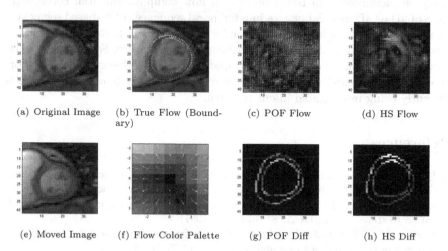

(a) Original Image   (b) True Flow (Boundary)   (c) POF Flow   (d) HS Flow

(e) Moved Image   (f) Flow Color Palette   (g) POF Diff   (h) HS Diff

Fig. 3. Comparison of results of the POF method in (c) and the HS method in (d), using the color palette in (f), when applied to cardiac magnetic resonance images depicting the left ventricle of the heart contracting, as seen between (a) and (e)

---

[2] http://www.cse.yorku.ca/~mridataset/

second time frames, resulting in two independent point-sets, and then computing a regional signed Hausdorff Distance which identifies a vector from each vertex of a first point set to the closest point on the edges of the segmentation contour connecting the second point set [8] (Fig. 3(b)). Only the computed optical flow values on the boundaries of the left ventricle were then compared against this ground truth to calculate RMSE; differences in the computed vectors are shown in Fig. 3(g) and Fig. 3(h). Again, the POF method performed better, with POF RMSE = 2.1 and HS RMSE = 2.4.

4   Conclusion

In this paper we present a new method for modeling and computing optical flow in images, using a probabilistic formulation. In our POF method, we use three different factors to constrain flow values, namely intensity, distance, and neighbor factors. We discuss its advantages over traditional optical flow methods in terms of its ability to be robust to changing pixel intensity. It also results in consistent flow values among neighboring pixels and within tracked objects, and yields smooth transitions along object boundaries. Formulating optical flow in a probabilistic setting also enables adding more constraints on flow values, should the need arise. Gibbs sampling would then favor flow values that satisfy all factors, including the new ones, better.

Our initial results suggest that the POF method may be effective in tracking cardiac structures and therefore could form the basis of a spatio-temporal image segmentation tool based on optical flow computation from consecutive pairs of 2D or 3D medical images in a temporal sequence. POF-based segmentation would address an important reason for dissatisfactory performance of many cardiac segmentation algorithms described in the literature. For the most part, they do not consider the temporal information reflecting change in cardiac morphology over the cardiac cycle as an integral part of their functionality. This is currently being investigated in our research.

References

1. Horn, B.K., Schunck, B.G.: Determining optical flow. In: 1981 Technical Symposium East, pp. 319–331. International Society for Optics and Photonics (1981)
2. Lucas, B.D., Kanade, T.: An iterative image registration technique with an application to stereo vision. IJCAI 81, 674–679 (1981)
3. Barron, J.L., Fleet, D.J., Beauchemin, S.S.: Performance of optical flow techniques. International Journal of Computer Vision 12, 43–77 (1994)
4. Koller, D., Friedman, N.: Probabilistic graphical models: principles and techniques. MIT press (2009)
5. Geman, S., Geman, D.: Stochastic relaxation, gibbs distributions, and the bayesian restoration of images. IEEE Transactions on Pattern Analysis and Machine Intelligence (6), 721–741 (1984)
6. van Laarhoven, P.J., Aarts, E.H.: Simulated annealing. Springer (1987)

7. Andreopoulos, A., Tsotsos, J.K.: Efficient and generalizable statistical models of shape and appearance for analysis of cardiac mri. Medical Image Analysis 12(3), 335–357 (2008)
8. Adhyapak, S.M., Menon, P.G., Mehra, A., Tully, S., Rao Parachuri, V.: Rapid quantification of mean myocardial wall velocity in ischemic cardiomyopathy by cardiac magnetic resonance: An index of cardiac functional abnormalities during the cardiac cycle. J. Clin. Exp. Cardiolog 5(288), 2 (2014)

Detection of Myocardial Perfusion Defects Using First Pass Perfusion Cardiac MRI Data

Stephen Kruzick[1,*], Ole Mengshoel[2,**], and Prahlad G. Menon[3,4,**]

[1] Carnegie Mellon University, Pittsburgh, PA, USA
[2] CMU Silicon Valley, Mountain View, CA, USA
[3] SYSU-CMU Joint Institute of Engineering, Pittsburgh, PA, USA
[4] SYSU-CMU Shunde International Joint Research Institute, Guangdong, China
pgmenon@andrew.cmu.edu

Abstract. First pass perfusion cardiac magnetic resonance imaging (FPP-CMR) presents a non-invasive method of detecting restricted blood flow to the myocardium, heart muscle tissue, early in development of coronary heart disease. This paper proposes simple classification methods applied to FPP-CMR data to detect regions of poor perfusion. Preliminary results show correspondence to regions of scar tissue detected from thresholding of late Gadolinium enhancement CMR imaging.

Keywords: cardiac magnetic resonance imaging, coronary heart disease, classification, Dice index, Gaussian naive Bayes, myocardium, perfusion.

1 Introduction

Modern technological advances in medical imaging, such as **cardiac magnetic resonance (CMR) imaging**, enable clinicians to non-invasively obtain important diagnostic information regarding patients. The digital data collected by these methods affords the opportunity to employ techniques from statistical signal processing for benefit of the diagnostic process. One of many medical applications that could benefit, the early detection of **coronary heart disease (CHD)** holds great interest in the medical imaging community. To that end, this paper focuses on detecting **ischemic** regions of the **myocardium** heart muscle that are receiving insufficient **perfusion**, supply of blood, using data from a specific CMR procedure called **first pass perfusion CMR (FPP-CMR)**.

Coronary heart disease develops when blockage of the arteries that serve the heart leads to insufficient blood perfusion in the myocardium. Heart disease may not lead to noticeable symptoms until after a significant amount of myocardial tissue is already scarred. However, the quality of myocardial perfusion can be an early indicator of developing heart disease. Additionally, the state of the art

* This research was conducted with government support under and awarded by the DoD, Air Force Office of Scientific Research, NDSEG Fellowship, 32 CFR 168a.
** This research is also funded in part by CMU-SYSU Collaborative Innovation Research Center and the SYSU-CMU International Joint Research Institute.

Y.J. Zhang and J.M.R.S. Tavares (Eds.): CompIMAGE 2014, LNCS 8641, pp. 248–254, 2014.
© Springer International Publishing Switzerland 2014

standard for diagnosing CHD is coronary angiography, an expensive and invasive catheterization process. Approximately 40% of coronary angiographies are performed on patients that do not require clinical intervention. Thus, prescreening with FPP-CMR, a non-invasive and less expensive technique, could reduce unnecessary coronary angiography procedures [1]. The difficulty of discriminating perfusion defects in FPP-CMR data by visual inspection and the value of clinician time consumed motivate development of automatic diagnosis tools.

This work describes simple features and models proposed for automatic classification, either supervised or unsupervised, of FPP-CMR data pixels according to perfusion quality in section 2. Results, tested on a small data set focusing on the left ventricle, appear in section 3. Concluding analysis follows in section 4.

2   Proposed Approach

Classification of myocardial pixels in FPP-CMR data by blood perfusion uptake curve shape in order to detect ischemic regions comprises the objective of this study. This section first describes the composition and origins of the two primary types of data, FPP-CMR and LGE-CMR, used in this work. It then proposes two feature sets computed from the FPP-CMR data which can then be used with a Gaussian naive Bayes model to obtain classifications. Finally, a method of comparing the results to scar regions detected in LGE-CMR data is given.

2.1   Data Examined

The primary data studied in this paper comes from **first pass perfusion cardiac magnetic resonance imaging (FPP-CMR)**. Clinicians obtain FPP-CMR data by introducing a **Gadolinium contrast agent** into the blood stream by intravenous injection, which then causes the blood to become highlighted in measurements taken by the MRI scanner. Regions of high blood content appear with greater intensity than regions of low blood content in the resulting images. The contrast agent eventually reaches the heart blood pool and the measurements of interest begin. These measurements continue to be taken as the blood with contrast agent perfuses the myocardial muscle tissue over the course of one **cardiac cycle**, a heart beat. Since this is the first cycle over which the blood and contrast agent perfuse the heart muscle, this procedure is called first pass perfusion. Thus, as blood perfuses the myocardial muscles, the recorded intensity corresponds to the strength of the perfusion [3]. Over multiple time samples, the MRI scanner records perfusion intensity images for several **slices** of the heart organized along the third axis, resulting in a three-dimensional description of blood perfusion over the time. Figure 1a shows FPP-CMR data for one patient.

Another source of data important in this study, **late Gadolinium enhancement cardiac magnetic resonance imaging (LGE-CMR)** serves a slightly different purpose. After waiting a relatively long period of time from the injection of the Gadolinium contrast agent, LGE-CMR data shows the remaining Gadolinium content of the heart in a single time sample of each of the slices.

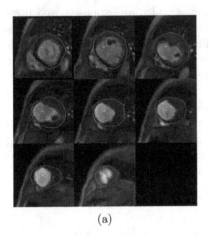 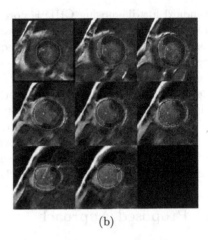

(a)   (b)

Fig. 1. Figure 1a shows FPP-CMR data for Patient 3 at a time sample near peak intensity. The blood chamber of the left ventricle is the bright spot in the middle. The surrounding annular region is the myocardium. Figure 1b shows LGE-CMR data for Patient 3. The yellow curves in the myocardium demark scar tissue detected in Medviso Segment [2] using Otsu's method of image thresholding.

For instance, LGE-CMR imaging could take place five minutes subsequent to FPP-CMR imaging at which time a single snapshot of intensity data is taken. Excess Gadolinium accumulates in scarred myocardial tissue, whereas it is flushed out of healthy myocardial tissue. Thus, LGE-CMR data highlights regions of the myocardium that have experienced scarring [4]. Regions of scarring generally should experience poor perfusion, though they may not be the only regions experiencing poor perfusion. Figure 1b shows an example of LGE-CMR data.

The data set available for this preliminary study is comprised of FPP-CMR data for three patients. Patient 1, for whom only FPP-CMR data is available, has ischemic regions that can be marked and used as training data for the ischemic class. Patient 2, also for whom only FPP-CMR data is available, has mostly healthy regions that can be marked and used as training data for the healthy class. Patient 3, for whom both FPP-CMR data and LGE-CMR data are available, has many diseased regions. Because the LGE-CMR data will be used to obtain an approximate ground truth against which FPP-CMR based classifications can be compared, the data from Patient 3 will be used for testing. This is a very small data set, so no general claims will be made about the performance quality of the data analysis methods described later.

2.2   Classification Methods

This paper classifies perfusion quality of individual pixels in the myocardial region M based on the curve shape of the corresponding intensity time series, using two separate feature sets which reflect the shape of the intensity curve.

The first feature set F_p is comprised of a transformed version of the individual intensity samples $I_p(t)$ of the pixel $p \in M$ at each time, normalized for scaling and offset differences between patients and equipment as in (1).

$$F_{p,t} = I'_p(t) = \frac{I_p(t) - \min_{\tau_1} (I_p(\tau_1))}{\max_{\tau_2} (I_p(\tau_2) - \min_{\tau_1} (I_p(\tau_1)))} \qquad (1)$$

The second feature set is a logistic curve fit of the normalized time series data. During the uptake region of the cardiac cycle, from first to maximum perfusion, the normalized intensity time series $I'_p(t)$ computed in (1) can be approximated as a **logistic** function g parameterized linearly with respect to time, which takes the form in (2) for parameter β_p.

$$I'_p(t) \approx g(\beta_{p,0} + \beta_{p,1}t) = \frac{1}{1 + e^{\beta_{p,0} + \beta_{p,1}t}} \qquad (2)$$

Coefficients β_p that describe the uptake interval are found by first transforming the data according to the **logit** function g^{-1}, inverse of the logistic function. Subsequently, a linear least squares fit yields values for the features $F_p = \beta_p$.

Programs were developed to use the above features under **Gaussian naive Bayes** model assumptions for classification of spatial pixels as healthy or ischemic. In this model, the features have Gaussian distributions conditionally independent of each other given only the pixel class, which itself is a random variable with values healthy and ischemic that has a categorical distribution. Both supervised learning from the Patient 1 and Patient 2 data sets and unsupervised clustering using the **expectation maximization (EM) algorithm** without labeled training data were implemented. The learned models were applied to classification of FPP-CMR data for Patient 3, for which LGE-CMR data was available, using **maximum a posteriori probability (MAP)** estimation.

2.3   Evaluating Success

Note that in Fig. 1a, which shows FPP-CMR data, and in Fig. 1b, which shows LGE-CMR data, the shapes and rotation of the myocardial region are not identical. Thus, a pixel to pixel comparison of the perfusion classifications, shown in Figs. 2a and 2b, and scar detections from LGE-CMR data, shown in Fig. 2c, is not possible. To address this problem, an angular reference is set, and the fraction of ischemic pixels in FPP-CMR data or scarred pixels in LGE-CMR data is computed for a number of angular sectors. The results can be displayed for visual comparison in a heat map as shown in Figs. 2d, 2e, and 2f of the results.

In order to produce a quantitative measure of how well these heat maps correspond, Otsu's method of image thresholding is first applied to the heat maps to identify sectors with significant amounts of scar or ischemic pixels present. Subsequently, the **Dice index** of the two thresholded heat maps can be

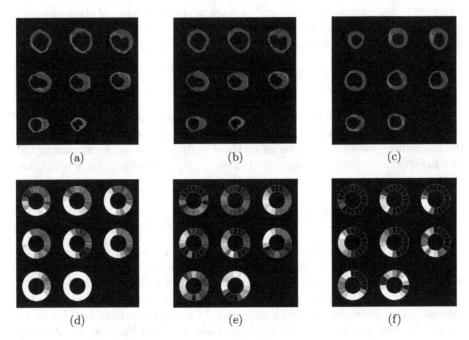

Fig. 2. Results for Patient 3 using unsupervised clustering with ischemic or scarred regions in red and healthy regions in blue. Figures 2a and 2d show results for time sample features. Figures 2b and 2e show results for logistic fit features. Compare to Figs. 2c and 2f, which pertain to LGE scar detection data. Similar plots are also available for the supervised learning approach.

computed as a similarity measure. Let S_{FPP} be the set of sectors with thresholded heat map showing significant poorly perfused regions and S_{LGE} be the set of sectors showing significant scarred regions. Then the Dice index, ranging from 0 to 1 with higher values indicating greater similarity, is given by (3).

$$D\left(S_{FPP}, S_{LGE}\right) = \frac{2\left|S_{FPP} \cap S_{LGE}\right|}{\left|S_{FPP}\right| + \left|S_{LGE}\right|} \tag{3}$$

3   Preliminary Results

Results from the classification program were computed for Patient 3 and are reported in three forms. Classification images are produced for the perfusion and scarring data, examples of which appear in Figs. 2a-2c. Angular sector detection ratio heat maps, like the examples in Figs. 2d-2f, are also provided. Finally, the sector heat maps are thresholded and Dice indices, located in Table 1, are

Table 1. Dice indices (Patient 3)

	Feature	
	Time Series	Logistic Fit
Supervised	.6500	.6479
Unsupervised	.6963	.5581

computed to provide a quantitative measure of similarity between the detected ischemic regions and scar regions.

There is a visible correspondence between regions of high ischemic perfusion pixels and regions of high scar tissue in the detection maps and sector heat maps for each of the feature type and supervision level. While unsupervised clustering using the intensity sample feature gave the highest Dice index, all methods were relatively close, and the data set size prevents a definite comparison.

4   Conclusions

Reliable automatic classification of poorly perfused regions of the myocardial heart muscle using FPP-CMR data would benefit the non-invasive early diagnosis of coronary heart disease. This paper has proposed simple classification methods using two different feature sets, pixel intensity time series and logistic fit parameters, with Gaussian naive Bayes model assumptions which can be used in supervised or unsupervised learning situations. FPP-CMR data based classifications for each of these feature and supervision type combinations were performed, and the results were compared against scar tissue detected by thresholding of LGE-CMR data. Angular sectors with high fraction of ischemic pixels generally correspond to those with high fractions of scar tissue pixels, which is visible in the heat maps produced and quantified in the Dice indices computed.

However, there are weaknesses of the methods presented that remain to be addressed and possible directions of expansion that could continue to be explored. Even if there is an overall correspondence with regions of scarring, the accuracy of the perfusion classification leaves improvement to be desired. More rigorous preprocessing using active shape models to deal with myocardial shape distortion may benefit the classification process. Also, improvements may be achieved by finding features and models that cluster more strongly, providing clearer distinction between poorly perfused pixels and normally perfused pixels, and are more comparable between different patients and different MRI scanning equipment. Regardless, the study should be extended to include many more patients from a more representative sample with both FPP-CMR data and LGE-CMR data. Then, the performance of the classifiers can be more fully examined.

References

[1] Patel, M., et al.: Low Diagnostic Yield of Elective Coronary Angiography. New England Journal of Medicine (March 2010)

[2] Heiberg, E., et al.: Design and validation of Segment–freely available software for cardiovascular image analysis. BMC Med. Imaging 10(1) (January 11, 2010), doi:10.1186/1471-2342-10-1. NOTE: Analysis was performed using Segment version 1.9 R2046 (http://segment.heiberg.se)

[3] Gebker, R., Schwitter, J., Fleck, E., Nagel, E.: How We Perform Myocardial Perfusion With Cardiovascular Magnetic Resonance. Journal of Cardiovascular Magnetic Resonance (2007)

[4] Kim, R., Shah, D., Judd, R.: How We Perform Delay Enhancement Imaging. Journal of Cardiovascular Magnetic Resonance (2003)

Numerical Simulation from Medical Images: Accurate Integration by Means of the Cartesian Grid Finite Element Method

Onofre Marco[1], Rubén Sevilla[2], Juan José Ródenas[1], and Manuel Tur[1]

[1] Centro de Investigación en Ingeniería Mecánica,
Universitat Politècnica de València, Spain
onmaral@upvnet.upv.es, {jjrodena,matuva}@mcm.upv.es
[2] College of Engineering,
Swansea University, Wales, UK
R.Sevilla@swansea.ac.uk

Abstract. Nowadays, when it comes to generation of patient-specific Finite Element model, there are two main alternatives. On the one hand, it is possible to generate geometrical models through segmentation, whereupon FE models would be obtained using standard mesh generators. On the other hand, we can create a Cartesian grid of uniform hexahedra in which the elements fit each pixel/voxel perfectly. In both cases, geometries will take part during the analysis either as complete models, in the first case, or as auxiliary entities, to apply boundary conditions properly for instance, in the second case. In any case, once the geometrical entities have been obtained from the medical image, the efficient generation of an accurate Finite Element model for numerical simulation in not trivial. The aim of this paper is to propose an efficient integration strategy, using Cartesian meshes, of 3D geometries defined by parametric surfaces, i.e. NURBS, obtained from medical images.

Keywords: Cartesian Grid FEM, Medical Imaging, NURBS, NEFEM.

1 Introduction

During the last years, the development of computers allowed researchers to spread the use of the Finite Element Method, broadly used for industrial applications, to other fields such as Medicine. In this field, we can find plenty of areas where numerical solutions are needed in order to solve problems that could improve the quality of life of patients.

The translation of complex CAD based geometrical models into conforming FE discretizations is computationally expensive. Immersed boundary methods do not require body-fitted meshes, but to embed the domain into a Cartesian grid, which is generated irrespective of the geometric complexity of the physical domain. In a Cartesian grid environment the auxiliary domain is a cube whose discretization into hexahedral elements of uniform size is trivial. Since the mesh is not conforming with the geometry, these methods require special

Y.J. Zhang and J.M.R.S. Tavares (Eds.): CompIMAGE 2014, LNCS 8641, pp. 255–260, 2014.

treatment of element integrals along the boundary. The accuracy of the results provided by these techniques depends on the accuracy of the integration process. In the literature we can find results showing the power of this method in both computational cost and accuracy[1].

From this point of view, we think the use of Cartesian grids is the most natural way to move from medical imaging to Finite Element Analysis due to its hierarchical structure[2]. In addition our approach will allow to calculate accurate numerical integration taking into account exact 3D models which is one of the aims of Isogeometric Analysis[3], technique still under development.

Hence, the methodology proposed in this paper includes an efficient integration procedure based on the NURBS-enhanced Finite Element Method (NEFEM)[4] which considers efficient strategies for numerical integration on elements affected by curved boundaries while at elements not intersecting the boundary classical isoparametric finite elements are used, preserving the efficiency of the FEM. This strategy will allow us to consider the actual boundary providing the exact element integrals (up to the accuracy of the numerical integration and round-off errors). In addition, the ideas supporting this approach are valid for any piecewise boundary parametrization, not only NURBS.

This contribution is the first step to achieve a method able to get real patient-specific material properties and accurate integration of geometries within the same framework. As application for this image/geometry interaction we can point out the simulation of prosthetic devices[5]. This kind of analysis will allow us to know the behaviour of different components under boundary conditions based on real human tissue information extracted from image-based Cartesian grid FEM models.

2   Method

Once the geometrical model has been created from a medical image, the first step of the method will consist in creating a Cartesian grid that completely covers the model. Later on, we need to find the intersections between the geometry and the Cartesian grid. With the intersections we can define integration subdomains needed to properly integrate the intersected elements. In order to do that, a strategy to identify intersection patterns has been implemented allowing the precalculation of sets of tetrahedra for the most common intersection patterns. Once we have the integration subdomains we will carry out the integration process.

2.1   Mesh Generation

To generate a Cartesian grid that embeds an arbitrary geometry we calculate a bounding box of the model in order to know the minimal dimensions required for the mesh. For each level of refinement, the embedding domain is partitioned in hexaedral elements of uniform size. One of the main benefits of the data structure adopted here is that the mappings of element in the Cartesian grid of any level are affine and, therefore, its Jacobian is constant. This property can be exploited to dramatically speed-up the computation of the elemental matrices. In Figures 1b, 1c and 1d we can see a CAD model of a human femur, obtained from a medical image by segmentation, immersed in a Cartesian grid.

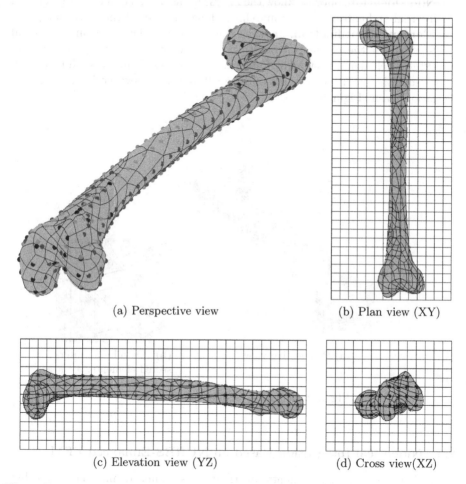

(a) Perspective view

(b) Plan view (XY)

(c) Elevation view (YZ)

(d) Cross view(XZ)

Fig. 1. Bone model intersected by a Cartesian grid. Coloured dots represent the intersections between the NURBS surfaces and the edges of the Cartesian grid.

2.2   Geometry/Mesh Intersection

Most of methods to evaluate the intersection between parametric surfaces and arbitrary lines were developed for ray-tracing, tasks related to the animation industry, where rendering CAD models is basic. The process used in this work consists of three steps:

- **Intersection of boundary with element edges**: we decided to use a basic Newton-Raphson algorithm to find the intersections between the edges of the elements from the approximation mesh and the surfaces. This way is efficient if we ensure the existence of intersections and good initial guess points. In Figure 1 we can see the femur model intersected by the axes.
- **Node location**: once we know the intersections we can differenciate between internal and external nodes marching along the axes of the Cartesian grid.
- **Element identification**: knowing the position of the nodes and the nodal topology of the elements to distinguish between intersected, internal and external elements is straight forward. As a result of this procedure we can remove the external elements and we will obtain a new mesh, called calculation mesh (Figure 2).

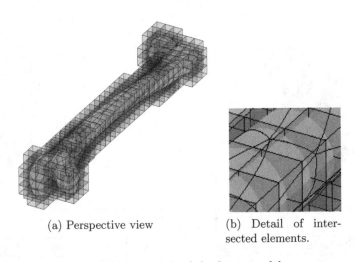

(a) Perspective view　　　(b) Detail of intersected elements.

Fig. 2. Calculation mesh of the femur model

2.3   Numerical Integration Based on NURBS-Enhanced FEM

As said before, internal elements are treated as standard finite elements, but the contribution from an intersected element requires special attention as the integral must be computed only over the portion of the intersected elements that lies inside the physical domain.

The strategy proposed here in order to perform the integration over the intersected elements consists of employing a tetrahedralization of this region. The proposed strategy is based on the Marching Cubes (MC) algorithm[6] which is widely used in computational graphics to represent approximations of surfaces as it is very efficient sorting out basic intersection patterns and creating linear surfaces between them. The usefulness of this algorithm for us comes from the possibility of identification of the most common intersection patterns and the creation of integration subdomains by Delaunay tetrahedralization that could be stored and reused for any intersected element with the same characteristics, see example in Figure 3a. For the special cases an exclusive tetrahedralization will be performed to ensure robustness.

Numerical integration on the intersected elements is then accomplished by integrating over each subdomain of the Delaunay tetrahedralization. In order to perform the integration over the subelements, the strategy proposed within the NURBS-Enhanced Finite Element Method (NEFEM) is adopted. A tetrahedral element T_e^F with a face on the physical boundary is parametrized using the mapping

$$\boldsymbol{\Psi} : \Lambda_e \times [0,1] \longrightarrow T_e^F$$
$$(\xi, \eta, \zeta) \longmapsto \boldsymbol{\Psi}(\xi, \eta, \zeta) := (1 - \zeta)\mathbf{S}(\xi, \eta) + \zeta\mathbf{x}_4, \tag{1}$$

where $\mathbf{S}(\Lambda_e)$ denotes the curved face of T_e^F on the boundary of the physical domain and $\mathbf{x}_4$ is the internal vertex of T_e^F. Analogously, a tetrahedral element T_e^E with an edge on the physical boundary is parametrized using the mapping

$$\boldsymbol{\Phi} : [\xi_1, \xi_2] \times [0,1]^2 \longrightarrow T_e^E$$
$$(\xi, \eta, \zeta) \longmapsto \boldsymbol{\Phi}(\xi, \eta, \zeta) := (1 - \zeta)(1 - \eta)\mathbf{C}(\xi) + (1 - \zeta)\eta\mathbf{x}_3 + \zeta\mathbf{x}_4. \tag{2}$$

where $\mathbf{C}([\xi_1, \xi_2])$ denotes the curved edge of T_e^E on the boundary of the physical domain and $\mathbf{x}_3$ and $\mathbf{x}_4$ are the two internal vertices of T_e^E.

Given these parametrizations, it is possible to perform the numerical integration over all the curved tetrahedral elements. To this end, we consider tensor products of triangle quadratures and one-dimensional Gaussian quadratures for the tetrahedrons with a face on the boundary of the physical domain, see Figure 3b.

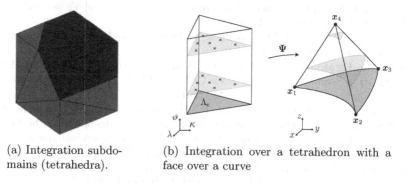

(a) Integration subdomains (tetrahedra).

(b) Integration over a tetrahedron with a face over a curve

Fig. 3. Integration process of intersected elements

For the tetrahedrons with an edge on the boundary of the physical domain, tensor products of one-dimensional Gaussian quadratures are employed. The number of integration points required in the parametric space of the parametric boundary representation will depend on the CAD technology employed. We have to note that for tetrahedra without edges or faces on the boundary integration will follow a standard isoparametric scheme.

3 Conclusions and Future Developments

There is a wide range of problems that arise, and we have to take into account, when trying to improve medical protocols or prosthetic technology. With this contribution we try to show a reliable alternative to integrate accurately geometrical models obtained from medical images, reducing this way the influence of the geometrical error in the FE analysis process. This paper represents an important contribution to our next step: to simultaneously consider, within a single FE model, both biological tissue models obtained by an image-based Cartesian grid FEM and prosthetic components, such as dental or hip implants.

Acknowledgements. With the support of the European Union Framework Program (FP7) under grant No. 289361 'INSIST', Ministerio de Economía y Competitividad of Spain (DPI2010-20542)(DPI2013-46317-R), FPI program (BES-2011-044080) and Generalitat Valenciana (PROMETEO/2012/023).

References

1. Nadal, E., Ródenas, J.J., Albelda, J., Tur, M., Tarancón, J.E., Fuenmayor, F.J.: Efficient Finite Element Methodology based on Cartesian grids: Application to structural shape optimization. Abstract and Applied Analysis (2013)
2. Giovannelli, L., Marco, O., Navarro, J.M., Giner, E., Ródenas, J.J.: Direct Creation of Finite Element Models from Medical Images using Cartesian Grids. In: Proceedings of IV ECCOMAS Thematic Conference on Computational Vision and Medical Image Processing, VipIMAGE (2013)
3. Cottrell, J.A., Hughes, T.J.R., Bazilevs, Y.: Isogeometric Analysis: Toward Integration of CAD and FEA Wiley (2009)
4. Sevilla, R., Fernández, S., Huerta, A.A.: NURBS-Enhanced Finite Element Method (NEFEM): a Seamless Bridge Between CAD and FEM. Archives of Computational Methods in Engineering 18(4), 441–484 (2011)
5. Ródenas, J.J., Giovannelli, L., Nadal, E., Navarro, J.M., Tur, M.: Creation of Patient Specific Finite Element Models of Bone-Prosthesis. Simulation of the Effect of Future Implants. In: Proceedings of IV ECCOMAS Thematic Conference on Computational Vision and Medical Image Processing, VipIMAGE (2013)
6. Lorensen, W.E., Cline, H.E.: Marching Cubes: A High Resolution 3D Surface Construction Algorithm. Computer Graphics 21(4), 163–169 (1987)

Nonlinear Transformation of the Distance Function in the Nearest Neighbor Image Recognition

Andrey V. Savchenko

National Research University Higher School of Economics,
Nizhny Novgorod, Russian
avsavchenko@hse.ru

Abstract. Conventional image recognition methods usually include dividing the keypoint neighborhood (for local features) or the whole object (for global features) into a grid of blocks, computing the gradient magnitude and orientation at each image sample point and uniting the orientation histograms of all blocks into a single descriptor. The query image is recognized by matching its descriptors with the descriptors of reference images. The matching is usually done by summation of distances between descriptors of corresponding blocks. Unfortunately, such approach does not lead to a correct distance between vector of points (histograms of each block) if popular square of Euclidean distance is used as a discrimination. To calculate the correct discrimination, we propose to sum the square roots (or, more generally, appropriate nonlinear transformation) of distances between block histograms. Such approach is experimentally examined in a face recognition problem with FERET and AT&T datasets. The results support the statement that the proposed approach provides higher accuracy (up to 5.5%) than state-of-the-art methods not only for the Euclidean distance but for other popular similarity measures (L_1, Kullback-Leibler, Jensen-Shannon, chi-squared and homogeneity-testing probabilistic neural network).

Keywords: Image recognition, face recognition, nearest neighbor, Scale-Invariant Feature Transform (SIFT), histogram of oriented gradients (HOG), probabilistic neural network, homogeneity testing, Jensen-Shannon divergence.

1 Introduction

Image recognition is a challenging problem [1] due to the variable appearance of the same object under different conditions (pose, illumination, scale, cluttered background, etc) [2] and the practical limitations on the computing efficiency of the implemented algorithms [3], [4]. It is well-known that the proper choice of the feature set and the similarity measure have a strong impact on the recognition accuracy and reliability [1]. Nowadays, conventional gradient orientation textured features have reached a certain level of maturity [1], [5]. Most popular are local invariant descriptors, e.g. SIFT [6] and SURF [3], [7], computed in

Y.J. Zhang and J.M.R.S. Tavares (Eds.): CompIMAGE 2014, LNCS 8641, pp. 261–266, 2014.

the neighborhoods of extracted keypoints (image points which differ from their immediate neighborhoods) [8]. To evaluate each local descriptor, the keypoint neighborhood is divided into a grid of uniformly spaced cells. Global descriptors, e.g., color histograms and HOG [8], [9], also give essentially perfect results, especially if the object of interest is previously detected by, e.g., Viola-Jones method [10]. Like for the local descriptor, the global one is calculated by dividing the whole object into a fixed-size grid, evaluating the descriptors (e.g., histogram) of each cell and combining them into a single feature vector [6], [11].

At the same time, the studies devoted to the proper choice of similarity measures are limited to the application of concrete distances (Euclidean, chi-squared, Mahalonbis, Bhattacharya, Kullback-Leibler (KL), Jensen-Shannon (JH), etc.) [12], [13] or various classifiers (nearest neighbors (NN), support vector machines, etc.) with experimental parameters selection [2], [4]. The similarity of the input and reference objects is estimated as a sum of distances between descriptors of corresponding cells in a grid. There are practically no studies of other ways to combine the distances between histograms of each block [4]. Inspired by the fact that the Euclidean distance between set of points should be computed as a sum of square roots of similarities between corresponding points, the presented paper explores the possibility to improve the recognition accuracy by summation of the nonlinearly transformed distances between corresponding blocks.

The rest of the paper is organized as follows: Section 2 introduces the proposed approach to sum up the nonlinear transformations (e.g., square root) of the histogram-based distances. In Section 3, we present the experimental results in the face recognition with FERET [1] and AT&T [2] datasets. Concluding comments are given in Section 4.

2   Materials and Methods

Let a set of $R > 1$ grayscale images $\{X_r\}, r \in \{1, ..., R\}$ be given. In image recognition it is required to assign a query image X to one of R classes specified by these reference images. At first, every image is put in correspondence with a set of feature descriptors [7], [9]. The common part of practically all modern algorithms is to divide the whole neighborhood into a regular grid of $K_1 \times K_2$ blocks, K_1 rows and K_2 columns, and separately evaluate the N bins-histogram $H^{(r)}(k_1, k_2) = \{h_1^{(r)}(k_1, k_2), ..., h_N^{(r)}(k_1, k_2)\}$ of appropriate simple features for each block $(k_1, k_2), k_1 \in \{1, ..., K_1\}, k_2 \in \{1, ..., K_2\}$, of the reference image X_r. The most popular image point's simple feature is the gradient orientation [8], [9] (sometimes, weighted with the gradient magnitude [4], [6]), though other features, such as color values, are also wide applicable. In this paper we assume, that each histogram $H^{(r)}(k_1, k_2)$ is normalized, so that it may be treated as a probability distribution [8]. The same procedure is repeated to evaluate the matrix of histograms $H(k_1, k_2) = \{h_1(k_1, k_2), ..., h_N(k_1, k_2)\}$ corresponding to the query image. The recognition is performed by any machine learning classifier

---

[1] http://www.itl.nist.gov/iad/humanid/feret/

[2] http://www.cl.cam.ac.uk/research/dtg/attarchive/facedatabase.html

[2], [7], [9]. Many of them, e.g., NN methods, SVM with radial kernel [2], are based on the calculation of distance between histograms of the query and reference images, especially, if the number of models in each class is low (in the worst case, single model per class). The distance is usually calculated as a summand of distances $\rho(H(k_1, k_2), H^{(r)}(k_1, k_2))$ between histograms of corresponding blocks [4], [6]. The most popular distance is the square of L_2 (Euclidean) [6], [8], which is implemented in the OpenCV library as a default matcher, though other distances, such as L_1, chi-squared, etc., are also useful [12], [13].

The major drawback of such approach is the loss of metric properties if conventional Euclidean distance is applied. Really, the correct way to calculate the distance between set of vectors is the following one

$$\rho^{(\Delta)}(X, X_r) = \sum_{k_1=1}^{K_1} \sum_{k_2=1}^{K_2} \varphi \left(\min_{\substack{|\Delta_1| \leq \Delta, \\ |\Delta_2| \leq \Delta}} \rho(H(k_1, k_2), H^{(r)}(k_1 + \Delta_1, k_2 + \Delta_2)) \right) \quad (1)$$

where $\varphi(\rho) = \sqrt{\rho}$. Here, we use the mutual alignment of the histograms in the Δ- neighborhood of each block [4] in order to take into account the small spatial deviations due to misalignment after keypoint or object detection. The state-of-the-art approach is equivalent to (1) if $\Delta = 0$. Though the miss of the square root calculation for the whole $\rho^{(\Delta)}(X, X_r)$ in (1) is reasonable, there is no sense of the usage of linear function $\varphi(\rho) = \rho$. As a matter of fact, in our experiments we found that various nonnegative monotonous functions $\varphi(\rho) = \rho^\alpha$ outperforms the conventional distance $(\varphi(\rho) = \rho)$ if $0 < \alpha < 1$, the best accuracy and computing efficiency was achieved with the square root $(\alpha = 0.5)$.

Though the computing efficiency of the proposed modification (1) is a little worse due to additional $K_1 \cdot K_2$ square root calculations, it provides higher accuracy than the classical approach $(\Delta = 0, \varphi(\rho) = \rho)$. This is related to the different weights of the blocks: the square root nonlinear transform smoothes down large contributions (values on the tail of the distance distribution) and, more important, overstates small contributions to the overall distance as it occurs in the Markov Random Fields clique potential functions [5]. The next section provides an experimental evidence to support this claim.

3   Experimental Results

The experimental study is devoted to the face recognition problem [7], [9]. Popular FERET and AT&T datasets were used. From FERET dataset all available 2720 face-to-face images of 994 persons were chosen. AT&T dataset contains 400 images of 40 different people. The faces were detected with the OpenCV library. The median filter with window size (3x3) was applied to remove noise in detected faces [15]. The number of bins in the gradient orientation histogram $N = 8$ [6]. As the performance issues are behind the key aspect of our paper, we used both our modification of the weighted HOG [15] and SIFT (one of the best local descriptors in terms of achieved accuracy) [6]. In the former case the faces were divided into 100 blocks ($K_1 = K_2 = 10$). Conventional grid $K_1 = K_2 = 4$ [6] was used in the latter case. The match of keypoints is accepted only if the distance ratio of the first NN and the second NN is lower than 0.8 [6].

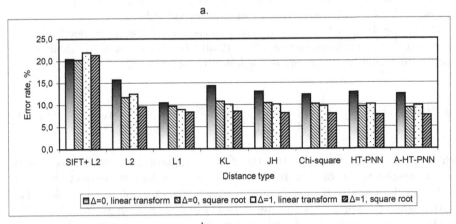

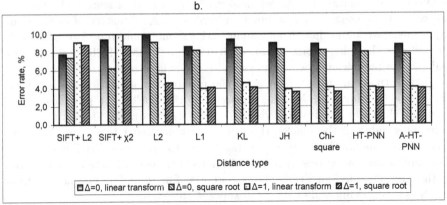

Fig. 1. Face recognition error rates: a. FERET dataset; b. AT&T dataset

To evaluate the distance (1), square root nonlinear transformation was applied $\varphi(\rho) = \sqrt{\rho}$, which is evaluated with an x86-assembler code to provide the best computational speed. The following neighborhood sizes were tested: $\Delta = 0$ and $\Delta = 1$. The following measures of similarity were used: state-of-the-art square of L_2, L_1, chi-squared distance, the KL discrimination, the

JH divergence, our homogeneity-testing probabilistic neural network (HT-PNN) [4], [14] and its simplification - approximate HT-PNN (A-HT-PNN):

$$\rho_{\text{A-HT-PNN}}(H, H^{(r)}) =$$

$$\sum_{i=1}^{N} \left(\frac{h_i(2(h_{K;i})^2 - (h_{K;i} + h_{K;i}^{(r)})^2)}{h_{K;i}(h_{K;i} + h_{K;i}^{(r)})} + \frac{h_i^{(r)}(2(h_{K;i}^{(r)})^2 - (h_{K;i} + h_{K;i}^{(r)})^2)}{h_{K;i}^{(r)}(h_{K;i} + h_{K;i}^{(r)})} \right) \quad (2)$$

where $h_{K;i}^{(r)} = \sum_{i=1}^{N} K_{ij} h_i^{(r)}, h_{K;i} = \sum_{i=1}^{N} K_{ij} h_i$ are the convolution of the HOGs with discrete Gaussian Parzen kernel K_{ij}; indices (k_1, k_2) are removed for simplicity.

The NN rule's accuracy was estimated by 20 times-repeated random sub-sampling validation. At first, the model database size R was fixed and the training set is filled by the randomly chosen photos from the dataset (1400 and 120 models in a training set for FERET and AT&T, respectively). Other photos formed the test set (1320 and 260 images for FERET and AT&T). It was required to put at least one photo of each person in both training and test set.

The average error rates are presented in Fig. 1. Here, first, the error rate of conventional summation of histogram distances ($\varphi(\rho) = \rho$) exceeds the error rate of the proposed approach ($\varphi(\rho) = \sqrt{\rho}$) not only for Euclidean distance, but for all explored similarity measures, both for conventional summation ($\Delta = 0$) and histograms alignment ($\Delta = 1$) and for either SIFT or HOG descriptors. Second, though the performance of the SIFT method is rather bad for FERET dataset, SIFT descriptors for AT&T are characterized with the best results (sometimes, 3%-higher accuracy than the HOG with the A-HT-PNN) if there is no alignment ($\Delta = 0$). Third, the conventional Euclidean distance is characterized with the worst accuracy. The lowest error rate is achieved with our A-HT-PNN for FERET and the JS divergence and chi-squared distance for AT&T. Fourth, the HOG's alignment ($\Delta = 1$) allows to decrease the error rate at 1-6%, though it does not work for SIFT as the grid size is low ($K_1 = K_2 = 4$). However, such improvement of the recognition accuracy is achieved only with the 10-times loss of performance. Fifth, the proposed nonlinear transformation does not always lead to the better accuracy (Fig. 1b), though the accuracy decrease is rather low (no more than 0.3%). For instance, it is preferable to use the conventional linear function $\varphi(\rho) = \rho$ for L_1 metric and, in some cases, for our HT-PNN.

4   Conclusion

Based on our experimental results we could draw the following conclusions. We explored the dependence of the image recognition quality on the distance calculation method which compares descriptors containing a grid of locally normalized histograms. We proposed to sum the nonlinear transformation of distances between corresponding blocks (1). It was shown that this slight modification of the conventional distance summation allows to increase the face recognition accuracy in most cases. For example, for FERET dataset we achieve the gain in accuracy up to 4% for the distance without block's alignment ($\Delta = 0$) and up to 2.9% for the distance (1) with $\Delta = 1$. It is necessary to emphasize that the loss in computational speed (0.1-0.3 ms) does not seem to be significant for the usage of our approach as the square root can be efficiently calculated.

To sum it up, this article highlights the need to properly combine the distances between histograms of each block in a grid. It was experimentally demonstrated that the summation of nonlinear distance transformation and looking for the best match in the neighborhood of each block (1) appears quite promising. The future work may be devoted to the application of our approach with more popular classifiers, e.g., the support vector machine with the radial kernel.

References

1. Sonka, M., Hlavac, V., Boyle, R.: Image Processing, Analysis, and Machine Vision, 4th edn. Cengage Learning (2014)
2. Theodoridis, S., Koutroumbas, C.: Pattern Recognition, 4th edn. Elsevier Inc. (2009)
3. Bay, H., Ess, A., Tuytelaars, T., Van Gool, L.: SURF: speeded up robust features. Computer Vision and Image Understanding 110(3), 346–359 (2008)
4. Savchenko, A.V.: Real-time image recognition with the parallel directed enumeration method. In: Chen, M., Leibe, B., Neumann, B. (eds.) ICVS 2013. LNCS, vol. 7963, pp. 123–132. Springer, Heidelberg (2013)
5. Prince, S.J.D.: Computer Vision: Models Learning and Inference. Cambridge University Press (2012)
6. Lowe, D.: Distinctive image features from scale-invariant keypoints. International Journal of Computer Vision 60(2), 91–110 (2004)
7. Bairagi, B.K., Das, S.C., Chatterjee, A., Tudu, B.: Expressions invariant face recognition using SURF and Gabor features. In: Third International Conference on Emerging Applications of Information Technology, pp. 170–173 (2012)
8. Dalal, N., Triggs, B.: Histograms of oriented gradients for human detection. In: Conference on Computer Vision and Pattern Recognition, pp. 886–893 (2005)
9. Albiol, A., Monzo, D., Martin, A., Sastre, J., Albiol, A.: Face recognition using HOG-EBGM. Pattern Recognition Letters 29(10), 1537–1543 (2008)
10. Viola, P., Jones, M.: Robust real-time face detection. International Journal of Computer Vision 57(2), 137–154 (2004)
11. Tuytelaars, T., Mikolajczyk, K.: Local invariant feature detectors: a survey. Foundations and Trends in Computer Graphics and Vision 3(3), 177–280 (2007)
12. Martins, A.F.T., Figueiredo, M.A.T., Aguiar, P.M.Q., Smith, N.A., Xing, E.P.: Nonextensive entropic kernels. In: 25th International Conference on Machine Learning, pp. 640–647 (2008)
13. Ahonen, T., Hadid, A., Pietikainen, M.: Face recognition with local binary patterns. In: European Conference on Computer Vision, pp. 469–481 (2005)
14. Savchenko, A.V.: Probabilistic neural network with homogeneity testing in recognition of discrete patterns set. Neural Networks 46, 227–241 (2013)
15. Savchenko, A.V.: Directed enumeration method in image recognition. Pattern Recognition 45(8), 2952–2961 (2012)

A New Method to Improve Quality
of Reconstructed Images in Tomography

Ahlem Ouaddah and Dalila Boughaci

University of Science and Technology Houari Boumediene USTHB,
Electrical Engineering and Computer Science Department,
El-Alia BP 32 Bab-Ezzouar,16111 Algiers, Algeria
{aouaddah,dboughaci}@usthb.dz

Abstract. This paper presents a new method to improve quality of reconstructed images in tomography.

A lot of methods to reconstruct images in tomography are proposed, but the filtered backprojection method (FBP) is broadly used in clinical setting. FBP is a fast method but the quality of reconstructed data is largely disputed, because of that, we propose an iterative, locally adaptive thresholding technique for removing star artifacts from reconstructed images by FBP method.

The validation of our approach consists to compare reconstructed images by our method with reconstructed one by FBP method using different models as Hoffman model.

1 Introduction

Quality of reconstructed images in tomography, especially in medical imaging, is very important, because they are used to detect and diagnostic diseases on a part or all human body.

The basic principle of this method is to reconstruct the object from some outside measured data [7,8].

This technical is used to give information about some parameters of the inside of the object as the attenuation of a light beam in medical imaging or polarization of seismic waves in geophysics [1,3].

The history of this approach, dates back to 1917 when the Austrian mathematician Johann Karl August Radon developed the Radon Transform [9], which consists to compute the projections of an object $f(x,y)$. The resulting projections are the integral of all points (x,y) that contributes for each projection P in each angle θ, as 1.

$$P(s, \theta) = \int_{-\infty}^{+\infty} \int_{-\infty}^{+\infty} f(x, y)\delta(s - x\cos\theta - y\sin\theta)dxdy \qquad (1)$$

where $\delta(.)$ is the function of Dirac and $s = x\cos\theta + y\sin\theta$.

Y.J. Zhang and J.M.R.S. Tavares (Eds.): CompIMAGE 2014, LNCS 8641, pp. 267–272, 2014.
© Springer International Publishing Switzerland 2014

Added to this transform, John Radon has proved that the reconstruction of the object $f(x,y)$ from its projections is possible and could be exact if we have an infinite number of projections, as 2, which is impossible in real case [2,6].

$$f(x, y) = \int_{-\infty}^{+\infty} P(s, \theta) \tag{2}$$

Various methods are proposed to reconstruct images from projections but the FBP method is largely used, because it's fast and easy to use [5].

For this reason, we propose a new method to enhance quality of produced images by FBP method.

Our aim is to improve identifying the distribution of physical parameter produced with computed tomography (CT).

2   Filtered Backprojection Method (FBP)

Filtered backprojection method is based on Fourier Transform [4], for each projection we apply Fourier Transform and introduce negative values to reduce stars artifacts and then amplify the high frequencies.

However, this method has an important condition to work on that it should be large number of projections, because in the opposite case, the artifacts persist and the result is the same if we have a higher activity in a slice of image. In general, FBP is used widely but the stars artifacts are not eliminated completely. For these reasons, we introduce a new method that removes the artifacts and upgrade the quality of reconstruction.

3   Our Method

In this section, we introduce our proposed method for improving quality of reconstructed images by FBP method in tomography.

3.1   Basic Principle

The adaptive technique is a succession of local enhancements based on grayvalues in the local neighborhood of each pixel.

The main principle of our method is to enhance regions of points (pixels) which have the same characteristics: in the same range of values which are adjacent. At the same time remove all false positive points corresponding to the artifacts. At the end, we produce an image with a high contrast between the pixels corresponding to the activity and the pixels which are not corresponding to any activity. The key information is that the pixels in the edges area differ strongly but not outside or inside of the edges. The main idea is to apply transformation on current pixel considering intensity distribution among its neighbors pixels of reconstructed image by FBP method.

3.2   Our Algorithm

The principle steps of our algorithm can be related as follows:

step 0   Produce initial image using FBP method
step 1   take each point $P(x,y)$ of the current image
step 2   through the matrix vertically
step 3   compute the rate of similarity between the current point
              $P(x,y)$ and the point $P(x+1,y)$
step 4   thresholding selection: if rate of similarity is less than thresh-
              old limit value A
step 5   enhance foreground point
step 6   remove background point
step 7   if threshold selection of the current point $P(x, y)$ is more
              than threshold limit value A
step 8   enhance the two values
step 9   remove false positive points and transform false negative
              points
step 10   loop to step 1 until all points are evaluated.

Fixed value A: Fixed value A which is 40% rate of similarity, corresponds to rate of similarity between the current point and its neighbors. The grayvalue of the current point has to be similar to the grayvalues of its neighbors points with 40% rate of similarity.

3.3   Image Segmentation Based on Classification

We can divide values of reconstructed images into two parts:

– the points corresponding to the activity (foreground)
– the points which not corresponding to any activity (background)

But in reconstructed image by FBP method, we can divide results into four parts:

– the points corresponding to the activity (foreground) with high probability
– the points corresponding to the activity (foreground) with low probability
– the points which not corresponding to any activity (background) with high probability
– the points which not corresponding to any activity (background) with low probability

Our aim is to detect sets of points corresponding to the distribution of physical parameter, enhance its values, detect false positives points and remove them at the same time. At the end, we will localize the right points corresponding to the distribution of physical parameter, which means a better localization of this physical phenomenon.

3.4   Threshold Clustering

The principle of clustering based method is to choose which part this current point depends: foreground or background part.

3.5   Amplification of Foreground Points

This operation is used to increase the contrast of all points supposed corresponding to the activity.

3.6   Thresholding False Positive Points

This threshold is used to detect and remove points which were taken wrongly as foreground points.

3.7   Similarity Rate

To detect each successive points (vertically) which have the same level of values: correspond to the same level of activity or not, we compute the rate between each point $P(x, y)$ and point $P(x + 1, y)$, we choose rate because it gives information about percentage of similarity and dissimilarity.

4   Results

To validate the proposed method, we developed synthetic phantoms and also we apply our method on real phantoms as Hoffman model.
    Results are presented in this section:
(a): represent the original image
(b): represent the reconstructed image by FBP method
(c): represent the reconstructed image by our method.

In this part, we describe quantitatively the quality of reconstructed images by our method and the FBP method. For each reconstructed image (Figure 1, Figure 2, Figure 3) we compute number of misplaced pixels (NMP) which means the number of wrong localization of physical parameter in the reconstructed image and its time of computation.

Table 1. Table of number of misplaced pixels (NMP) and computation time needed for each reconstruction using FBP method and ours

Image test	size	FBP method		Our method	
		NMP	time(s)	NMP	time(s)
Image test 01	29x33	981	0.039	10	8.59
Image test 02	50x63	3138	0.17	70	88.89
Image test 03	128x128	13916	0.35	490	790.36

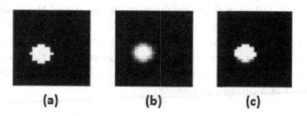

Fig. 1. Optimization of reconstructed image test 01

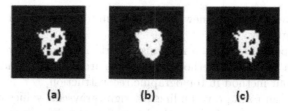

Fig. 2. Optimization of reconstructed image test 02

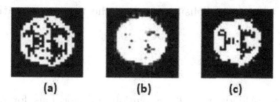

Fig. 3. Optimization of reconstructed image test 03

5 Discussion

The given results in (Figure 1,Figure 2,Figure 3) show clearly that the proposed algorithm improves reconstruction. Comparing to the FBP method, our process gives better results of images reconstruction.

As shown in Table 1, our method succeeds to upgrade the quality of reconstructed images compared to FBP approach.

However the search process in our method is time consuming compared to the reconstruction process in FBP. FBP fails in finding good quality of reconstructed images comparing with our method.

Comparing NMP of reconstructed images by our process and FBP process, we can say that our method is an efficient and promising method. The average of the NMP value of reconstructed images by FBP approach is 50 times more than the NMP value of reconstructed images by our approach.

This is due to the good exploration of the search space and using the basic idea to separate the background to the foreground searching the similarity between each pixels and his neighbors pixels, enhance each point of object and remove each point corresponding to the background, which allows to locate each good point corresponding to the right position of the physical parameter.

The time of computation depends directly on the size of the image and as we see in Table 1, the time of computation of our process is large enough compared to the time of computation using FBP process. However, the progress in parallel programming, gives us the possibility to use it in reducing time computing and knowing that our principal aim is to improve quality of reconstructed images, we conclude that is a promising method.

6   Conclusion

In this paper we proposed a new method to improve quality of reconstructed images in tomography.

To asses our proposed method in terms of performance, we have implemented and compared it with FBP method. The results are promising and demonstrate the benefits of our method in tomographic reconstruction.

Further, we plan to improve finding the right grayscale values of each point, because the principle aim of our method is to find the right position of physical parameter in image.

We plan also to use parallelism to reduce the time computation of our approach.

References

1. Bosman, P.A.N., Alderliesten, T.: Evolutionary algorithms for medical simulations: a case study in minimally-invasive vascular interventions. In: Proceedings of the 2005 Workshops on Genetic and Evolutionary Computation (GECCO 2005), pp. 125–132 (2005)
2. Bruyant, P.: Analytic and iterative reconstruction algorithms in SPECT. J. Nucl. Med. 43, 1343–1358 (2002)
3. Dines, K.A., Lytle, R.J.: Computerized Geophysical Tomography. Proceedings of the IEEE 67, 1065–1073 (1979)
4. Duhamel, P., Vetterli, M.: Fast Fourier transforms: a tutorial review and a state of the art. Signal Processing 19, 259–299 (1990)
5. Fessler, J.: Analytical Tomographic Image Reconstruction Methods, ch. 3 (November 19, 2009)
6. Herman, G.T.: Image Reconstruction from Projections. Academic Press, New York (1980)
7. Jain, A.K.: Image reconstruction from projections. In: Kailath, T. (ed.) Fundamentals of Digital Image Processing, pp. 431–475. Prentice-Hall, Englewood Cliffs (1989)
8. Kak, A.C., Slaney, M.: Principles of Computerized Tomographic Imaging. Society of Industrial and Applied Mathematics (2001)
9. Radon, J.: On the determination of functions from their integrals along certain manifolds (in German). Math. Phys. Klass. 69, 262–277 (1917)

A General Framework for Nonlinear Regularized Krylov-Based Image Restoration

Serena Morigi[1], Lothar Reichel[2], and Fiorella Sgallari[1]

[1] Department of Mathematics, University of Bologna, Bologna, Italy
{serena.morigi,fiorella.sgallari}@unibo.it
[2] Department of Mathematical Sciences, Kent State University, Kent, USA
reichel@math.kent.edu

Abstract. This paper introduces a new approach to computing an approximate solution of Tikhonov-regularized large-scale ill-posed problems with a general nonlinear regularization operator. The iterative method applies a sequence of projections onto generalized Krylov subspaces using a semi-implicit approach to deal with the nonlinearity in the regularization term. A suitable value of the regularization parameter is determined by the discrepancy principle. Computed examples illustrate the performance of the method applied to the restoration of blurred and noisy images.

1 Introduction

We consider solution methods for minimization problems of the form

$$\min_{x \in \mathbb{R}^n} \left\{ \|Ax - b\|_2^2 + \mu \|\mathcal{L}(x)\|_2^2 \right\},\tag{1}$$

where $A \in \mathbb{R}^{m \times n}$, $b \in \mathbb{R}^m$, $x \in \mathbb{R}^n$, and $\mathcal{L} : \mathbb{R}^n \to \mathbb{R}^s$ is a linear or nonlinear operator. In particular, in this paper, we applied model (1) to the restoration of images, where the vector x represents the desired unknown image and the available noise- and possibly blur-contaminated image is represented by the vector b. Thus

$$b = \hat{b} + e,\tag{2}$$

where $\hat{b}$ is the unknown error-free vector associated with b, and e represents the error. The first term in (1) is commonly referred to as the *fidelity term* and the second term as the *regularization term*. The operator $\mathcal{L}$ is chosen to yield a computed solution with some known desired features. The scalar $\mu > 0$ is a regularization parameter. Its purpose is to balance the influence of the fidelity and regularization terms on the computed solution in a suitable manner.

In image restoration applications, A is a blurring operator which is generally severely ill-conditioned and may be singular. The purpose of the regularization term is to be able to determine a useful solution of (1) of moderate norm.

When $\mathcal{L}$ is a linear operator represented by a regularization matrix $L \in \mathbb{R}^{s \times n}$, the minimization problem (1) is the classical Tikhonov-regularized linear

Y.J. Zhang and J.M.R.S. Tavares (Eds.): CompIMAGE 2014, LNCS 8641, pp. 273–279, 2014.
© Springer International Publishing Switzerland 2014

least-squares problem, and assuming that $\text{rank}([A \quad L]^T) = n$ the problem (1) has the unique solution

$$x_\mu = \left(A^T A + \mu L^T L\right)^{-1} A^T b \tag{3}$$

for any $\mu > 0$. Here and below the superscript ^{T} denotes transposition. For large-scale problems and a fixed $\mu > 0$, an approximation of x_μ can be determined by applying an iterative method, such as LSQR, to (3). However, generally, a suitable value of the parameter μ is not known a priori and has to be determined during the solution process. Many methods for the selection of an appropriate regularization parameter μ require the normal equations for (3) to be solved repeatedly for many different values of the parameter μ. A popular strategy for the selection of μ is based on the discrepancy principle, which assumes that an estimate ϵ of the norm of the error e in the vector b in (2) is available. A vector $\widetilde{x}_\mu$, such that

$$\|A\widetilde{x}_\mu - b\| = \delta := \eta\epsilon, \quad \epsilon \approx \|e\| \tag{4}$$

holds, is said to satisfy the discrepancy principle. Here $\eta > 1$ is a user-specified constant, whose size depends on the accuracy of the estimate ϵ of $\|e\|$.

When L is the identity matrix, denoted by I, the Tikhonov regularization problem (1) is said to be in *standard form* and the solution can be computed efficiently by, e.g., partial Golub–Kahan bidiagonalization of A; see, e.g., [1,2,3]. The computed approximation $\widetilde{x}_\mu^k$ lives into a Krylov subspace

$$\mathcal{K}_k(A^T A, A^T b) = \text{span}\{A^T b, (A^T A)A^T, \dots, (A^T A)^{k-1} A^T b\} \tag{5}$$

for some $k \geq 1$.

Golub–Kahan bidiagonalization also can be applied when $L \neq I$, provided that the regularization problem can be transformed to standard form without too much effort by applying the *A-weighted pseudoinverse* of L; see [4] for details.

As an alternative, a scheme that projects L into the Krylov subspace (5) and determines an approximate solution of (1) in this subspace is described in [6]. We will refer to this Krylov subspace approach to the problem (1) as KS.

Methods based on reducing both A and L by generalized Arnoldi-type or Golub–Kahan-type methods are discussed in [7,9]. An efficient iterative algorithm for the solution of large-scale Tikhonov regularization problems (1) with linear regularizing operators $\mathcal{L}$ and automatic selection of the regularization parameter μ is proposed in [8].

This work presents an extension of the algorithm in [8] which can be applied to the solution of (1) for general nonlinear operators $\mathcal{L}$ which are well-assessed in image restoration. By using a semi-implicit approach we replace (1) by

$$\min_{x \in \mathbb{R}^n} \left\{ \|Ax - b\|_2^2 + \mu \|\mathcal{L}(x, x_*)\|_2^2 \right\}, \tag{6}$$

where x_* is a known approximation, e.g. the result of a previous step in an iterative procedure. Therefore, the nonlinear operator $\mathcal{L}$ becomes a linear function of x. We refer to this method as the GKS method, which will be described in the following section.

2   The GKS Method

The method proposed in [8] is designed for the solution of large-scale Tikhonov regularization problems (1) with a general linear regularization operator $\mathcal{L}$ and determines the regularization parameter $\mu > 0$ by the discrepancy principle [5]. The method determines a sequence of orthogonal projections of generalized Krylov subspaces onto subspaces of low dimension; the operator $\mathcal{L}$ is unchanged at each iteration.

In the proposed GKS extension, we assume $\mathcal{L}(x)$ to be a nonlinear regularization operator, such as those describe in subsection 2.1, which is updated at each iterative step and contributes to enlarge the generalized Krylov subspace. The GKS method is initialized with a user-chosen subspace $\mathcal{V}_0 \subset \mathbb{R}^n$ of low dimension $l \ll n$. In the numerical section we let $\mathcal{V}_0 = \mathcal{K}_l(A^T A, A^T b)$ for $l \leq 3$. Let the columns of the matrix $V_0 \in \mathbb{R}^{n \times k}$ form an orthonormal basis for the space $\mathcal{V}_0$.

Assume that an estimate $\delta > 0$ for the l_2-norm of the noise in b is available. The discrepancy principle (4) is then applied to determine a suitable value of $\mu = \mu_k$ for each iteration $k = 0, 1, \ldots$ and compute the solution $x^{(k)}$ of the Tikhonov minimization problem (6) restricted to the subspace $\mathcal{V}_k$. This subspace is spanned by the orthonormal columns of the matrix V_k. Thus, $x^{(k)}$ is computed as follows:

$$y^{(k)} = \arg \min_{y \in \mathbb{R}^{l+k}} \left\{ \|AV_k y - b\|_2^2 + \mu_k \|L_{k-1} V_k y\|_2^2 \right\}, \quad x^{(k)} = V_k y^{(k)}, \qquad (7)$$

where L_{k-1} denotes the discretization of the nonlinear operator $\mathcal{L}$ linearized at the approximate solution $x_\mu^{(k-1)}$, which was computed at the previous iteration step. Define the $n \times n$ matrix

$$T(\mu_k) := A^T A + \mu_k L_{k-1}^T L_{k-1} . \qquad (8)$$

The solution $y^{(k)}$ of the reduced minimization problem (7) can be determined by solving the corresponding normal equations,

$$V_k^T T(\mu_k) V_k \, y = V_k^T A^T b , \qquad (9)$$

for $y^{(k)}$. The associated approximate solution $x^{(k)}$ of the original unreduced problem (1) is given by $x^{(k)} = V_k y^{(k)}$.

Following the approach in the nonlinear Arnoldi method also used in [8], the subspace $\mathcal{V}_k$ is expanded to $\mathcal{V}_{k+1}$ by adding a new basis vector v_{new} to $\mathcal{V}_k$. This basis vector is determined by normalizing the residual $r^{(k)}$ of the unreduced problem (1). Thus,

$$v_{\text{new}} = \frac{r^{(k)}}{\|r^{(k)}\|_2}, \quad r^{(k)} = T(\mu_k) x^{(k)} - A^T b . \qquad (10)$$

Notice that the residual vector $r^{(k)}$ is parallel to the gradient of the functional minimized in the original unreduced problem (1) evaluated at $x^{(k)}$. In the absence of round-off errors, $r^{(k)}$ is orthogonal to the search space $\mathcal{V}_k$. To enforce orthogonality in the presence of round-off errors, the residual $r^{(k)}$ can be re-orthogonalized against $\mathcal{V}_k$ before normalization.

We remark that the space $\mathcal{V}_k$ is a Krylov subspace only in very special situations. Since the regularization parameter μ_k is updated during the iterations, so is the matrix $T(\mu_k)$. Therefore, the space $\mathcal{V}_k$, in general, is not a Krylov subspace when $L \neq I$. For this reason, the search space $\mathcal{V}_k$ is referred to as a generalized Krylov subspace.

2.1   Choice of the Regularization Operator $\mathcal{L}$

Nonlinear PDE-based methods have been applied successfully to noise-removal [11]. In the continuous setting, a popular general nonlinear diffusion model determines a denoised image w from a noise-contaminated image b by solving

$$\frac{\partial w}{\partial t} = \mathrm{div}(g(|\nabla w|)\nabla w), \quad w(x, 0) = b. \tag{11}$$

According to the definition of the diffusivity function g, that are, i.e.

$$g_{PM}(s) := 1/(1 + s^2/\rho^2), \quad g_{TV}(s) := 1/s, \quad g_{Lap}(s) := 1/s, \tag{12}$$

we get the well-known Perona Malik (PM) [11], Total Variation (TV) [10], and Laplacian (Lap) restoration models.

The regularization matrix L_{k-1} at the iteration k of the iterative method GKS is obtained by the linearization of the right hand side of (11) that is, by evaluating g at $|\nabla w|$ using w from the previous time-step i, i.e.,

$$\mathcal{L}(w^{(i)}) \approx \mathrm{div}(g(|\nabla w^{(i-1)}|)\nabla w^{(i)}). \tag{13}$$

Discretization of (13) gives the matrix $L_{k-1} \in \mathbb{R}^{n^2 \times n^2}$ with, generically, five nonvanishing entries in each row. Spatial partial derivatives are approximated by central finite differences; see [11] for details.

After a few time steps i (5 in the computed examples at most), the regularization matrix L_{k-1} is updated to obtain the new regularization matrix. In the numerical section, we compare results obtained when the matrix L is defined by the different choices in (12). We will denote these matrices by L_{PM}, L_{TV}, and L_{Lap}, respectively.

3   Numerical Examples

This section illustrates the performance of the proposed GKS approach described in Section 2 when applied to the restoration of gray scale images test, barbara, peppers, and cameraman. These images are represented by arrays of 256×256 pixels stored column-wise in vectors in $\mathbb{R}^n$ with $n = 65536$.

The images are synthetically corrupted by blur and noise. Let the vector $x \in \mathbb{R}^n$ represent the original, unavailable blur- and noise-free image. A block Toeplitz with Toeplitz blocks blurring matrix $A \in \mathbb{R}^{n \times n}$ is generated with the

Table 1. Comparison of the KS and GKS algorithms applied to the images `test` and `cameraman` corrupted by fixed Gaussian noise with $\sigma = 10$

blur		Reg.	SNR$_0$	Its		SNR		SNR$_0$	Its		SNR	
band	sigma	L		KS	GKS	KS	GKS		KS	GKS	KS	GKS
					test					cameraman		
3	1	L_{Lap}	2.61	6	6	11.29	11.10	3.77	7	6	11.36	11.66
		L_{PM}		3	7	11.61	11.81		8	8	11.76	12.00
		L_{TV}		6	3	11.30	11.44		11	2	11.42	11.76
5	1.5	L_{Lap}	3.80	6	9	8.98	10.60	4.80	10	10	9.99	10.66
		L_{PM}		12	8	10.25	10.42		12	9	10.65	10.80
		L_{TV}		10	3	9.92	10.63		13	2	10.07	10.34

function `blur` in MATLAB. This function has the parameters `band` and `sigma`, which determine the half-bandwidth of each Toeplitz block in A and the standard deviation of the underlying Gaussian point spread function, respectively.

We compare the quality of the restorations determined by the GKS and KS methods by measuring the Signal-to-Noise Ratio SNR; larger SNR-values generally indicate more accurate restorations. In the Tables the SNR-values of the initial contaminated images are tabulated in the column labelled SNR$_0$.

Computational efficiency is measured in terms of the total number of iterations, *Its* in the Tables, required by the algorithms to satisfy the following stopping criterion. The number of iterations of the KS and GKS algorithms are terminated as soon as the relative error $\|x^{(k)} - x^{(k-1)}\|/\|x^{(k)}\|$ of the computed approximate solution $x^{(k)}$ drops below a user-specified threshold which for the reported experiments is $\tau = 5 \cdot 10^{-4}$.

The overall computational cost for *Its* iterations with the GKS algorithm is dominated by the count of arithmetic floating point operations required to evaluate $4Its$ matrix-vector products (MVP); each MVP with T is computed by evaluating one MVP with each one of the matrices L, L^T, A and A^T; cf. (8). Moreover, at each iteration, we computate a new regularization matrix L. This is not expensive due to the sparsity of L. The dominant computational cost for each iteration with the KS method is limited to 2 MVPs. The parameter η in (4) is 1.05.

Table 1 reports results for the restorations of the test images `test` and `cameraman` degraded by Gaussian blur with different parameters `band` and `sigma`, and a fixed Gaussian noise with $\sigma = 10$. Specifically, we considered the three regularization operators L_{Lap}, L_{PM}, and L_{TV} defined in Section 2.1. Table 1 illustrates the good performance of the GKS approach in terms of both accuracy of the restorations and computational effort. Figures 1 and 2 show restorations obtained by the GKS and KS algorithms when applied to the test images `test` and `cameraman`. The degraded images in Figures 1(b) and 2(b) were obtained from the original blur- and noise-free images in Figures 1(a) and 2(a), respectively, by applying Gaussian blur with parameters `band` = 5 and `sigma` = 1.5, for `test` and `band` = 5 and `sigma` = 2.0 for `cameraman`. The noise is Gaussian with

$\sigma = 10$ and the regularization operator is L_{TV} for both images. Figures 1(c),2(c) and Figures 1(d),2(d) depict restorations obtained with the GKS and KS methods, respectively. For both test images, the GKS method yields a slightly more accurate restoration than the KS method both in terms of visual quality and SNR-value.

Table 2. Comparison of the GKS and KS algorithms using $L = L_{TV}$; the images have been contaminated by Gaussian blur with **band** = 5 and **sigma** = 2.0

Image	noise	SNR$_0$	Its		SNR	
	σ		KS	GKS	KS	GKS
	5	1.74	10	2	12.40	12.58
peppers	10	1.60	13	3	10.84	11.26
	15	1.38	9	3	9.78	10.65
	20	1.08	8	3	8.87	8.81
	5	-0.33	4	2	10.54	10.80
cameraman	10	-0.39	16	3	9.20	9.81
	15	-0.49	36	2	8.37	9.30
	20	-0.63	36	3	7.71	7.90
	5	-0.37	6	2	7.96	8.13
barbara	10	-0.50	4	3	7.15	7.38
	15	-0.71	6	3	6.47	6.97
	20	-0.99	7	3	5.88	6.64

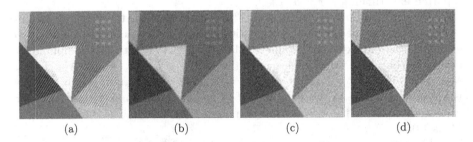

(a)   (b)   (c)   (d)

Fig. 1. Restoration results:(a) original, (b) corrupted (SNR = 3.80), (c) restored by KS (SNR = 9.92), (d) restored by GKS (SNR = 10.63)

In Table 2, we consider the restoration of three different images corrupted by Gaussian blur with **band** = 5 and **sigma** = 2.0 (second column), and by additive zero-mean white Gaussian noise with different standard deviations σ. The benefits of the GKS algorithm using the L_{TV} regularization operator can be observed both in terms of computational effort and quality of the restored images (SNR).

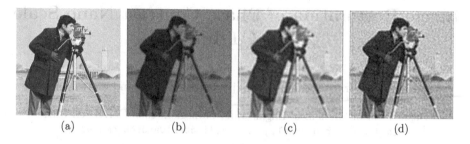

(a)   (b)   (c)   (d)

Fig. 2. Restoration results: (a) original (b) corrupted ($SNR_0 = -0.39$), (c) restored by KS ($SNR = 9.30$) ,(d) restored by GKS ($SNR = 9.81$)

4   Conclusions

The proposed scheme is an extension to the method in [8] and allows nonlinear regularization operators. This has been realized by a semi-implicit strategy based on updating the regularization matrix L at every iteration step. We have shown that this approach requires fewer iterations than application of a standard Krylov subspace method and produces restored images of higher quality.

Acknoledgement. Research supported in part by NSF grant DMS-1115385.

References

1. Björck, Å.: A bidiagonalization algorithm for solving large and sparse ill-posed systems of linear equations. BIT Numer. Math. 28, 659–670 (1988)
2. Calvetti, D., Reichel, L.: Tikhonov regularization of large linear problems. BIT Numer. Math. 43, 263–283 (2003)
3. Calvetti, D., Morigi, S., Reichel, L., Sgallari, F.: Tikhonov regularization and the L-curve for large, discrete ill-posed problems. J. Comput. Appl. Math. 123, 423–446 (2000)
4. Eldén, L.: A weighted pseudoinverse, generalized singular values, and constrained least squares problems. BIT Numer. Math. 22, 487–502 (1982)
5. Engl, H.W., Hanke, M., Neubauer, A.: Regularization of Inverse Problems. Kluwer, Dordrecht (1996)
6. Hochstenbach, M.E., Reichel, L.: An iterative method for Tikhonov regularization with a general linear regularization operator. J. Integral Equations Appl. 22, 463–480 (2010)
7. Hochstenbach, M.E., Reichel, L., Yu, X.: A Golub–Kahan-type reduction method for matrix pairs (submitted for publication)
8. Lampe, J., Reichel, L., Voss, H.: Large-scale Tikhonov regularization via reduction by orthogonal projection. Linear Algebra Appl. 436, 2845–2865 (2012)
9. Reichel, L., Sgallari, F., Ye, Q.: Tikhonov regularization based on generalized Krylov subspace methods. Appl. Numer. Math. 62, 1215–1228 (2012)
10. Rudin, L., Osher, S., Fatemi, E.: Nonlinear total variation based noise removal algorithms. Physica D 60, 259–268 (1992)
11. Weickert, J., Romeny, B.M.H., Viergever, M.A.: Efficient and reliable schemes for nonlinear diffusion filtering. IEEE Trans. Image Processing 7, 398–410 (1998)

Image Restoration of Phase Contrast Nano Scale X-ray CT Images

Arjun Kumar, Pratiti Mandal, Yongjie Jessica Zhang, and Shawn Litster

Department of Mechanical Engineering, Carnegie Mellon University, USA
{arjun.kumar,pmandal,jessicaz,litster}@andrew.cmu.edu

Abstract. Zernike phase contrast is a technique useful for nano-scale X-ray imaging of materials with a low absorption coefficient. It enhances the image contrast using a phase ring. However, it also creates artifacts that hinder the use of traditional techniques for X-ray computed tomography (CT) image segmentation. We propose an image restoration method that models the phase contrast optics and minimizes an energy function. Though similar techniques have been used for visible light microscopy, this method deals with more spacious samples using an effective edge detection method. This paper demonstrates the removal of artifacts in multiple slices of phase contrast X-ray CT images and the potential in using this technique to aid CT image segmentation.

Keywords: Nano scale X-ray computed tomography, phase contrast optics, image restoration, image segmentation.

1 Introduction

X-ray CT images can be very effective in differentiating the density and absorption coefficient of the materials being imaged. However, materials for a lot of engineering and medical applications, such as polymers, carbon structures and soft tissues, often have a low atomic number (Z) and offer negligible contrast relative to their surroundings. In addition, many of these materials have sub-micron features of interest that require nano-scale resolution X-ray CT (nanoCT). The use of lens-based X-ray optics, that achieve resolutions as high as 30-50 nm [1], makes Zernike phase contrast the most suitable technique for nanoCT [2].

The key component of Zernike phase contrast is the phase ring. Initially, the sample phase shifts the incoming wave due to the change in refractive index [3]. However, this difference in phase is minimal and provides insufficient image contrast. The phase ring increases the contrast by phase shifting the surrounding waved by $\pi/2$. However, a fraction of the diffracted wave leaks onto the phase ring and is also phase shifted by $\pi/2$. As a result, dark artifacts appear where the magnitude of the particle wave is lower than that of the surrounding wave [4]. Specifically, the thin dark region around a sample is known as halo, and the low contrast within is known as shade-off. Due to these artifacts, standard segmentation techniques produce inaccurate results.

Y.J. Zhang and J.M.R.S. Tavares (Eds.): CompIMAGE 2014, LNCS 8641, pp. 280–285, 2014.

Though current trends are changing, the use of phase contrast imaging is far more prevalent in biological visible light than in X-ray microscopy [5]. Yin et al. [4] reviewed the drawbacks of previous methods that automate the segmentation of phase contrast microscopy images. They restore artifact-free images based on a derived model of the microscope optics to produce quick and accurate segmented results. For X-ray microscopy, current efforts, like [3] and [6], focus on retrieving the phase shift for each radiograph by modelling the refractive index of the object. Other interesting methods that tackle the same issue include frequency harmonics [7], regularization techniques [8] and optics modeling [9]. However, a lot of these attempts verified their theoretical work using simulations and not acquired images. Lastly and importantly, for Zernike phase contrast, phase retrieval algorithms often perform poorly [10]. They are directed for other phase contrast imaging techniques, the most common one being interferometry [2].

Our work aims to deconvolve the nanoCT images to eliminate the artifacts and easily generate accurate segmented results. To that end, we model the optics of a nanoCT machine in Section 2. The modelling of this combination of components to set up an inverse problem is a new technique for Zernike phase contrast in nanoCT. We present the energy function and describe the robust edge detection method used to solve the inverse problem in Section 3. We use slices from two CT images obtained from the nanoCT (UltraXRM-L200, Xradia Inc., Pleasanton, CA) for testing and show their results in Section 4. Finally, we close with conclusions and future directions in Section 5.

2   Derivation of Imaging Model

The components of a nanoCT machine are linear shift-invariant systems. We derive the kernel $h(x, y)$ that convolves each X-ray radiograph into one with artifacts. This derivation uses the model of diffraction. Diffraction in the nanoCT typically occurs in the Fresnel regime [11]. Hence, the diffracted wave through an aperture is given by [12],

$$U(x, y, z) = U(x', y', 0) * \frac{e^{ikz}}{i\lambda z} e^{\frac{ik}{2z}(x'^2 + y'^2)}$$
$$= U(x', y', 0) * K(g_a, z), \tag{1}$$

where k is the wave number and λ is the wavelength of the X-ray. z is the distance between the aperture plane and plane of interest. x and y are the coordinates at the plane of interest; x' and y' are the coordinates at the aperture plane. The coordinates x, y and z are defined in Figure 1. Finally, $U(x', y', 0)$ describes the wave at the aperture plane and $(x', y') \in g_a$ defines the aperture domain.

We derive the final kernel by modelling the effect each component in the nanoCT has on the waveforms. These operations are shown in Figure 1 and most of them take the form of Eq. 1. The intensity of the radiograph at the detector is given by the magnitude square of the difference between the surrounding and diffracted wave. Since the phase shift of the diffracted wave due to the sample is small, we make a linear approximation to derive the kernel $h(x, y)$. In this study,

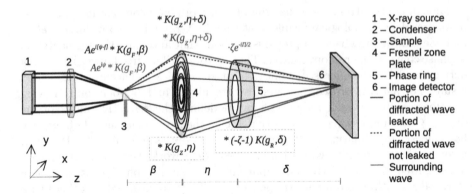

Fig. 1. Flow chart of the operations applied on the waves, where f is the sample, g_F is the field of view, g_z is the aperture of the Fresnel zone plate (FZP), g_R is the outer ring domain. The FZP focuses the waves by means of diffraction to achieve high resolution [1]. Since the phase ring in this study uses negative phase contrast, the phase ring shifts the waves by $-\pi/2$.

we apply the the negative of this kernel to virtual slices of the image instead of the acquired radiographs. Quantifying the error induced by this approximation is the focus of future work. However, since the artifacts also appear in virtual slices, we argue that this is a good approximation. We use the negative of the derived kernel because the reconstructor displays the attenuation coefficient of the sample, which is inversely related to the intensity of a radiograph.

3   Energy Function Minimization

With the optical model derived above, we set up an inverse problem such that

$$g = Hf + C, \tag{2}$$

where g is the input image, f is the artifact-free image and H is an ill-conditioned matrix. Solving this problem by matrix inversion is highly sensitive to noise. Hence, our algorithm proposes the minimization of an energy function [4], written as

$$O(f) = \|Hf - g\|_2^2 + \omega_s f^T L f + \omega_r \|\Lambda f\|_1, \tag{3}$$

where ω_s and ω_r are weighting parameters. The second term is the spatial smoothness regularization, which performs edge-preserving smoothing. The third term is the sparsity regularization term, where Λ is a diagonal positive matrix, whose values corresponding to dark pixels should be high and vice versa for bright pixels.

Λ in Eq. 3 is important in making this algorithm robust [13] and effective for spacious structures. We initialize this matrix by interpolating the image from the sample boundary. The gradient magnitude of Figure 3(a) is shown in Figure 2(a).

As it is evident, the edges of the object have varying magnitudes due to the fickle nature of the artifacts. We tackle this issue by segmenting the gradient magnitude image using Otsu's method. We output three or four classes, which correspond to the homogeneous regions, noise, fine features and strong boundaries of the image. The latter two classes are shown in Figure 2(b) and (c). Unfortunately, the artifacts also exist in the class shown in Figure 2(b). They are eliminated, as shown in the resulting control points in Figure 2(d), if the corresponding edge is also represented by the class shown in Figure 2(c).

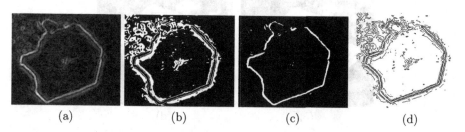

(a)   (b)   (c)   (d)

Fig. 2. Construction of a set of control points for the virtual slice shown in Figure 3(a). (a) Gradient magnitude image; segmented class of (b) fine features; (c) strong boundaries; and (d) resulting control points.

We then create an image g_c, whose value at each non-control point is set to the mean of the intensities at the closest N_c control points. If $g' = \alpha g_c + (1-\alpha)g$, where α is an user defined input, we initialize Λ, yielding

$$\Lambda^{init} = diag\left(e^{\frac{-(g'-\mu)}{\sigma}}\right),\qquad(4)$$

where μ and σ are the mean and standard deviation of the image g.

4   Results and Discussion

In this section, we display the algorithm performance on a virtual slice of two different particles, shown in Figures 3(a) and 4(a), and segment them by thresholding. The particle shown in Figure 3(a) is a dust particle out of a combustion chamber. Firstly, the restored image shows the contrast this method generates making a simple segmentation technique, like thresholding, viable. The segmentation of the restored image captures the actual boundary of the object with good accuracy. It also captures the particles at the top left corner of the image with good specificity. There are a few, small erroneous segmented regions around them. The biggest drawback of the result is the blurring of fine details, especially the hole in the middle of the particle. This could be improved with further morphological operations.

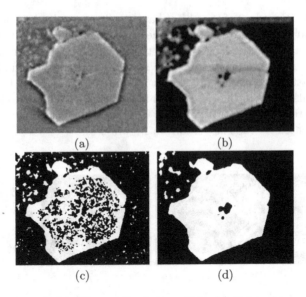

Fig. 3. Performance of algorithm on the dust particle. (a) Original image; (b) restored image; (c-d) Otsu thresholding of the original and restored images, respectively.

The particle in Figure 4(a) is a fiber coated with Polytetrafluoroethylene (PTFE). The increase in contrast is more predominant in this case. This is a harder object to segment due to the intricate PTFE structure coated on the fiber. Due to the weak boundaries of the PTFE, the algorithm creates artifacts at its vicinity in the restored image. However, the contrast is sufficient to accurately differentiate the object, as shown in Figure 4(d). The errors can be further reduced by improving the search method for the control points. In this example, fine details, such as the gap between the holes, are also blurred.

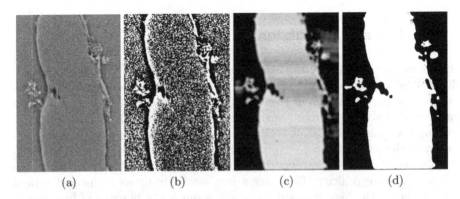

Fig. 4. Performance of algorithm on the fiber. (a) Original image; (b) restored image; (c-d) Otsu thresholding of the original and restored images, respectively.

5   Conclusion and Future Work

Preliminary results show that modelling phase contrast optics, specific to the imaging conditions, and the design of an optimal objective function can restore Zernike phase contrast CT images from a nanoCT machine. The advantage of modelling the optics is the ease of extension to different applications, instruments and experimental objectives. Our thorough construction of the energy function can make this algorithm robust for many samples. The increased contrast and the absence of false edges allow us to accurately segment nanoCT images. This method needs to extend to 3D images and include a strong verification of the kernel derivation. Another useful study is the comparison of this method to effective segmentation algorithms, for speed and accuracy.

References

1. Chen, Y.T., Chen, T.Y., Yi, J., Chu, Y.S., Lee, W.K., Wang, C.L., Margaritondo, G.: Hard x-ray Zernike microscopy reaches 30 nm resolution. Optics Letters 36(7), 1269–1271 (2011)
2. Withers, P.J.: X-ray nanotomography. Materials Today 10(12), 26–34 (2007)
3. Maksimenko, A., Ando, M., Hiroshi, S., Yuasa, T.: Computed tomographic reconstruction based on X-ray refraction contrast. Applied Physics Letters 86(12), 124105 (2005)
4. Yin, Z., Kanade, T., Chen, M.: Understanding the phase contrast optics to restore artifact-free microscopy images for segmentation. Medical Image Analysis 16, 1047–1062 (2012)
5. Lider, V.V., Kovalcuk, M.V.: X-ray phase-contrast methods. Crystallography Reports 58(6), 769–787 (2013)
6. Mayo, S.C., Davis, T.J., Gureyev, T.E., Miller, P.R., Paganin, D., Pogany, A., Stevenson, A.W., Wilkins, S.W.: X-ray phase-contrast microscopy and microtomography. Optics Express 11(19), 2289–2302 (2003)
7. Wu, J., Chen, J.: A phase retrival algorithm for X-ray phase contrast imaging. Optik 124, 864–866 (2013)
8. Köhler, T., Brendel, B., Roessl, E.: Iterative reconstruction for differential phase contrast imaging using spherically symmetric basis functions. Medical Physics 38(8), 4542–4545 (2011)
9. Pavlov, K.M., Kewish, C.M., Davis, J.R., Morgan, M.J.: A variant on the geometrical optics approximation in diffraction enhanced tomography. Journal of Physics D: Applied Physics 34(10A), A168 (2001)
10. Tkachuk, A., Duewer, F., Cui, H., Feser, M., Wang, S., Yun, W.: X-ray computed tomography in Zernike phase contrast mode at 8 keV with 50-nn resolution using Cu rotating anode X-ray source. Zeitschrift fur Kristallographie 222, 650–655 (2007)
11. Zoofan, B., Kim, J.-Y., Rokhlin, S.I., Frankel, G.S.: Phase-contrast X-ray imaging for nondestructive evaluation of materials. Journal of Applied Physics 100(1), 014502 (2006)
12. Born, M., Wolf, E.: Principles of Optics, 6th ed. Pergamon Press (1980)
13. Snyder, W.E., Qi, H.: Machine Vision. Cambridge Press (2004)

Predictive Modeling for 2D Form Design

Erhan Batuhan Arisoy, Gunay Orbay, and Levent Burak Kara*

Department of Mechanical Engineering
Carnegie Mellon University
Pittsburgh, Pennsylvania 15213, USA
{earisoy,gorbay,lkara}@andrew.cmu.edu

Abstract. In product design, designers often generate a large number of concepts in the form of sketches and drawings to develop and communicate their ideas. Concrete concepts typically evolve through a progressive refinement of initially coarse and ambiguous ideas. However, a lack of suitable means to visualize the emerging form at these early stages forces the designer to constantly maintain and negotiate an elusive mental image. To assist this process, we describe a predictive modeling technique that allows early, incomplete 2D sketches to be transformed into suggestive complete models. This helps designers take a sneak peek at the potential end result of a developing concept, without forcing them to commit to the suggestion. We demonstrate and discuss preliminary results of our technique on 2D shape design problems.

Keywords: CAD, predictive modeling, conceptual design.

1 Introduction

Recent developments in computer-aided design (CAD) have led to a large number professional software packages for different modeling needs. These packages all share a common goal, that is, to enable design of sophisticated geometries with less effort and prior experience. Nevertheless, most of these professional tools still require acquaintance with the underlying geometrical representations and related modeling operations and lack of suitable means to quickly visualize the emerging design ideas forces the designer to constantly maintain the mental image without any visual reference. To enhance this process, we propose a predictive form modeling method that converts early, incomplete drawings into suggestive complete models to establish visual references.

The main challenge in the proposed work is being able to interpret incomplete sketches to find a complete geometric model biased toward simpler interpretations, aligned with Occam's Razor theorem [12]. Our proposed technique has following specific contributions:

1. Generating a suggestive prediction for the intended geometry from user drawn strokes

---

* Corresponding author.

Y.J. Zhang and J.M.R.S. Tavares (Eds.): CompIMAGE 2014, LNCS 8641, pp. 286–291, 2014.

2. Enabling early visualization of the intended geometry for rapid evaluation and refinement decisions
3. Creating a feedback mechanism to check feasibility of the developed concept under proposed constraints

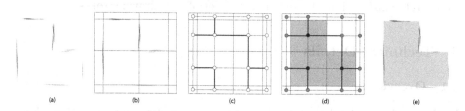

Fig. 1. The inner workings of our preliminary predictive drawing tool. (a) The input is a set of strokes that are grouped as they are drawn by the user. (b) The strokes are converted into geometric entities that partition the drawing plane. (c) The resulting partitions are represented as a graph structure. (d) The graph structure allows calculation of a region that is blocked by the input strokes (e) and visualized for the user.

In a typical scenario, our method takes as input a set of 2D sketches with 2D coordinate values and performs stroke clustering and beautification. In the next step, each stroke is treated as an infinitely long line which partitions the drawing plane into two regions and our method seeks to identify a union of these regions generated by every stroke as the prediction for the intended geometry through a genetic algorithm (GA).

2 Related Work

Researchers have extensively studied line drawings and their utilization in a wide variety of application areas ranging from non-photorealistic rendering techniques to 3D reconstruction. However, these line drawings typically involve roughly drawn overlapping strokes that require a separate analysis to identify salient curves and regions. To this end, Grabli *et al.* [2] and Wilson *et al.* [3] proposed line omission techniques where original strokes with less effectiveness scores are eliminated from the input set. Similarly, Barla and Sheh [4] developed simplification schemes based on perceptual and spatial grouping. In addition to sketch beautification and simplification, Sezgin [6] and Fu [7] focused on recognition and utilization of 2D user drawings and proposed tools designed to detect symbol networks from user drawings and convert them into engineering diagrams. Similarly, researchers teased out the importance of drawing order in sketches and Tversky and Suwa presented that the drawing order gives clues to the mental organization of the human brain [1]. Likewise, Novik and Tversky [8] supported this argument such that the drawing order reflects how the designers construct a concept in his mind. In addition to these studies, a multitude of tools are proposed for rapid 3D reconstruction using rough 2D sketches. Zeleznik [9] proposed a modeling tool which seeks to fit 3D primitives by grouping user drawn strokes. Igarashi [10,5] utilized user drawn strokes for initial model generation and its deformation. The main advantage of the proposed system is bringing a higher level of prediction capability such that the prediction depends not only on one to one relationships but also on the entire set of user drawn strokes.

3   Technical Details

3.1   Overview

In this work, we develop and utilize a novel prediction approach that allows early, incomplete sketches to be transformed into suggestive geometries and our approach consists of 3 main steps: (1) generation of input curve set, its simplification and beautification, (2) construction of an undirected graph structure and (3) definition of an objective function and its minimization on the constructed graph and visualization of the results.

3.2   Preprocessing of the Input Strokes

In this step, an automatic stroke grouping algorithm groups and separates the input strokes into distinct clusters of curves and each stroke is analyzed using two geometric pairwise stroke features. The first feature is the closest distance between the two strokes, and the second is the angle difference between the tangents that are drawn at the points that yield the closest distance between the strokes. After grouping, each stroke group is further analyzed and every stroke in the sketch is represented as line segments, arcs or circles.

3.3   Construction of Graph Structure

In our formulation, every user-drawn stroke is treated as an infinite line which partitions input domain into two different regions where our algorithm will assign either a positive or negative label for each region where positive assignments represent inclusions to the domain and negative assignments mean subtractions from the domain. We assign a probability on each extended line E_i such that they have a maximum value of 1 at the center position (C_x, C_y) of the representing stroke S_i and decreases as we move on E_i. Actually, we place a Gaussian distribution centered at (C_x, C_y) with mean 0 and variance depending on the length of S_i using equation (1). Figure 2 demonstrates the extension of beautifed user drawn strokes with corresponding probability assignments.

$$N(x) = e^{-(x-\mu)^2/2\sigma^2} \; where \; \sigma = \frac{\|E_i\|}{5} \; and \; \mu = 0 \tag{1}$$

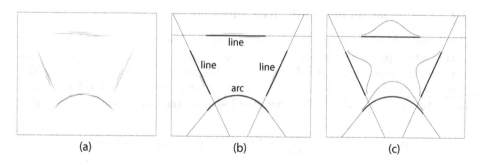

Fig. 2. The extension of the geometric entities to partition the drawing plane. (a) A given sketch, is first converted into a set of line or arc segments. (b) The lines and arcs are then extended at their end points in the tangent directions. (c) The extended lines attain weights according to a Gaussian kernel defined as a function of the segments length (*i.e.* influence).

Graph Structure. Our graph model $G(V, E_d)$ consists of nodes N and undirected edges E_d connecting nodes to each other. In our problem setting, each node represents a partition created after the infinite extension of a stroke S_i in the image domain and each edge acts as the boundary existing between two partitions. Figure 3 demonstrates the conversion from partitioned image domain to the graph structure G. After creation of complete graph G, our algorithm calculates a probability for each edge based on the probability weights assigned in the stroke extension phase. The probability values exist on the extended lines enable us to have a metric to measure how likely the boundary between two partitions is a contour or not. This value is calculated by taking the mean of the corresponding probability values assigned on that portion of the extended line.

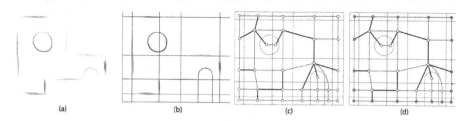

Fig. 3. The conversion of a sketch into a graph and the initial value assignments. (a) A given sketch is first converted into regions (b) by extending the identified lines, arcs, and circles. (c) Each resulting graph is represented as a node in the graph, while each adjacent region forms a link between their associated nodes. Here, the links that correspond to region boundaries that coincide with the original segments, are labeled as *constrained links*. (d) Initially, the regions that touch the drawing plane boundary are labeled as empty space.

3.4   Optimization and Objective Function

Our approach seeks to find the right combination of region labels through an optimization procedure where our objective function in Eqn. 2 consists of two main terms. First term, called assumed probability for an edge, represents the likelihood of an edge to be a part of the user drawn stroke intended for contour generation and second term is calculated based on the initial label assignments.

$$objective function = \sum_{k=1}^{m} \sum_{i=1}^{n_k} (assumed weight_{ki} - real weight_{ki}) \qquad (2)$$

where m is the total number of nodes (i.e. number of partitions) and n_k is the number of first ring neighbors of the kth node. Since our candidate solutions can be easily represented using chromosomes, we employ genetic algorithm to minimize our objective function using five steps explained in [11].

3.5   Results and Implementation Details

The interface of our algorithm is implemented in C++ and the optimization part is performed in MATLAB environment. Curve sets are generated using a graphics tablet interface. In all cases the domain is quantized into an $N \times N$ uniform grid. An important user adjustment parameter is the variance of the Gaussian distribution used in probability assignments on infinite lines. Users might prefer higher covariance values which increases the effect of the user drawn strokes or vice versa. The motivation is if the covariance is chosen very high, even a very short user drawn line will be treated as a very important contour separating inside form from the outside. The designer can modify this parameter according to his drawing style. Figure 4 illustrates two examples generated using proposed methodology where the domain size is 600 by 600 and covariance parameters are selected as 10. The optimization converged in 5 steps under 2 seconds. In terms of technicality, our main technical challenge is the fast increasing number

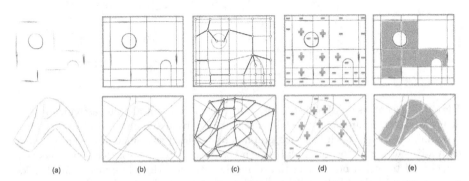

Fig. 4. Examples generated using proposed methodology. (a) 2D input drawings. (b) Extended lines and domain partitioning. (c) Corresponding graph structures. (d) Labels obtained via optimization. (e) Predicted solid regions.

of partitions with the introduction of each additional stroke to the domain. Since each added partition expands dimension of the solution space and slows down the optimization. However, for most of the test cases, our GA method reaches global minimum in less than 50 iterations under 10 seconds. Furthermore, image based representation prevents us from dealing small area partitions and detection of neighborhood information using pixel data.

3.6   Conclusion and Future Work

In this paper we proposed a computer tool for early design stages which allows designers to take a sneak peek at the potential end results of an evolving design form. Our approach has been different than previous studies such that it can handle with both incomplete and higher genus geometries. We believe that future CAD tools will improve their auto complete or snap features to support more general prediction problems.

References

1. Tversky, B., Suwa, M.: Thinking with sketches. Tools for Innovatio 1(9), 75–85 (2009)
2. Grabli, S., Durand, F., Sillion, F.: Density measure for line-drawing simplification. In: Proceedings of the 12th Pacific Conference on Computer Graphics and Applications, PG 2004, pp. 309–318 (2004)
3. Wilson, B., Ma, K.-L.: Rendering complexity in computer-generated pen-and-ink illustrations. In: Proceedings of the 3rd International Symposium on Non-Photorealistic Animation and Rendering, NPAR 2004, pp. 129–137. ACM (2004)
4. Barla, P., Thollot, J., Sillion, F.X.: Geometric clustering for line drawing simplification. In: ACM SIGGRAPH 2005 Sketches, SIGGRAPH 2005. ACM (2005)
5. Nealen, A., Igarashi, T., Sorkine, O., Alexa, M.: Fibermesh: designing freeform surfaces with 3D curves. ACM Trans. Graph. 26(3), 41 (2007)
6. Sezgin, T.M., Stahovich, T., Davis, R.: Sketch based interfaces: early processing for sketch understanding. In: ACM SIGGRAPH 2006 Courses, SIGGRAPH 2006. ACM (2006)
7. Fu, L., Kara, L.B.: Neural network-based symbol recognition using a few labeled samples. Computers & Graphics 35(5), 955–966 (2011)
8. Novick, L., Tversky, B.: Cognitive constraints on ordering operations: The case of geometric analogies. Journal of Experimental Psychology: General 116(1), 50 (1987)
9. LaViola, J., Zeleznik, R.: Mathpad2: A system for the creation and exploration of mathematical sketches. Proceedings of SIGGRAPH 23, 432–440 (2004)
10. Igarashi, T., Matsuoka, S., Tanaka, H.: Teddy: a sketching interface for 3D freeform design. In: Proceedings of SIGGRAPH 1999, p. 21. ACM (1999)
11. Goldberg, D.: Genetic algorithms in search, optimization, and machine learning. Addison-wesley (1989)
12. Blumer, A., Ehrenfeucht, A., Haussler, D., Warmuth, M.K.: Occam's razor. Information processing letters 24(6), 377–380 (1987)

Computational Image Modeling for Characterization and Analysis of Intracellular Cargo Transport

Kuan-Chieh Chen[1,2], Minhua Qiu[1,2,4], Jelena Kovacevic[1,2,3], and Ge Yang[1,2]

[1] Department of Biomedical Engineering
[2] Center for Bioimage Informatics
[3] Department of Electrical Engineering, Carnegie Mellon University,
Pittsburgh, PA 15213, USA
{kuanchic,jelenak,geyang}@andrew.cmu.edu
[4] Genomics Institute of the Novartis Research Foundation, San Diego, CA 92121, USA
minhua.qiu@gmail.com

Abstract. Active intracellular cargo transport is essential to survival and function of eukaryotic cells. How this process is controlled spatially and temporally so that the right cargo is delivered to the right destination at the right time remains poorly understood. To address this question, it is essential to characterize and analyze the molecular machinery and spatiotemporal behavior of intracellular transport. To this end, we developed related computational image models. Specifically, to study the molecular machinery of intracellular transport, we developed anisotropic spatial density kernels for reconstruction and segmentation of related super-resolution STORM (stochastic optical reconstruction microscopy) images. To study the spatiotemporal behavior of intracellular transport, we developed hidden Markov models and principal component analysis for representation and analysis of movement of individual transported cargoes. We validated and benchmarked the image models using simulated and actual experimental images. The models and related computational analysis methods developed in this study are general and can be used for studying molecular machinery and spatiotemporal dynamics of other cellular processes.

Keywords: image modeling, intracellular transport, spatiotemporal dynamics, super-resolution imaging, STORM imaging, spatial density estimation, hidden Markov model, principal component analysis.

1   Introduction

The inner environment of eukaryotic cells is highly dynamic and heterogeneous yet exquisitely organized. A basic principle of the organization is to compartment the intracellular environment into membrane-enclosed organelles. However, this creates a logistics problem because materials must be transferred between the organelles [1]. Cells solved this problem by utilizing an intracellular cargo transport system [2], which in many ways resembles the vehicular transport system of our cities.

Y.J. Zhang and J.M.R.S. Tavares (Eds.): CompIMAGE 2014, LNCS 8641, pp. 292–303, 2014.

Intracellular cargo transport is essential to survival and function of eukaryotic cells. This is especially evident in neurons, whose structure and function are highly polarized. A hallmark of the polarized structure of neurons is their long and thin axons, which in humans can extend for more than one meter at a diameter of a few micrometers. Because material synthesis and degradation are carried out mostly in the neuronal cell body, a wide variety of cargoes essential to the survival and function of neurons must be actively transported between the cell body and synaptic terminals [3]. Indeed, transport defects have been strongly implicated in the development of many human neurodegenerative diseases such as Alzheimer's disease [4].

A basic requirement for intracellular cargo transport is to deliver the right cargo to the right destination at the right time. This relies on spatial and temporal control of movement of individual cargoes. How this is achieved within cells remains largely unknown. To answer this question, it is essential to study the molecular machinery of intracellular transport as well as spatial and temporal behavior of transported cargoes. In related biological studies, the machinery and behavior of intracellular transport were often visualized using fluorescence microscopy techniques. It became evident from these studies that both are highly complex. Correspondingly, objects in images of intracellular transport exhibit highly complex structure and dynamics. Understanding the complex structure and dynamics of these image objects is essential to understanding the spatial and temporal control of intracellular transport. To achieve this goal, computational modeling of the image objects is essential.

In this paper we present our research results on using computational image modeling for characterization and analysis of intracellular transport. In the first part of the paper, we present results on using computational modeling of super-resolution STORM images for nanometer resolution characterization and analysis of molecular machinery of intracellular transport. In the second part of the paper, we present results on using computational modeling of time-lapse images for characterization and analysis of spatiotemporal behavior of intracellular transport.

1.1   Computational Image Modeling for Studying Molecular Machinery of Intracellular Transport

Active intracellular transport of cargoes is driven by molecular motors that walk along cytoskeletal filaments such as microtubules. Cargoes, molecular motors, and cytoskeletal filaments are therefore key components of the molecular machinery of intracellular transport. Dimensions of these components are often on the nanometer scale. Conventional fluorescence microscopy cannot fully resolve their structures because its resolution is limited to ~200nm by diffraction of visible light (Fig. 1A-B). This imposes a fundamental limitation on studying molecular machinery of intracellular transport. To overcome this limitation, we used STORM (stochastic optical reconstruction microscopy) [5], a super-resolution imaging technique that provides resolutions up to ~20nm. Because STORM relies on stochastic excitation of fluorophores [5], the resulting images of cellular structures are characterized by discontinuously distributed particles (Fig. 1C-D), which are significantly different from the typically continuous region objects in conventional microscopy images (Fig. 1A-B). Computational image models are required for representing the spatial distribution of such particles so that the underlying molecular machinery of intracellular transport can be characterized and analyzed. In this study, we developed kernel-based spatial density models for reconstruction and segmentation of such particle images.

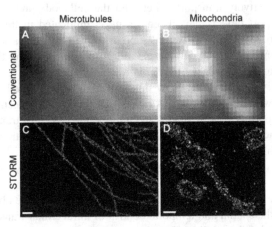

Fig. 1. Conventional fluorescence microscopy images versus super-resolution STORM images of microtubules and mitochondria, one among many different types of intracellular cargoes. (A, C) Conventional and STORM images of microtubules, respectively; (B, D) Conventional and STORM images of mitochondria, respectively. Scale bars: 500nm.

1.2   Computational Image Modeling for Studying Spatiotemporal Behavior of Intracellular Transport

In this study we focus on a specific model system of intracellular cargo transport (Fig 2A): the transport of amyloid precursor protein (APP) vesicles within axons of Drosophila third instar larvae. Vesicles are small intracellular cargoes that are enclosed by a lipid bilayer membrane. Drosophila has been used extensively to model human neurodegenerative diseases. The long and straight axons of Drosophila larvae (Fig. 2A) simplify imaging and data analysis and provide a powerful experimental system for studying intracellular cargo transport. To follow the movement of individual vesicles with high spatial resolution, we developed a single particle tracking method that recovers complete cargo trajectories at nanometer resolution (Fig. 2B-C) [6]. Recovered trajectories revealed complex spatiotemporal behavior of transported cargoes, such as pauses between movements, switches in movement directions, and changes in movement velocities [6]. In this study, we developed hidden Markov models (HMMs) [7] and principal component analysis (PCA) [8] for characterization and analysis of cargo behavior.

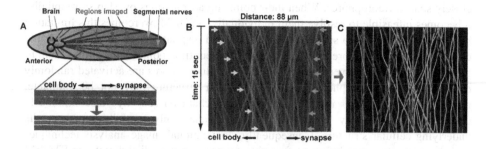

Fig. 2. Imaging and tracking axonal cargo transport in Drosophila third instar larvae. (A) Upper panel: regions selected for imaging. Middle panel: one frame from a time lapse video of APP vesicle transport. Lower panel: a band (5 pixels between green curves) following the axon (marked in cyan) is taken from each frame. (B) Bands from all frames were placed sequentially to generate a kymograph, a map of vesicle movement along the axon over time. Yellow and green arrows point to trajectories of two vesicles moving towards the synapse and the cell body, respectively. (C) Trajectories recovered by single particle tracking software were randomly colored and overlaid onto the kymograph for visual inspection.

1.3   Organization of the Paper

The rest of the paper is organized as follows: Section 2 presents results on using spatial density kernel based image models for reconstruction and segmentation of STORM images of molecular machinery of intracellular transport, specifically microtubules and mitochondria of mammalian BS-C-1 cells. Section 3 presents results on using hidden Markov models (HMMs) and principal component analysis (PCA) for representation and analysis of behavior of transported cargoes, specifically APP vesicles in neurons of Drosophila third instar larvae. Section 4 concludes with a summary as well as an outlook on ongoing work.

2   Computational Image Modeling for Studying Molecular Machinery of Intracellular Transport

2.1   Image Data Collection

Fluorescently labeled microtubules and mitochondria in fixed BS-C-1 cells were imaged using a Nikon N-STORM microscope with a 100×/1.41NA oil objective lens. Images were captured using an Andor Ultra 897 EMCCD camera, with a pixel size of 16 μm. Image collection was controlled using Nikon Element software. Image reconstruction was performed using custom software.

2.2   Spatial Density Kernel Models for Reconstruction of STORM Images

Resolution of conventional fluorescence microscopy is limited by diffraction of visible light to ~200nm. This resolution limit results from simultaneous excitation of closely spaced fluorophores. When their point spread functions overlap substantially, it becomes infeasible to resolve them individually. STORM overcomes this limitation by randomly activating a small fraction of the total population of fluorophores so that closely spaced fluorophores are activated at different time points. This allows them to be resolved separately over time. Since different fluorophores are activated randomly over time while fluorophore labeling of cellular structure may not be complete, reconstructed STORM images are usually characterized by discontinuously distributed particles. By themselves, these particles only partially represent the underlying cellular structure. Consequently, conventional image analysis techniques such as segmentation techniques often give poor results if applied directly to STORM images due to lack of information (see Fig. 4 & 5 for examples). Solving this problem requires computational image models to fully extrapolate or reconstruct the underlying cellular structure. This extrapolation or reconstruction can also be considered as smoothing of STORM images.

In this study, we consider the distributed particles as random samples of an unknown continuous spatial density function that represents the underlying cellular structure. We propose to estimate this spatial density function using kernel based multivariate density estimation [9]. Specifically, we estimated the 2D spatial density function at location x using the following equation

$$\hat{p}(x) = \frac{1}{N} \sum_{i=1}^{N} K(x, x_i) \tag{1}$$

where $x_1, x_2, \ldots, x_N$ are the N nearest neighbors in the STORM image, and $K(\cdot)$ is a kernel function.

We started with a commonly adopted isotropic Gaussian kernel

$$K_i(x, x_i) = \frac{1}{2\pi\sigma^2} \exp\left(-\frac{\|x - x_i\|^2}{2\sigma^2}\right) \tag{2}$$

where σ is the standard deviation and a measure of kernel size. In this study, we chose σ empirically to be within the range of 10~50 nm to account for uncertainty of fluorophore position detection as well as incompleteness of cell structure labeling. Although this isotropic kernel based estimation approach is simple and straightforward to implement, it has several limitations. First, the estimation becomes unreliable when the distribution of particles becomes highly directional, as is for example the case near boundaries of objects. Second, even when the spatial distribution of particles is omnidirectional, the estimation becomes inaccurate when the distribution is spatially inhomogeneous. Third, since the same kernel size σ needs to be used over the image, empirical tuning is often required to reconcile variations in particle distribution within different image regions.

To overcome these limitations, we proposed an adaptive anisotropic kernel based approach in which we use the following anisotropic Gaussian kernel:

$$K_a(x, x_i) = \frac{1}{2\pi \det\left(\Sigma_{x_i}\right)} \exp\left(-\frac{1}{2}(x - x_i)^T \Sigma_{x_i}^{-1}(x - x_i)\right) \tag{3}$$

where the local covariance matrix Σ_{x_i} at x_i is estimated using the following equation:

$$\Sigma_{x_i} = \frac{1}{N}\sum_{j=1}^{N}\left(x_j - x_i\right)\left(x_j - x_i\right)^T \qquad (4)$$

where $x_1, x_2, ... x_N$ are the N nearest neighbors. N is typically chosen within 10~30 to balance the localization and reliability of estimation. We first used a simple example to compare the performance of isotropic kernels versus adaptive anisotropic kernels for spatial density estimation (Fig. 3A-D). A qualitative visual assessment confirmed that the anisotropic kernels outperform the isotropic kernels substantially.

To characterize the molecular machinery of intracellular transport, the corresponding image objects in reconstructed images must be segmented. Here, we used STORM images reconstructed from the estimation of spatial density function for segmentation. This also allowed us to further compare quantitatively performance of isotropic kernels versus anisotropic kernels in reconstruction of STORM images. As discussed previously, the kernel-based estimation of spatial density function also provides a way for smoothing raw STORM images. This allowed us to use a simple density thresholding scheme for image segmentation. We empirically modeled the density distribution of actual image objects by finding the non-zero density bins from the spatial histogram. The density threshold was set by finding the pth percentile of the spatial densities. We found p to be within the range of 1~15. We tested our segmentation method on both simulated and actual STORM images.

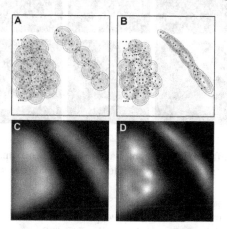

Fig. 3. Spatial density estimation using isotropic kernels versus adaptive anisotropic kernels. (A, B) Isotropic kernels and adaptive anisotropic kernels, respectively, overlaid on data points sampled from a curvilinear feature and a blob feature. (C, D) Estimated spatial density function images using isotropic kernels and adaptive anisotropic kernels, respectively.

2.3   Segmentation of Simulated STORM Images

Simulated STORM images were generated for microtubules and mitochondria, two key components of the molecular machinery of intracellular transport. Assuming a uniform fluorophore labeling density in object regions, we simulated random activation of fluorophores at two densities: 1,000 and 2,000 activations in an image region of 2560nm×2560nm. Random background noise was added under different signal to noise ratios (SNRs), which was set to 20 dB in this paper. To provide a reference for comparison, we used an active contour algorithm for segmentation of simulated STORM images [10]. We found that boundaries of image objects segmented using this algorithm were very sensitive to missing particles due to random fluorophore activation (Fig. 4).

We then applied the previously described density thresholding algorithm for segmentation of images reconstructed using isotropic kernels and adaptive anisotropic kernels, respectively. Compared to the active contour segmentation, thresholding of images reconstructed using isotropic kernels provided better performance but still suffered from over-segmentation as well as false segmentation of background noise (Fig. 4; Table 1). Thresholding of images reconstructed using anisotropic kernels provided overall the best result. In particular, it performed robustly against random variations of activated fluorophores and provided more accurate segmentation for both sample structures.

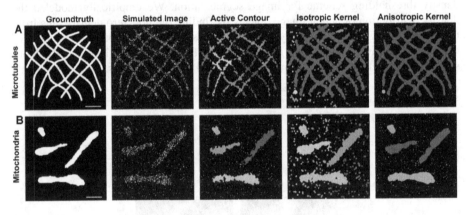

Fig. 4. Comparison of different image segmentation algorithms on simulated STORM images. Segmentation results are shown in random colors and overlaid onto simulated images. Scale bars: 500nm.

For quantitative comparison, we adopted performance metrics used in [11]: area similarity (AS), precision (P), and recall (R). AS measures the overlap of segmentation results relative to the ground truth. P is the ratio between the total number of correctly segmented objects to the total number of segmented objects. R is the ratio between the total number of correctly segmented objects to the total number of objects in the ground truth. Calculated metrics were averaged over all objects and all images and listed in Table 1. It is clear that thresholding of images reconstructed using anisotropic kernels provided overall the best result, especially in minimizing over-segmentation, as measured by precision P.

Table 1. Performance metrics of segmentation on simulated STORM images

	Microtubules			Mitochondria		
	AC	IKDES	AKDES	AC	IKDES	AKDES
AS	0.64	0.75	**0.79**	0.90	0.88	**0.90**
P	0.01	0.02	**0.37**	0.30	0.44	**0.96**
R	1.00	1.00	**1.00**	1.00	1.00	**1.00**

AC: active contour segmentation

IKDES: isotropic kernel based density estimation segmentation

AKDES: anisotropic kernel based density estimation segmentation

2.4   Segmentation of Actual STORM Images

We also compared the three segmentation algorithms on actual STORM images of microtubules and mitochondria in fixed BS-C-1 cells. Fig. 5 shows results in a region of 4000nm×4000nm. Similar to the case of simulated images, the active contour segmentation produced fragmented clusters of particles while the isotropic kernel based method suffered from over-segmentation as well as false segmentation of background noise. The adaptive anisotropic kernel based segmentation reliably identified image object boundaries and performed robustly against background noise.

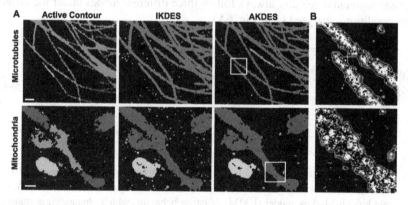

Fig. 5. Comparison of different image segmentation algorithms on actual STORM images. (A) Comparison of different image segmentation algorithms. (B) Comparison of segmented image object boundaries in regions corresponding to boxed regions in column 3 of panel A, where green, blue, and red contours show active contour, IKDES, and AKDES results. Scale bars: 500nm.

3   Computational Image Modeling for Studying Spatiotemporal Behavior of Intracellular Transport

3.1   Image Data Collection

Axonal transport of vesicles carrying amyloid precursor protein tagged with YFP (APP-YFP) was imaged in axons within segmental nerves of dissected Drosophila third instar larvae under different genetic modifications of kinesin and dynein subunits. Each time-lapse movie was collected for 20 seconds at 11 frames per second using a Nikon Ti-E inverted microscope with a 100×/1.41NA oil objective lens and a Photometric CoolSnap HQ2 camera. Movie collection was controlled using Nikon Element software.

3.2   Computational Modeling of Vesicle Movement

Complete trajectories of vesicles were recovered at nanometer resolution using custom software [6]. At any time, individual vesicles may reside in one of the following states: moving towards a distal synaptic terminal (anterograde movement; denoted by *A*), moving towards the neuronal cell body (retrograde movement; denoted by *R*), or pausing (denoted by *P*). A vesicle may switch between movement and pause and between anterograde and retrograde movement.

To characterize vesicle movement, we first calculated and analyzed segmental velocities of individual vesicles. A *segment* is a part of the trajectory of a vesicle in which it moves consistently in one direction. It is usually a part of the trajectory between two pauses, two direction reversals, or a pause and a directional reversal. The segmental velocity is the average velocity of a vesicle within the given segment. Using model-based clustering [12], we determined that anterograde as well as retrograde segmental velocity always follow three different modes under the different genetic conditions analyzed [13] (Fig. 6A).

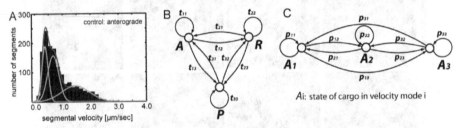

Fig. 6. Computational modeling of vesicle behavior. (A) Velocities of cargoes moving towards the synaptic terminal follow three modes (red: total distribution. cyan: individual modes). (B) A coarse scale hidden Markov model (HMM) of cargo behavior, which characterizes transitions between anterograde movement *R*, retrograde movement *R*, and pause *P*. (C) A fine scale hidden Markov model (HMM) of cargo behavior, which characterizes transitions between different anterograde velocity modes.

To characterize and analyze vesicle behavior, we used hidden Markov models [7, 14]. Depending on the research questions to be addressed, we modeled vesicle behavior at two levels. The coarse scale model (Fig. 6B) characterizes transition of cargo between pause (*P*) and anterograde movement (*A*) and retrograde movement (*R*). A fine scale model (Fig. 6C) allows us to determine the transition probabilities between different anterograde (or retrograde) velocity modes.

Here we give an example of estimating probabilities of transition between different anterograde velocities modes in wild-type (*wt*) animals versus animals with genetic modification of kinesin (kinesin heavy chain, $khc^8/+$) and dynein (dynein intermediate chain, *GEN-DIC/+*), where $P_1 = p_{11} + p_{22} + p_{33}$ (Fig. 6C) is the probability of no mode change, $P_2 = p_{12} + p_{21} + p_{23} + p_{32}$ is the probability of shifting to neighboring states (i.e. $I \leftrightarrow II$, $II \leftrightarrow III$) and $P_3 = p_{13} + p_{31}$ is the probability of mode jump (i.e. $I \leftrightarrow III$). All computations were performed using the PMTK (Probabilistic Modeling Toolkit for MATLAB/Octave) package. The results, listed in Table 2, indicate that genetic modifications of molecular motors can influence transitions between different velocity modes. In this specific case, genetic reductions of kinesin and dynein reduced probabilities of switching between velocity mode I and mode II.

Table 2. Estimated transition probabilities between different anterograde velocity modes

	P_1	P_2	P_3
wt	0.59	0.38	0.03
khc^8/+	0.79	0.20	0.01
GEN-DIC/+	0.79	0.18	0.03

3.3   Principal Component Analysis for Comprehensive Characterization of Cargo Behavior

In the previous section, we analyzed segmental velocities of transported vesicles. However, comprehensive characterization of transport behavior requires additional descriptors. Table 3 shows representative descriptors of vesicle behavior under three categories: movement, pause, and switch (i.e. reversal in movement direction). Descriptors under each category characterize vesicle behavior from different perspectives. Detailed definitions of these descriptors are given in [13].

Table 3. Representative descriptors of vesicle behavior

Anterograde movement descriptor	Abbreviation	Retrograde movement descriptors	Abbreviation
anterograde net velocity	aNetV	retrograde net velocity	rNetV
anterograde instantaneous velocity	aInstV	retrograde instantaneous velocity	rInstV
anterograde segmental velocity	aSegV	retrograde segmental velocity	rSegV
anterograde duration weighted segmental velocity	aDWSegV	retrograde duration weighted segmental velocity	rDWSegV
anterograde net run-length	aNet RL	retrograde net run-length	rNet RL
anterograde total run-length	aTotRL	retrograde total run-length	rTotRL
anterograde segmental pause frequency	aSegPF	retrograde segmental pause frequency	rSegPF
anterograde total pause duration	aTotPD	retrograde total pause duration	rTotPD
switch frequency*	SF	switch frequency**	SF

*,**: switch frequency are used as descriptors for both anterograde and retrograde movement.

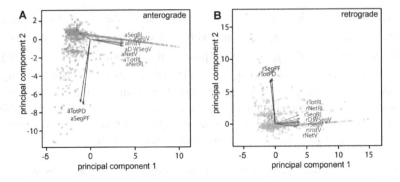

Fig. 7. Principal component analysis of cargo behavior descriptors. (A) anterograde descriptors and principal component, calculated based on n= 1745 measurements from 18 animals. (B) retrograde descriptors and principal components, calculated based on n= 1745 measurements from 18 animals.

Here two basic questions should be addressed. First, do descriptors under the same category provide the same information? Second, what are the relations between descriptors under different categories? To answer these questions, we used principal component analysis (Fig. 7 A-B). It showed that different descriptors under the same category, represented in Fig.7 using the same color, are highly correlated and thus provide similar information. For example, for both anterograde and retrograde movement, velocity descriptors and run-length descriptors are highly correlated and provide similar information, indicating that fast moving vesicles tend to travel long distances. On the other hand, descriptors under different categories are nearly orthogonal and thus uncorrelated. For example, pause descriptors are orthogonal and thus uncorrelated with movement descriptors, suggesting that pauses are likely caused by mechanisms different from those driving movement. Similarly, switch frequency are largely orthogonal to pause and motion descriptors, indicating that switches in movement are likely mediated by different mechanisms.

4   Summary and Outlook

In this study we developed and applied computational image models for studying the molecular machinery and spatiotemporal behavior of intracellular transport. Our results demonstrated the power of these models in representing complex cellular structure and dynamic behavior. The models and related computational analysis methods are general and applicable to studies of other cellular processes. We are addressing several limitations of this study in ongoing work. First, the anisotropic kernel cannot be used to model structures that spatially overlap with each other. We are addressing this limitation using Gaussian mixture models. Second, the hidden Markov models only describe ensemble cargo behavior. It does not directly represent spatial behavior of individual cargoes. We are addressing this limitation by developing statistical models that explicitly describe cargo spatial behavior. Third, the axonal transport process is essential one dimensional whereas intracellular transport in non-polarized cells is two dimensional. We are extending our current one-dimensional cargo behavior models for two-dimensional intracellular transport.

Acknowledgments. We gratefully acknowledge support from the US National Science Foundation through grants 1017278 (J.K.), and DBI-1149494, DBI-1052925, MCB-1052660 (G.Y).

References

1. Wickner, W., Schekman, R.: Protein translocation across biological membranes. Science 310, 1452–1456 (2005)
2. Vale, R.D.: The molecular motor toolbox for intracellular transport. Cell 112, 467–480 (2003)
3. Brown, A.: Axonal transport of membranous and nonmembranous cargoes: a unified perspective. J. Cell Biol. 160, 817–821 (2003)
4. De Vos, K.J., Grierson, A.J., Ackerley, S., Miller, C.C.J.: Role of axonal transport in neurodegenerative diseases. Annu. Rev. Neurosci. 31, 151–173 (2008)
5. Rust, M.J., Bates, M., Zhuang, X.: Sub-diffraction-limit imaging by stochastic optical reconstruction microscopy (STORM). Nat. Meth. 3, 793–796 (2006)
6. Qiu, M., Yang, G.: Nanometer resolution tracking and modeling of bidirectional axonal cargo transport. In: Proc. IEEE Int. Symp. Biomedical Imaging (ISBI), Barcelona, Spain, pp. 992–995 (2012)
7. Rabiner, L.R.: A tutorial on hidden Markov models and selected applications in speech recognition. Proc. IEEE 77, 257–286 (1989)
8. Jolliffe, I.T.: Principal Component Analysis. Springer (2002)
9. Scott, D.W.: Multivariate Density Estimation. John Wiley & Sons (1992)
10. Chan, T.F., Vese, L.A.: Active contours without edges. IEEE Trans. Image Processing 10, 266–277 (2001)
11. Chen, K.C.J., Yu, Y., Li, R., Lee, H.-C., Yang, G., Kovacevic, J.: Adaptive active-mask image segmentation for quantitative characterization of mitochondrial morphology. In: 2012 19th IEEE Int. Conf. Image Processing (ICIP), pp. 2033–2036 (2012)
12. Fraley, C., Raftery, A.E.: Model-based clustering, discriminant analysis and density estimation. J. Am. Stat. Assoc. 97, 611–631 (2002)
13. Reis, G.F., Yang, G., Szpankowski, L., Weaver, C., Shah, S.B., Robinson, J.T., Hays, T.S., Danuser, G., Goldstein, L.S.B.: Molecular motor function in axonal transport in vivo probed by genetic and computational analysis in Drosophila. Mol. Biol. Cell 23, 1700–1714 (2012)

Element Stiffness Matrix Integration in *Image-Based* Cartesian Grid Finite Element Method

Luca Giovannelli, Juan J. Ródenas, José M. Navarro-Jimenez, and Manuel Tur

Centro de Investigación en Ingeniería Mecánica - CIIM,
Universitat Politècnica de València, Spain
lugio3@upv.es, {jjrodena,matuva}@mcm.upv.es, navarrojim22@gmail.com

Abstract. Patient specific Finite Element (FE) simulations are usually expensive. Time consuming geometry creation procedures are normally necessary to use standard FE meshing software, while direct pixel-based meshing techniques typically lead to a large number of degrees of freedom hence introducing a high computational cost. *Image-based* Cartesian grid Finite Element Method (*image-based* cgFEM) allows accurate models to be automatically obtained with a low computational cost without the necessity of defining geometries. In cgFEM the image is directly immersed into a Cartesian mesh which is h-adapted on the basis of the pixel value distribution. A hierarchical structure of nested Cartesian grids guarantees the efficiency of the process. In each element, the material elastic properties are heterogeneous, therefore a critical aspect of *image-based* cgFEM is the integration of the element stiffness matrices which homogenize the material elastic behavior at the element level. This paper compares accuracy and computational cost of different integration strategies: pixel direct integration schemes (Riemann sum and subdomain Gauss quadrature) and recovery based schemes (Least Squares fitting and Superconvergent Patch Recovery).

Keywords: Cartesian grid, Finite Element, Medical Simulation, Patient Specific Simulation.

1 Introduction

Medical imaging has a key role in patient-specific treatment, [1], as shown by the great amount of publications on this topic. Intense research has been devoted to find new ways of taking advantage of the information provided by medical images. As a consequence, a large number of new applications based on the use of numerical simulation tools have been proposed in many different fields such as the prediction of bone fracture risk, [2], the reduction of surgery invasiveness, [3], prosthesis selection, [4], and the evaluation of bone quality parameters for the detection of osteoporosis, [5]. Many applications in which it is necessary to compute mechanical quantities of biological structures in a patient specific framework are at the crossroads between these image based applications and the area

Y.J. Zhang and J.M.R.S. Tavares (Eds.): CompIMAGE 2014, LNCS 8641, pp. 304–315, 2014.

of computational mechanics, traditionally linked to industrial production. This is the case of bone mechanics for instance. A rich literature exists about creation of numerical models derived from computational mechanics from medical images for specific applications, such as, for instance, [6]. Most of these techniques use the Finite Element Method (FEM), as this is the most spread numerical tool for structural simulation. Traditional patient specific medical FEM applications can be classified into two main categories [7]. We call the methods belonging to the first one *image-based*, since they take advantage of the regular spatial distribution of the pixels/voxels to directly assign a Finite Element (FE), usually hexahedral, to each of them. The first step is usually a segmentation procedure to select the pixels of interest; afterwords the mesh creation is straightforward. This technique automatically provides uniform structured meshes which present some advantages from the point of view of information treatment due to the similarities between all the elements. In addition, if local material properties have to be taken into account, information transfer between image and mesh is very easy due to the biunivocal correspondence between elements and pixels. The main price to pay for using this method is the great amount of degrees freedom of the final problem, which can be computationally very expensive.

The second family, which we call *geometry-based*, uses procedures to create CAD models from image data. Afterwords, the modeling and simulating processes used are exactly the same as in standard FEM problems. On one hand this means that the tools and techniques used for FE modeling in structural analysis can be easily extended to the patient specific problem. Doing so, problems with a reasonable number of degrees of freedom can usually be obtained. On the other hand, some typical modeling problems related to complex geometries may appear. On this point note that in usual structural simulations, the phases of adapting CAD models to FE domain discretization and meshing are responsible on average for about 80% of all the time cost, [8].

The main drawback of the *geometry-based* methods is not in modeling and simulation, yet in the creation of the CAD model from the original image. This process requires cumbersome and time consuming techniques of segmentation and geometry creation which can be seldom completely automatic, hence resulting in high costs in terms of highly specialized man-hours. In addition, including local information into the simulation involves a considerable computational cost, in the general case, for FE models thus obtained, as the mesh and bitmap topologies are totally independent.

Recently, in order to overcome the limits of both *image-* and *geometry-based* procedures, advanced FE methods, formerly developed for lightening the meshing and remeshing burden in standard geometrical problems, have been extended to this area, such as the Extended Finite Element Method (XFEM) [9] or the Finite Cell Method (FCM) [10].

Our proposal is an advanced FE method for performing linear elasticity analyses in the case the problem data are available in the form of bitmaps. We call this method *image-based* Cartesian grid Finite Element Method (*image-based* cgFEM). cgFEM provides meshes characterized by a reasonable number of degrees of freedom, as in the *geometry-based* procedures, but, at the same time, no CAD model to mesh has to be created and all the local pixel information can be used, as in *image-based* procedures, [11]. It has points in common especially with FCM, since both methods create regular square/hexahedral meshes directly inside the bitmap and, as a consequence, have to use special techniques for enforcing Dirichlet boundary condition on surfaces which cut the elements. The main difference is in the mesh refinement procedures. FCM enhances the FE solution by performing p-refinement, that is by increasing the polynomial order of the shape functions used for interpolating the displacement field and has to deal with their proper integration, while, in contrast, in cgFEM the model is refined via local local h-adaptivity, hence reducing the element size on the basis of the evaluation of the variability of the pixel value field.

As in usual FEM, in *image-based* cgFEM it is necessary to compute the integral (1) for each element of the mesh in order to be able to assemble the element stiffness matrices $\mathbf{k}^e$ into the problem global stiffness matrix $\mathbf{K}$.

$$\mathbf{k}^e = \int_{\Omega} \mathbf{B}^T \mathbf{D} \mathbf{B} \mathrm{d}\Omega \tag{1}$$

In (1), whose evaluation is performed by numerical integration, $\mathbf{B}$ is the matrix relating strains and nodal displacements and $\mathbf{D}$ is the Hook's law matrix which relates strains and stresses in linear elasticity. As opposed to usual FEM, in which only $\mathbf{B}$ depends on the position, in *image-based* cgFEM the $\mathbf{D}$ matrix also does. This is due to the fact that, in general, the material inside each element is not homogeneous. This heterogeneity is only sampled at the centers of the pixels, therefore, in order not to lose information, it is necessary to take into account all the pixels during the simulation. In cgFEM this information is included by considering all the pixels for homogenizing the elastic properties at the element level. As a consequence each element contains a number of pixels, hence significantly reducing the number of degrees of freedom because in the final model there are significantly less elements than pixels, in contrast to the classical *image-based* methods. The aim of the previous adaptivity process is avoiding excessive homogenization of the material properties inside each element. Due to the specific features of the procedure, the numerical integration is not standard. In this paper, we propose and compare different strategies for evaluating the integral (1) in the context of image-based cgFEM. They can be divided in two classes:

- Strategies based on the direct use of the whole image information
  - Riemann Sum (RS) based technique
  - Integration subdomain Gauss quadrature (ISGQ)
- Strategies based on the reconstruction of a continuous elastic property distribution inside each element
  - Least Square fitting (LS) to the pixel field in each element
  - Superconvergent Patch Recovery (SPR) fitting to the pixel field in the set of elements connected to each vertex node

After this introduction, in Section 2 the *image-based* cgFEM technique, the different integration techniques and the test problem are presented followed by the numerical results in Section 3. Finally, Section 4 is devoted to the discussion of the results and the formulation of the conclusions.

2   Method

2.1   *Image-Based* cgFEM

FE modeling in linear elasticity consists mainly of three steps: domain discretization, stiffness matrix calculation and imposition of the boundary conditions. In cgFEM, a hierarchical structure of nested Cartesian grids is used for making meshing and *h*-refinement efficient, [12]. This consists of a series of Cartesian grids in which the first one, so called *0 level*, only consists of one single element coinciding with the bounding box which contains the domain of interest, see Figure 1. The *i*-level grid is then obtained by splitting each element of the $(i-1)$-level in two in each direction, therefore it contains $2^{d \times i}$ elements, in which d represent the problem dimensionality. The final mesh is created by assembling elements from different levels. This is computationally efficient because the elements are related by parenthood and neighborhood relations known in advance, therefore the amount of data to store decreases. The FE mesh, thus obtained, has hanging nodes at which the displacement field continuity has to be enforced by using Multi Point Constraints (MPC). The level difference between two adjacent elements is enforced not to be more of one level.

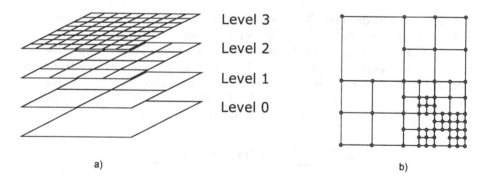

Fig. 1. a) First levels of the hierarchical structure of nested Cartesian grids; b) Example of non-conforming Finite Element mesh with cgFEM

At the beginning of the simulation, the image is reshaped, usually adding *dummy* pixels, so that its dimensions, measured in pixels, are powers of two along each direction. This guarantees that, in the hierarchical structure of Cartesian grids, a number of levels exist in which all the elements contain an integer number of pixels. This makes the process of structuring the image into the mesh straightforward. The second step is to h-refine the mesh by evaluating the pixel value distribution in each element. For this purpose two possible indicators of the pixel distribution are used: the ratio between the element and the whole image value range or the coefficient of variation, the ratio between the image value standard deviation and its mean value have been considered. The h-refinement process simply consist of recursively subdividing the elements whose value of the indicator considered for the refinement is higher than a prescribed threshold value. Once the problem has been discretized, the element stiffness matrix (1) is numerically calculated by using (2).

$$\mathbf{k}^e = \sum_{i=1}^{IP} \mathbf{B}^T(\boldsymbol{\xi}_i)\mathbf{D}(\boldsymbol{\xi}_i)\mathbf{B}(\boldsymbol{\xi}_i) \mid \mathbf{J}(\boldsymbol{\xi}_i) \mid w_i \tag{2}$$

In which the number of the integration points IP, their positions $\boldsymbol{\xi}_i$ (corresponding in 2D with the vector (ξ_i, η_i), in 3D with (ξ_i, η_i, τ_i)), the Jacobian $\mid \mathbf{J}(\boldsymbol{\xi}_i) \mid$, the weights and the material property values $\mathbf{D}(\boldsymbol{\xi}_i)$ depend on the quadrature rule chosen.

2.2   Pixel Based Integration Methods

In this group of integration strategies, no treatment of the image is performed and the values of $\mathbf{D}$ introduced in (2) are directly the ones associated to the pixels.

Integration Subdomain Gauss quadrature (ISGQ). A first approach consists of considering the pixels as element integration subdomains in which the values of $\mathbf{D}$ are constant over the subdomain, therefore a proper Gauss integration has to be performed in each pixel. As a result the number of integration points IP required in each element is $NP \times GIP$, where NP is the number of pixels contained in the element and GIP the number of integration points required by the Gauss quadrature for an homogeneous domain.

$$\mathbf{k}^e = \sum_{j=1}^{Pixels} \sum_{i=1}^{IP} \mathbf{B}^T(\boldsymbol{\xi}_i)\mathbf{D}_j\mathbf{B}(\boldsymbol{\xi}_i) \mid \mathbf{J}_{ij}(\boldsymbol{\xi}_i) \mid w_i \tag{3}$$

Riemann Sum Based Integration (RS). The second approach consists of implementing Riemann sum hence locating one constant weight integration point at the center of each pixel.

$$\mathbf{k}^e = \sum_{i=1}^{IP} \mathbf{B}^T(\boldsymbol{\xi}_i)\mathbf{D}_i\mathbf{B}(\boldsymbol{\xi}_i)PA_i \tag{4}$$

in which PA_i is the measure of the pixel area in global coordinates.

2.3   Recovered Image Integration Methods

In this second group, a continuous material property field is used to interpolate the values of the pixels, therefore the proper Gauss quadrature (5) is used.

$$\mathbf{k}^e = \sum_{i=1}^{GP} \mathbf{B}^T(\boldsymbol{\xi}_i)\mathbf{D}(\boldsymbol{\xi}_i)\mathbf{B}(\boldsymbol{\xi}_i) \mid \mathbf{J}_{ij}(\boldsymbol{\xi}_i) \mid w_i \tag{5}$$

Least Square Recovery (LS). Least Square techniques provides a polynomial interpolation $f(\boldsymbol{\xi}_i) = \mathbf{p}(\boldsymbol{\xi}_i)\mathbf{a}$ of the material property field in each element. This is, in general, discontinuous at the interface between two adjacent elements and is obtained by minimizing the function Π (6) with respect to each one of the polynomial coefficients a_i (7), which leads to a linear system of equations that is used to evaluate $\mathbf{a}$.

$$\Pi = \sum_i^{Pixels} (PV_i - f(\boldsymbol{\xi}_i))^2 = \sum_i^{Pixels} (PV_i - \mathbf{p}(\boldsymbol{\xi}_i)\mathbf{a})^2 \tag{6}$$

$$\frac{\partial \Pi}{\partial a_i} = 0 \tag{7}$$

In the following, for simplicity, we only consider that p represents a bilinear polynomial basis.

Superconvergent Patch Recovery (SPR). The SPR recovery [13] uses a Least Square polynomial fitting to the values of the pixels contained in a patch. A patch is the set of the elements which share the same node. The fitted polynomial is then used to evaluate the material property value at the common node of the patch $\mathbf{D}_i$. These nodal values are then used for calculating the values at the Gauss points by FE interpolation, see (8)

$$\mathbf{D}(\boldsymbol{\xi}_i) = \sum_j^{Nodes} N_j(\boldsymbol{\xi}_i)\mathbf{D}_j \tag{8}$$

The resulting field is continuous over the whole mesh.

2.4   Reference Problems

The different integration techniques have been compared on two reference problems. For the sake of simplicity we use two 2D images of a phalanx and a metacarpal which we call Problem 1 (P1) and Problem 2 (P2), Figures 2 b) and d) respectively. They were extracted from different the X-ray images expressed in grey scale (with values from 0 to 255), see Figures 2 a) and c).

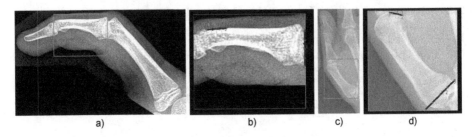

Fig. 2. a) P1: finger X-ray; b) P1: phalanx from Figure 2 a); c) P2: thumb X-ray; b) P2: metacarpal from Figure 2 c)

In both reference problems, the relation between the pixel values and the material elastic properties were assigned by associating data from the literature, [14] and [15], to certain values of the gray scale. Young's modulus values of 0, 645, 14000 and 14200 MPa and Poisson's ratio values of 0, 0.43, 0.3 and 0.3 were associated to the gray scale values of of 0, 150, 190 and 255 respectively. For the rest of the gray scale, linear interpolation was used.

3   Numerical Results

In both P1 and P2, our reference solution corresponds to the energy norm evaluated considering one element per pixel in the image, considering also 4 integration points per element (pixel) to ensure that the numerical integration (1) is exact. Our goal is to check which of the integration methods provides the energy norm values closest to the reference solution at the minimum computational cost. To do so, we will first check the evolution of the solution obtained with each one of the different techniques, considering uniform mesh refinement with meshes with 8×8, 4×4, 2×2 and 1×1 pixels per element. Then we will select the most accurate technique to evaluate further improvements in computational cost associated to h-adaptive mesh refinement. Figure 3 shows the FE energy norm, $\sqrt{\int_\Omega \sigma \mathbf{D}^{-1} \sigma dV}$, of the reference problems for increasingly refined homogeneous meshes. Figures 3 a) and b) represent the energy norm versus the total number of degrees of freedom for P1 and P2. Figures 3 c) and d) show the energy norm versus the total number of integration points. Note that both parameters, number of degrees of freedom and integration points, are relevant for the computational efficiency because, on the one hand, the computational cost required for solving the system of equations associated to the FE problem depends on the number of degrees of freedom and, on the other hand, the effort associated to the creation of the system of equations increases with the number of integration points. In Figures 3 e) and f) the difference with the energy norm of the reference solution is used as a measure of the error. The blue line in Figures 3 represent the ISGQ, in which the integration subdomains are treated with the proper Gauss quadrature of four integration points. It converges smoothly to the

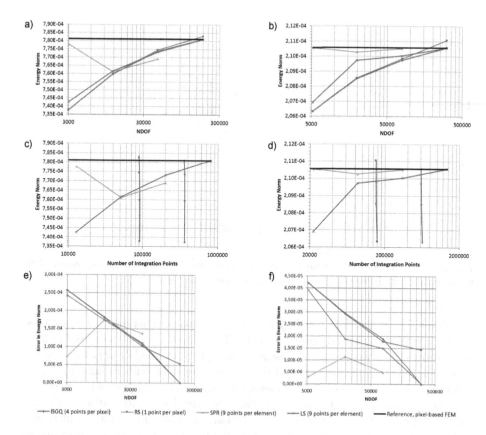

Fig. 3. a) P1: Energy Norm vs Degrees of freedom; b) P2: Energy Norm vs Degrees of freedom; c) P1: Energy Norm vs Integration points; d) P2: Energy Norm vs Integration points; d) P1: Error vs Degrees of Freedom; d) P2: Error vs Degrees of Freedom

reference solution since its finest mesh corresponds with the reference solution. The number of integration points involved is high and does not depend on the mesh. The results obtained by using RS integration are shown in red in Figure 3. Its behavior is very close to the previous one showing values similar to the ISGQ case as far as at least 4 integration points are contained in each element. In the most refined mesh the RS technique coincides with a reduced integration of one Gauss point and, as a consequence, the error suddenly increases. Note that for coarser meshes, the method provides almost the same accuracy as ISGQ with 1/4 of the integration points. In contrast to the other integration schemes proposed, the SPR, the green line, shows a behavior extremely dependent on the problem. In P1 the accuracy it provides is lower than that of the other methods, while in P2 it is surprisingly higher. In both P1 and P2, it provides very low values of the error in the coarser mesh, but with an unstable error reduction in the finer meshes. This unstable and image dependent behavior makes SPR unreliable for this application despite its high performance in the field for which it

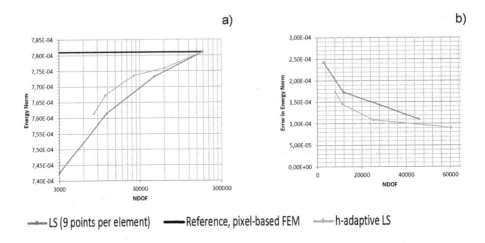

Fig. 4. a) H-adaptive refinement vs uniform refinement. Evolution of energy norm with mesh refinement; b) Evolution of the error in energy norm.

was developed, stress field recovery for error estimation. This technique provides continuous fields along adjacent elements. This characteristic smooths the material property between different tissues leading to very good or very bad results depending on the characteristics of the image gray level field. Finally, the integration of the LS interpolation, violet curve, shows the best behavior: it is not only characterized by higher accuracy than the pixel-based integration methods, converging correctly to the reference solution, but over a certain element size it is also cheaper from the point of view of the number of integration points. As opposed to SPR, the results obtained with SPR look stable and predictable. This good behavior is probably due to the fact that the bilinear LS interpolation of the material properties is consistent with the linear shape functions used for the FE interpolation of the displacement field. In addition the method filters the image high frequency noise taking into account only the low frequencies. Hence, in the process only the most important information is taken into account with a reduced number of degrees of freedom. Since the LS based integration technique proved to be the best one in the reference problems, it was used to obtain the results shown in Figure 4. Figure 4 shows the behavior of cgFEM h-adaptive models with respect to the uniform refined one. The analysis was performed on P1, see Figures 2 b). In the results shown in Figure 4 the h-adaptivity is guided by the evaluation of the pixel value variability. In particular a threshold for the maximum variability allowed in each element is used to guide the element splitting. The ratio between the pixel value range at the element and the range of the whole image is used as a measure of the variability. The h-adapted meshes corresponding to the points on the yellow curve in Figure 4 are shown in Figures 5 a), b), c) and d). They were obtained for the threshold values of 0.3125, 0.2344, 0.1562 and 0.0781 respectively. The maximum mesh level allowed was level 8 in a) and b) and level 9 in c) and d). During the h-adaptive process, the elements

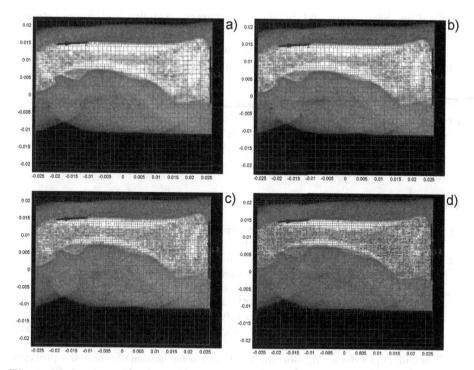

Fig. 5. Meshes created during the *h*-adaptive strategy corresponding to the yellow curves in Figure 4

which share a side with the element to split are checked and in the case a difference of more than one level is detected, the element dimensions are balanced by splitting. As a consequence, the number of degrees of freedom is only increased where it is useful for taking into account the effect of the material heterogeneity and for balancing the mesh. Figure 4 shows a relevant difference in the number of degrees of freedom, and hence in the computational cost, between the two methods for similar accuracies. This results suggest that, if used together with the proper integration method, *h*-refined *image-based*cgFEM models can be used for increasing patient specific simulation efficiency.

4   Conclusions

The *image-based* cgFEM technique has been presented and different techniques for the integration of element stiffness matrices evaluated from medical images have been compared. There are negligible differences between RS and ISGQ, which is computationally more expensive. The former only provides less accurate results for elements containing one single pixel. Both methods have a constant number of integration points independent from the mesh. The use of SPR provides unstable convergence curves with a hardly predictable level of error very dependent on the input image. It showed not to be a reliable method for this application. From the point of view of accuracy, stability and computational cost, the best results were obtained by LS. This was also used together with an heterogeneity based h-adaptive technique to show the higher accuracy and efficiency with respect to the uniform refinement.

Acknowledgements. With the support of the European Union Framework Program (FP7) under grant agreement No. 289361 'Integrating Numerical Simulation and Geometric Design Technology (INSIST)', Ministerio de Economía y Competitividad of Spain (DPI2013-46317-R) and Generalitat Valenciana (PROMETEO/2012/023).

References

1. Neal, M.L., Kerckhoffs, R.: Current progress in patient-specific modeling. Briefings in Bioinformatics 11(1), 111–126 (2010)
2. Grassi, L., Schileo, E., Taddei, F., Zani, L., Juszczyk, M., Cristofolini, L.: Accuracy of finite element predictions in sideways load configurations for the proximal human femur. Journal of Biomechanics 45(2), 394–399 (2012)
3. Viceconti, M., Lattanzi, R., Antonietti, B., Paderni, S., Olmi, R., Sudanese, A., Toni, A.: CT-based surgical planning software improves the accuracy of total hip replacement preoperative planning. Medical Engineering & Physics 25(5), 371–377 (2003)
4. Bongini, D., Carfagni, M., Governi, L.: Hippin: a semiautomatic computer program for selecting hip prosthesis femoral components. Computer Methods and Programs in Biomedicine 63(2), 105–115 (2000)
5. Alberich-Bayarri, A., Marti-Bonmati, L., Sanz-Requena, R., Belloch, E., Moratal, D.: In vivo trabecular bone morphologic and mechanical relationship using high-resolution 3-T MRI. American Journal of Roentgenology, AJR 191(3), 721–726 (2008)
6. García-Aznar, J.M., Bayod, J., Rosas, A., Larrainzar, R., García-Bógalo, R., Doblaré, M., Llanos, L.F.: Load transfer mechanism for different metatarsal geometries: A finite element study. Journal of Biomechanical Engineering 131(2) (2009)
7. Viceconti, M.: A comparative study on different methods of automatic mesh generation of human femurs. Medical Engineering and Physics 20, 1–10 (1998); Medical Engineering and Physics 22(5), 379–380 (2000)
8. Cottrell, J.A., Hughes, T.J.R., Bazilevs, Y.: Isogeometric Analysis: Toward Integration of CAD and FEA, 1st edn. Wiley (2009)
9. Lian, W.D., Legrain, G., Cartraud, P.: Image-based computational homogenization and localization: Comparison between X-FEM/levelset and voxel-based approaches. Computational Mechanics 51(3), 279–293 (2013)
10. Ruess, M., Tal, D., Trabelsi, N., Yosibash, Z., Rank, E.: The finite cell method for bone simulations: verification and validation. Biomechanics and Modeling in Mechanobiology 11(3-4), 425–437 (2012)
11. Giovannelli, L., Marco, O., Navarro, J.M., Giner, E., Ródenas, J.J.: Direct Creation of Finite Element Models from Medical Images using Cartesian Grids. In: Computational Vision and Medical Image Processing, IV ECCOMAS Thematic Conference on Computational Vision and Medical Image Processing, VipIMAGE (2013)

12. Nadal, E.: On the use of Cartesian Grid Finite Element codes in structural optimization (October 2012)
13. Zienkiewicz, O.C., Zhu, J.Z.: The superconvergent patch recovery and a posteriori error estimates. part 1: The recovery technique. International Journal for Numerical Methods in Engineering 33(7), 1331–1364 (1992)
14. Viceconti, M., Bellingeri, L., Cristofolini, L., Toni, A.: A comparative study on different methods of automatic mesh generation of human femurs. Medical Engineering & Physics 20(1), 1–10 (1998)
15. Kim, H., Jürgens, P., Weber, S., Nolte, L.P., Reyes, M.: A new soft-tissue simulation strategy for cranio-maxillofacial surgery using facial muscle template model. Progress in Biophysics and Molecular Biology 103(2-3), 284–291 (2010)

Pixel Based Meshfree Modeling of Skeletal Muscles

Ramya Rao Basava[1], Jiun-Shyan Chen[1], Yantao Zhang[1], Shantanu Sinha[2],
Usha Sinha[3], John Hodgson[4], Robert Csapo[2], and Vadim Malis[2]

[1] Department of Structural Engineering, University of California San Diego,
San Diego, CA, USA
{rbasava,js-chen,y5zhang}@ucsd.edu
[2] Department of Radiology, University of California San Diego, San Diego, CA, USA
{shsinha,rcsapo}@ucsd.edu, vadmalis@gmail.com
[3] Department of Physics, San Diego State University, San Diego, CA, USA
usinha@mail.sdsu.edu
[4] Department of Physiological Sciences, University of California Los Angeles,
Los Angeles, CA, USA
jhodgson@ucla.edu

Abstract. This paper introduces the meshfree Reproducing Kernel Particle Method (RKPM) in conjunction with a stabilized conforming nodal integration for 3D image-based modeling of skeletal muscles. This approach allows for construction of simulation model based on pixel data obtained from medical images. The model consists of different materials and muscle fiber direction obtained from Diffusion Tensor Imaging (DTI) is input at each pixel point. The reproducing kernel (RK) approximation also allows a representation of material heterogeneity with smooth transition. A multiphase multichannel level set based segmentation using Magnetic Resonance Images (MRI) and DTI formulated under a modified functional has been integrated into RKPM framework. The use of proposed methods for modeling the human lower leg is demonstrated.

Keywords: Image-based modeling, Meshfree modeling, 3D skeletal muscle model construction, Muscle force production, Individual muscle segmentation.

1   Introduction

In the conventional Finite Element (FE) approach, the meshes need to be conformed to muscle geometry, which increases the complexity of mesh construction. Generally muscles have a complex architecture and poorly built meshes can easily lead to significant errors in FE analysis due to mesh distortion. Abrupt changes of topology in the muscle cross sections could also result in failure in FE mesh generation. Additionally, muscle material is anisotropic in nature due to the presence of muscle fibers. In FE modeling, one way to introduce the anisotropy is to approximate the fiber directions by interpolating from some pre-defined templates as described in [1]. The fiber directions obtained in this way could generate noticeable discretization errors in the simulation models. In this work, we develop an image based meshfree modeling technique based on a Reproducing Kernel Particle Method (RKPM)[2, 3]. The fiber direction

Y.J. Zhang and J.M.R.S. Tavares (Eds.): CompIMAGE 2014, LNCS 8641, pp. 316–327, 2014.

obtained from DTI data [4, 5] and the material properties are defined at pixel points and are directly used as input into meshfree modeling. Since no mesh is required in meshfree methods, the complexity related with meshes in finite element method is avoided. The Reproducing Kernel (RK) approximation also allows for a smooth transition of material properties at the interfaces between different materials in the muscle. The skeletal muscle is represented as a nearly incompressible hyperelastic material following [6]. RKPM has been used to simulate extremely large deformation of rubber like hyperelastic material by Chen et al. in [3, 7].

Additionally in this paper we propose a method for the segmentation of individual muscles which have different fiber orientation. Automatically segmenting individual muscle components from MRI poses a difficult problem as the boundaries between different muscles are not clearly distinguishable. The most popular method used for this segmentation is to introduce prior knowledge into the segmentation process through registration [8] of images or statistical learning techniques [9, 10, 11, 12]. The idea proposed in this work is to use the MRI intensities in combination with the muscle fiber direction obtained from DTI, to segment individual muscles. A combined multiphase multichannel method of segmentation is used to implement this idea [13, 14]. The multichannel method incorporates the MRI and fiber direction in different channels, and a multiphase framework is required to segment connected regions in an image.

The remaining sections of the paper are arranged as follows. Section 2 gives the review of the RK approximation and the smooth transition between heterogeneous materials using RK approximation is demonstrated. In section 3 the variational formulation of hyperelasticity discretized by RKPM is introduced. The details of the proposed DTI enhanced multiphase multichannel level set segmentation of muscles and full RKPM model construction from images are given in Section 4. Section 5 discusses the results obtained from the meshfree pixel based modeling. In section 6 conclusions are given.

2   Reproducing Kernel (RK) Approximation

In meshfree modeling the problem domain is discretized with a set of arbitrarily distributed points (nodes) as shown in Fig. 1(a). Each point I is associated with an open cover ω_I which defines the locality of the approximation defined on ω_I. In the present modeling the pixel coordinates of the geometry are obtained from the images and are used as nodes for discretizing the domain for the meshfree modeling. The RK shape functions are constructed based on a set of points and are used to approximate the displacement field governed by the equilibrium equation or equation of motion of a solid [2, 3]. The derivation of the RK shape function is given in the following paragraph.

Let $\alpha = \alpha_1 \alpha_2 ... \alpha_d$ represent the multi-dimensional index notation where d is the spatial dimension, and $|\alpha| = \alpha_1 + \alpha_2 + ... + \alpha_d$. The following notations are used:

$$\mathbf{x}^\alpha = \mathbf{x}_1^{\alpha_1} \mathbf{x}_2^{\alpha_2} ... \mathbf{x}_d^{\alpha_d}, \ (\mathbf{x} - \mathbf{x}_I)^\alpha = (\mathbf{x}_1 - \mathbf{x}_{1I})^{\alpha_1} (\mathbf{x}_2 - \mathbf{x}_{2I})^{\alpha_2} ... (\mathbf{x}_d - \mathbf{x}_{dI})^{\alpha_d} \quad (1)$$

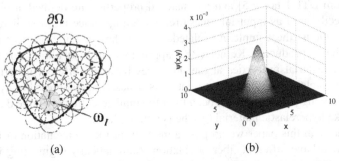

Fig. 1. (a) Domain discretization in meshfree modeling (b) Reproducing Kernel Shape Function

Consider a domain Ω in d dimensional space $\mathbb{R}^d$ which is discretized by a set of NP nodes given by $\{\mathbf{x}_I \mid \mathbf{x}_I \in \Omega\}_{I=1}^{NP}$. The RK approximation of a function u is given by:

$$u^h(\mathbf{x}) = \sum_{I=1}^{NP} \Psi_I(\mathbf{x})\, d_I \tag{2}$$

where $\Psi_I(\mathbf{x})$ is the RK shape function of node I, d_I is the coefficient at node I and $u^h(\mathbf{x})$ is the approximated function. The RK shape function is expressed as:

$$\Psi_I(\mathbf{x}) = C(\mathbf{x} : \mathbf{x} - \mathbf{x}_I)\, \phi_a(\mathbf{x} - \mathbf{x}_I) \tag{3}$$

where $\phi_a(\mathbf{x} - \mathbf{x}_I)$ is a kernel function which determines the locality of the approximation by its compact support measured by 'a' and the smoothness of the approximation, for example, a cubic B-spline function is twice differentiable. The term $C(\mathbf{x} : \mathbf{x} - \mathbf{x}_I)$ is a correction function expressed as

$$C(\mathbf{x} : \mathbf{x} - \mathbf{x}_I) = \sum_{|\alpha|=0}^{n} (\mathbf{x} - \mathbf{x}_I)^\alpha \mathbf{b}_\alpha(\mathbf{x}) = \mathbf{H}^T(\mathbf{x} - \mathbf{x}_I)\, \mathbf{b}(\mathbf{x}) \quad \text{in } \mathbb{R}^d \tag{4}$$

where n is the order of the basis functions, $\mathbf{H}^T(\mathbf{x} - \mathbf{x}_I) = \{(\mathbf{x} - \mathbf{x}_I)^\alpha\}_{|\alpha|=0}^{n}$ is a vector containing all the monomial basis functions, and $\mathbf{b}_\alpha(\mathbf{x})$ is an unknown vector which is determined by the following n^{th} order consistency conditions:

$$\sum_{I=1}^{NP} \Psi_I(\mathbf{x})\, \mathbf{x}_I^\alpha = \mathbf{x}^\alpha; \quad |\alpha| = 0,\dots,n \tag{5}$$

The above equation is used to obtain $\mathbf{b}(\mathbf{x}) = \mathbf{M}^{-1}(\mathbf{x})\, \mathbf{H}(0)$, where $\mathbf{M}$ is called the moment matrix and is given by:

$$\mathbf{M}(\mathbf{x}) = \sum_{I=1}^{NP} \mathbf{H}(\mathbf{x} - \mathbf{x}_I)\, \mathbf{H}^T(\mathbf{x} - \mathbf{x}_I)\, \phi_a(\mathbf{x} - \mathbf{x}_I) \tag{6}$$

Finally, the RK shape function can be re-written as:

$$\Psi_I(\mathbf{x}) = \mathbf{H}^T(0)\, \mathbf{M}^{-1}(\mathbf{x})\, \mathbf{H}(\mathbf{x} - \mathbf{x}_I)\, \phi_a(\mathbf{x} - \mathbf{x}_I) \tag{7}$$

Example of RK shape function constructed at node (5,5) of a domain defined by $\Omega \in [0,10] \times [0,10]$ is given in Fig. 1(b).

It has been shown in many studies [15] that the change of material property from skeletal muscle to tendon material is a smooth transition. Heterogeneous material modeling using FE method results in jumps in material properties, stresses and strains across the element boundaries and at the material interfaces. On the contrary, in the proposed meshfree RKPM analysis the material properties are assigned to the nodes, and at interfaces, material properties transition can be smoothed by using meshfree RK approximation with a desired degree of continuity, which avoids the abrupt jumps of stresses and strains. This material smoothing at interfaces is illustrated in the following example. Consider a region $[0, 10]$ with $x = 5$ defining interface between two materials and the Young's modulus (E) is given by: $E = 30$ for region $[0, 5)$ and $E = 5$ for region $[5, 10]$. As can be seen in Fig. 2, finite element approximation exhibits sharp discontinuity while the RK approximation shows smooth transition in representing the material property across the material interface. Further, the size of the transition zone can be adjusted by changing the support size (d) in RK approximation.

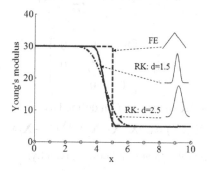

Fig. 2. 1D comparison of RK and FE approximations of the Young's modulus

3   Meshfree RKPM Formulation for Hyperelasticity

In this section, a 3D RKPM formulation is developed to solve the nonlinear elastic problem, in which penalty method is used to impose the Dirichlet boundary conditions and stabilized conforming nodal integration is employed to perform the numerical integration. The energy functional for this formulation is given by:

$$U = \int_{\Omega_x} W(\mathbf{u})d\Omega - \int_{\Omega_x} \rho_0 u_i b_i d\Omega - \int_{\partial\Omega_x^h} u_i h_i d\Gamma + \frac{\beta}{2} \int_{\partial\Omega_x^g} (u_i - g_i)^2 d\Gamma \qquad (8)$$

where, ρ_0 is mass density, $\mathbf{b}$ is body force per mass, $\mathbf{h}$ is prescribed surface traction on $\partial\Omega_x^h$, β is the penalty number and $\mathbf{g}$ is prescribed displacement on $\partial\Omega_x^g$. Taking the variation of equation (8), the stationary condition is achieved:

$$\int_{\Omega_X} \delta F_{ij} P_{ij} d\Omega + \beta \int_{\partial\Omega_X^g} \delta u_i u_i d\Gamma$$
$$= \int_{\Omega_X} \rho_0 \delta u_i b_i d\Omega + \int_{\partial\Omega_X^h} \delta u_i h_i d\Gamma + \beta \int_{\partial\Omega_X^g} \delta u_i g_i d\Gamma \tag{9}$$

where, F is the deformation gradient and P is the first Piola-Kirchhoff stress. Due to the geometric and material nonlinearities, Newton's method is used to solve the nonlinear equations and linearization of (9) is required. Let n and v denote the current load step counter and iteration step counter, the prescribed traction on the Neumann boundary and the prescribed displacement for the Dirichlet boundary for the $(n+1)^{th}$ load step are given. The linearized equation is given by:

$$\int_{\Omega_X} \delta F_{ij} (\mathbb{C}_{ijkl})_{n+1}^v \Delta F_{kl} d\Omega + \beta \int_{\partial\Omega_X^g} \delta u_i \Delta u_i d\Gamma = \int_{\Omega_X} \rho_0 \delta u_i (b_i)_{n+1} d\Omega$$
$$+ \int_{\partial\Omega_X^h} \delta u_i (h_i)_{n+1} d\Gamma + \beta \int_{\partial\Omega_X^g} \delta u_i [(g_i)_{n+1} - (u_i)_{n+1}^v] d\Gamma - \int_{\Omega_X} \delta F_{ij} (P_{ij})_{n+1}^v d\Omega \tag{10}$$

where $\mathbb{C}_{ijkl}$ is the first elasticity tensor. The displacement vector and its variation are approximated by RK shape functions as follows:

$$\mathbf{u} = \sum_I \mathbf{N}_I \mathbf{d}_I, \delta\mathbf{u} = \sum_I \mathbf{N}_I \delta\mathbf{d}_I \tag{11}$$

where

$$\mathbf{N}_I = \begin{bmatrix} \Psi_I & 0 & 0 \\ 0 & \Psi_I & 0 \\ 0 & 0 & \Psi_I \end{bmatrix} \tag{12}$$

Here Ψ is the Lagrangian RK shape function defined as:

$$\Psi_I(\mathbf{X}) = C(\mathbf{X}:\mathbf{X}-\mathbf{X}_I) \phi_a^X (\mathbf{X}-\mathbf{X}_I) \tag{13}$$

and the kernel ϕ_a^X is called the 'material kernel' given by:

$$\phi_a^X (\mathbf{X}-\mathbf{X}_I) = \phi_a^X \left(\frac{|\mathbf{X}-\mathbf{X}_I|}{a} \right) \tag{14}$$

The material kernel function deforms with the material deformation as illustrated in Fig. 3. The incremental deformation gradient in vector form is given by:

$$\Delta\mathbf{F} = \sum_I \mathbf{B}_I \Delta\mathbf{d}_I \tag{15}$$

where

$$\mathbf{u}^T = [u_1 \quad u_2 \quad u_3]$$
$$\mathbf{d}_I^T = [d_{1I} \quad d_{2I} \quad d_{3I}]$$
$$\mathbf{F}^T = [F_{11} \quad F_{22} \quad F_{33} \quad F_{12} \quad F_{21} \quad F_{13} \quad F_{31} \quad F_{23} \quad F_{32}]$$
$$\mathbf{B}_I^T = \begin{bmatrix} \Psi_{I,1} & 0 & 0 & \Psi_{I,2} & 0 & \Psi_{I,3} & 0 & 0 & 0 \\ 0 & \Psi_{I,2} & 0 & 0 & \Psi_{I,1} & 0 & 0 & \Psi_{I,3} & 0 \\ 0 & 0 & \Psi_{I,3} & 0 & 0 & 0 & \Psi_{I,1} & 0 & \Psi_{I,2} \end{bmatrix} \tag{16}$$

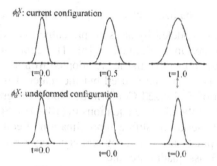

Fig. 3. Material kernel function

Here $\Psi_{I,j} = \partial\Psi_I / \partial X_j$. Taking the material derivative of the Lagrangian RK shape function is straight forward. The following matrix equation is obtained:

$$\mathbf{K}_{IJ}\Delta\mathbf{d}_J = f_I^{\text{ext}} - f_I^{\text{int}} \tag{17}$$

where

$$\mathbf{K}_{IJ} = \int_{\Omega_X} \mathbf{B}_I^T \mathbf{C}_{IJ}\mathbf{B}_J d\Omega + \beta \int_{\partial\Omega_X^g} \mathbf{N}_I^T\mathbf{N}_J d\Gamma$$

$$f_I^{\text{int}} = \int_{\Omega_X} \mathbf{B}_I^T\mathbf{P}d\Omega \tag{18}$$

$$f_I^{\text{ext}} = \int_{\Omega_X} \rho_0\mathbf{N}_I^T\mathbf{b}d\Omega + \int_{\partial\Omega_X^h} \mathbf{N}_I^T\mathbf{h}d\Gamma + \beta\int_{\partial\Omega_X^g} \mathbf{N}_I^T(\mathbf{g}-\mathbf{u}_{n+1}^v)d\Gamma$$

and

$$\mathbf{P} = \begin{bmatrix} P_{11} & P_{22} & P_{33} & P_{12} & P_{21} & P_{13} & P_{31} & P_{23} & P_{32} \end{bmatrix}^T$$

$$\mathbf{b} = \begin{bmatrix} b_1 & b_2 & b_3 \end{bmatrix}^T, \mathbf{h} = \begin{bmatrix} h_1 & h_2 & h_3 \end{bmatrix}^T, \mathbf{C}_{IJ} = \partial^2 W / \partial\mathbf{F}_I\partial\mathbf{F}_J \tag{19}$$

A transversely isotropic hyperelastic model is employed to represent the skeletal muscle. The strain energy density function for this model is decoupled into isotropic and anisotropic parts as defined below:

$$W_{\text{muscle}} = W_{\text{matrix}}(\bar{I}_1, \bar{I}_2, J) + W_{\text{fiber}}(\lambda) \tag{20}$$

where W_{matrix} is energy stored within muscle matrix where the material is homogeneous and isotropic, W_{fiber} is the energy stored within muscle fiber and this introduces anisotropy in the model, $\bar{I}_1, \bar{I}_2$ are the reduced invariants of right Cauchy-Green strain tensor, and $\lambda = \sqrt{\mathbf{N}\cdot\bar{\mathbf{C}}\cdot\mathbf{N}}$ is the reduced deviatoric stretch ratio along fiber direction where $\mathbf{N}$ is the fiber direction. A quadratic polynomial type strain energy density function for W_{matrix} as employed in [6] is used in this study. For the fiber part, the energy density function is defined as follows:

$$\lambda\frac{\partial W_{\text{fiber}}}{\partial\lambda} = \sigma_{\max}\frac{\lambda}{\lambda_0}(\alpha f_{\text{active}} + f_{\text{passive}}) \tag{21}$$

where λ_0 is the stretch ratio at optimal length, $\sigma_{\max}$ is the maximum isometric stress, α is the activation factor which represents the level of activation in the muscle, and

f_{active} and f_{passive} are the normalized active and passive fiber forces respectively. Connective tissue and fat are modeled by an isotropic cubic hyperelastic model with the strain energy density function as defined in [6]. The calibrated values of material constants for muscle and connective tissue are adopted from [6]. For the fat, the same material model as connective tissue is used but the material parameters are adopted from [16]. The method of Stabilized Conforming Nodal Integration (SCNI) [17, 18, 19], is used for integrating the discrete equations in (18)-(19). SCNI ensures quadratic rate of convergence in Galerkin meshfree approximation of equilibrium equation, and it achieves greater computational efficiency and accuracy for meshfree method compared to conventional Gauss quadrature rules.

4   Model Construction from Images

For individual muscle segmentation the idea proposed in this work is to use the muscle fiber direction which is obtained from the lead Eigen Vector (EV) of the DTI data at each pixel point, along with the MRI as input for segmentation and it is implemented using a combined multiphase multichannel level set based segmentation method as will be described below. The EV data which consist of a vector at each pixel point is obtained in 3 images where each image gives one of the vector components. For the purpose of segmentation the EV data is scaled suitably to match the range of intensities of the MRI. Each of the images, that is, MRI, e_1, e_2 and e_3 components of the EV data are taken as 4 channels for segmentation. As the final segmentation has 7 major muscles to be identified in the image, 3 level set functions are used for segmentation. The functional for the 3 level sets, 4 channels segmentation is given by [13, 14]:

$$\Pi(c_p^i,\phi_1,\phi_2,\phi_3)=\sum_{K=1}^{3}\mu_K\int_\Omega\delta(\phi_K)|\nabla\phi_K|\,d\mathbf{x}+\sum_{p=1}^{8}\left(\int_{\Omega_p}\frac{1}{4}\sum_{i=1}^{4}\left(\lambda_p^i(u_o^i(\mathbf{x})-c_p^i)^2\right)d\mathbf{x}\right) \quad (22)$$

where $u_o^i(\mathbf{x})$ denotes the pixel intensity in the ith channel at point $\mathbf{x}$, p denotes the number of regions that can be segmented and c_p^i denotes the unknown constants which represents the mean value of intensity in the region Ω_p of ith channel. c_p^i can be obtained by minimizing equation (22) with respect to each c_p^i keeping all other variables constant. The 3 Euler Lagrange equations for curve evolution can be obtained by minimizing the above functional with respect to ϕ_1,ϕ_2,ϕ_3 respectively keeping c_p^i constant. These are solved using a semi-implicit finite difference scheme. The important parameter to consider in the formulation (22) is the λ terms which are the weights for the forcing term. If the value of λ is decreased it allows for slightly more variance of intensities in the region to be segmented and vice versa. Fig. 4 shows the segmentation result for one of the MRI slices by taking $\lambda=0.02$. The human Medial Gastrocnemius (MG) muscle is segmented using the proposed method from 33 images and compared with manual segmentation as shown in Fig. 5.

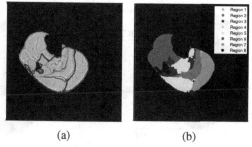

(a)   (b)

Fig. 4. Multiphase Multichannel segmentation of MRI and EV data (a) Final contours obtained from segmentation (b) Final segmented regions

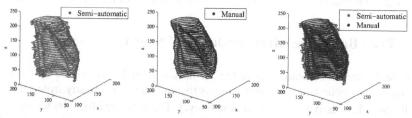

Fig. 5. Comparison of Semi-automatic and Manual segmentations of Medial Gastrocnemius muscle of human lower leg

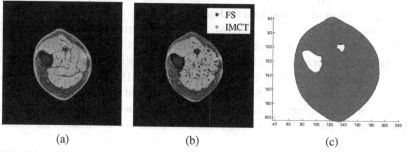

(a)   (b)   (c)

Fig. 6. (a) Outer contours and Bone contours obtained from segmentation (b) FS, IMCT points overlapped on MRI (c) Interior points

The following methodology is developed for constructing the full model of the human lower leg from medical images. The given data for segmentation includes MRI, binary segmented images for Intramuscular Connective Tissue (IMCT) and Intra-Muscular Fat Saturation (FS), muscle fiber direction given by three EV images. The Chan-Vese level set segmentation method [20] is used for extracting boundaries of the bones and the outer boundary of the lower leg from each MRI as shown in Fig. 6(a). The interior points of boundary contours are obtained as shown in Fig. 6(c). The FS and IMCT points extracted from binary images (Fig. 6(b)) are subtracted from these interior points to obtain an image (say image1). The points which have EV data are chosen as the muscle points in image1 and the remaining interior points are assigned as fat since they constitute the outer subcutaneous fat layer. The final image obtained with all the different materials points sorted is shown in Fig. 7(a). This procedure is repeated for every image (slice) and the 3D pixel based model is constructed by stacking the slices as shown in Fig. 7(b).

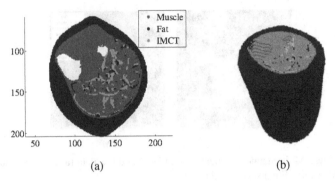

Fig. 7. (a) Fine model (b) 3D model constructed from 25 images, has 73,659 nodes

5   Pixel Based Meshfree Modeling of Skeletal Muscle

Example 1: Isometric contraction of the 3D muscle model is simulated by fixing the top and bottom boundaries and increasing activation factor α linearly from 0 to 1, so that the muscle is activated to its maximum level. The generated force by the muscle is calculated at the end cross section. Fig. 8 shows the displacement field in vector plots at sample planes and Fig. 9(a) and (b) show the distribution of stress at final configuration. To study the effect of IMCT in force generation, two different models are constructed. The first model is obtained as described previously. For the second model, the IMCT points in the first model are replaced by muscle material and the muscle fiber direction at these points are interpolated from neighboring muscle points. Fig. 9(c) shows the force generation at difference stages of activation. In model 2 the muscle volume is increased by 5.6% due to the replacement of IMCT. This results in an increase of force production by 4.8%. This shows an almost linear relationship between increase in muscle volume and force production. Also this example illustrates the effect on resultant force generation when connective tissue is considered in the model.

Example 2: To study the effect of aging on force generation, two models of the Medial Gastrocnemius (MG) were manually segmented as shown in Fig. 10(a) and (b). The MG is surrounded by an outer layer of connective tissue which is the aponeurosis, and the axial length of the muscle in both models is the same. The amount of different material components in the young and the old model are given in Table 1. The force generation at maximum activation shows that the younger model generates much bigger force than the older model (Fig. 10(c)). The effective force generated per total volume for the younger model is 0.5452 N/cm^3 and for the old model is 0.3534 N/cm^3. This shows that the amount of non-contractile tissue certainly effects the force production. Also the muscle volume of the older model is about 37% lesser than the younger model but the force generation in the older model drops by around 45% compared to the young model. There is a non-proportional decrease in force production due to decrease in muscle volume.

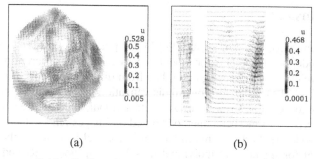

(a)   (b)

Fig. 8. Displacement field at final configuration on (a) Transverse plane at z = 5 cm (b) sagittal plane at y = 10.1 cm

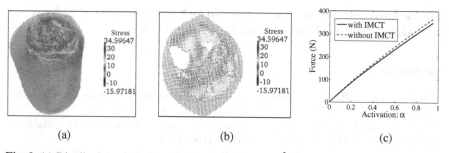

(a)   (b)   (c)

Fig. 9. (a) Distribution of maximum principal stress (N/cm^2) at final configuration (b) At transverse planes z = 5.0 cm (c) Comparison of force generation between the two models with and without IMCT

Table 1. Example 2: Young vs Old Model Results comparison

	Young model	Old model
Muscle(cm^3)	98.9	61.89
Fat(cm^3)	2.8	6.10
IMCT(cm^3)	24.49	38.66
F$_{max}$ (N)	68.8	37.7

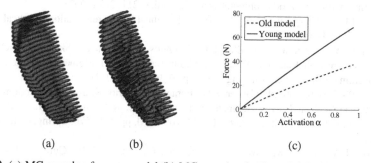

(a)   (b)   (c)

Fig. 10. (a) MG muscle of young model (b) MG muscle of old model: blue nodes are connective tissue points, green nodes are muscle points and red nodes are fat saturation points (c) Comparison of force generation versus activation level between young and old models

6   Conclusions

In this work, an image based meshfree RKPM computational framework is developed for muscle modeling. A method for model construction with different material components is developed by extracting pixel data from different images. The pixel points can be directly used as nodes for domain discretization in the meshfree modeling, and the fiber direction obtained from the DTI data is input directly at each pixel point. These characteristics of meshfree methods based on images render it suitable for subject specific modeling. Further a multiphase multichannel level set method with modified functional for segmenting individual muscles using both MRI and DTI data is proposed. A preliminary study on how the amount of connective tissue in the muscles can affect the force generation is performed using the proposed methods.

Acknowledgements. This study was supported by National Institute of Arthritis and Musculoskeletal and Skin Diseases Grant 5R01-AR-053343-07.

References

1. Blemker, S.S., Delp, S.L.: Three-Dimensional Representation of Complex Muscle Architectures and Geometries. Annals of Biomedical Engineering, 661–673 (2005)
2. Liu, W.K., Jun, S., Zhang, Y.F.: Reproducing Kernel Particle Methods. International Journal for Numerical Methods in Fluids 20, 1081–1106 (1995)
3. Chen, J.S., Pan, C., Wu, C.T., Liu, W.K.: Reproducing kernel particle methods for large deformation analysis of non-linear structures. Computer Methods in Applied Mechanics and Engineering, 195–227 (1996)
4. Bihan, D.L., Mangin, J.-F., Poupon, C., Clark, C.A., Pappata, S., Molko, N., Chabriat, H.: Diffusion Tensor Imaging: Concepts and Applications. Journal of Magnetic Resonance Imaging 13, 534–546 (2001)
5. Sinha, U., Yao, L.: In vivo diffusion tensor imaging of human calf muscle. Journal of Magnetic Resonance Imaging, 87–95 (2002)
6. Chi, S.W., Hodgson, J.A., Chen, J.S., Edgerton, V.R., Shin, D.D., Roiz, R.A., Sinha, S.: Finite element modeling reveals complex strain mechanics in the aponeuroses of contracting skeletal muscle. Journal of Biomechanics 43(7), 1243–1250 (2010)
7. Chen, J.S., Pan, C., Wu, C.T.: Large deformation analysis of rubber based on a reproducing kernel particle method. Computational Mechanics, 211–227 (1997)
8. Maintz, J.B.A., Viergever, M.A.: A survey of medical image registration. Medical Image Analysis 2(1), 1–36 (1998)
9. Baudin, P.-Y., Azzabou, N., Carlier, P.G., Paragios, N.: Automatic Skeletal Muscle Segmentation Through Random Walks and Graph-Based Seed Placement. In: International Symposium on Biomedical Imaging 2012, pp. 1036–1039 (2012)
10. Baudin, P.-Y., Azzabou, N., Carlier, P.G., Paragios, N.: Prior Knowledge, Random Walks and Human Skeletal Muscle Segmentation. In: Ayache, N., Delingette, H., Golland, P., Mori, K. (eds.) MICCAI 2012, Part I. LNCS, vol. 7510, pp. 569–576. Springer, Heidelberg (2012)
11. Prescott, J.W., Best, T.M., Swanson, M.S., Haq, F., Jackson, R.D., Gurcan, M.N.: Anatomically Anchored Template-Based Level Set Segmentation: Application to Quadriceps Muscles in MR Images from the Osteoarthritis Initiative. Journal of Digital Imaging 24(1), 28–43 (2011)

12. Neji, R., Fleury, G., Deux, J.F., Rahmouni, A., Bassez, G., Vignaud, A., Paragios, N.: Support Vector Driven Markov Random Fields Towards DTI Segmentation of the Human Skeletal Muscle. In: International Symposium on Biomedical Imaging, pp. 923–926 (2008)
13. Vese, L.A., Chan, T.F.: A Multiphase Levelset Framework for Image segmentation using the Mumford and Shah model. International Journal of Computer Vision 50(3), 271–293 (2002)
14. Chan, T.F., Sandberg, B.Y., Vese, L.A.: Active Contours without Edges for Vector-Valued Images. Journal of Visual Communication and Image Representation 11, 130–141 (2000)
15. Tidball, J.G.: Myotendinous junction: morphological changes and mechanical failure associated with muscle cell atrophy. Experimental and Molecular Pathology 40(1), 1–12 (1984)
16. McKnight, A.L., Kugel, J.L., Rossman, P.J., Manduca, A., Hartmann, L.C., Ehman, R.L.: MR elastography of breast cancer: preliminary results. American Journal of Roentgenology 178(6), 1411–1417 (2002)
17. Chen, J.S., Wu, C.T., Yoon, S., You, Y.: A stabilized conforming nodal integration for Galerkin mesh-free methods. International Journal for Numerical Methods in Engineering, 435–466 (2001)
18. Chen, J.S., Yoon, S., Wu, C.T.: Non-linear version of stabilized conforming nodal integration for Galerkin mesh-free methods. International Journal for Numerical Methods in Engineering, 2587–2615 (2002)
19. Puso, M.A., Chen, J.-S., Zywicz, E., Elmer, W.: Meshfree and Finite Element Nodal Integration methods. International Journal for Numerical Methods in Engineering 74, 416–446 (2008)
20. Chan, T.F., Vese, L.A.: Active Contours without edges. IEEE Transactions on Image Processing 10(2), 266–277 (2001)

Modelling of Bioimpedance Measurements: Application to Sensitivity Analysis

Alexander A. Danilov[1], Vasily K. Kramarenko[2], and Alexandra S. Yurova[3]

[1] Institute of Numerical Mathematics, Russian Academy of Sciences,
Moscow 119333, Russia
a.a.danilov@gmail.com
[2] Moscow Institute of Physics and Technology, Dolgoprudny, 141700, Russia
[3] Lomonosov Moscow State University, Department of Computational Mathematics
and Cybernetics, Moscow, 119991, Russia

Abstract. A technology for high-resolution efficient numerical modeling of bioimpedance measurements is considered that includes 3D image segmentation, adaptive unstructured tetrahedral mesh generation, finite-element discretization, and the analysis of simulation data. The first-order convergence of the proposed numerical methods on a series of unmatched meshes and roughly second order convergence on a series of nested meshes are shown. Sensitivity field distributions for a conventional tetrapolar, as well as eight- and ten-electrode measurement configurations are obtained.

Keywords: bioelectrical impedance analysis, FEM, sensitivity analysis, mesh generation.

1 Introduction

Measurements of the electrical impedance of biological tissue in response to applied alternating current provide a number of non-invasive, harmless, portable, and relatively low cost techniques for use in medical and biological studies [4,7,10]. An example is the application of bioelectrical impedance analysis (BIA) for the in vivo human body composition assessment [13,14]. The same measurement and similar methodological principles apply in impedance cardiography (ICG) for the assessment of central hemodynamics and also in impedance plethysmography (IPG) for the evaluation of peripheral vascular function [4]. In contrast to electrical impedance tomography aimed at visualization of the internal body structure (see, e.g., [3,10]), little amount of electrodes is used in BIA, ICG and IPG. But the spectrum of electrode types, their properties and configurations used (local, whole-body, segmental, polysegmental), as well as of the measurement frequencies, is wide. This inspires optimization of bioimpedance measurements for specific purposes. Since a real human body represents complex non-homogeneous and non-isotropic medium with variable cross-section area, the fundamental questions arose about the nature and relative contribution of various organs and tissues to the bioimpedance signal. The latter, as well as the problem of measurement optimization, was studied by means of impedance simulations using computerized models

Y.J. Zhang and J.M.R.S. Tavares (Eds.): CompIMAGE 2014, LNCS 8641, pp. 328–338, 2014.

of real human anatomy (see, e.g., [1,12,19]). Similar approach is also used in radiography, nuclear medicine, radiation protection and other research areas [2,18].

Modeling of sensitivity distributions for various measurement schemes requires solving a number of computational problems using high-resolution anatomically accurate 3D models [24]. Our aim was to describe unstructured mesh generation and computational modeling procedures for bioimpedance measurements, to characterize the convergence of the suggested numerical method, and to illustrate sensitivity field distributions for a conventional and segmental bioimpedance measurement schemes using anatomically accurate 3D model of the human body from Visible Human Project (VHP)[17].

2   Mathematical Model

As described in [7], the electrical fields generated during bioimpedance measurements are governed by the equation

$$\text{div}(\mathbf{C}\nabla U) = 0 \quad \text{in} \quad \Omega \tag{1}$$

with the boundary conditions

$$(\mathbf{J}, \mathbf{n}) = \pm I_0/S_\pm \quad \text{on} \quad \Gamma_\pm \tag{2}$$

$$(\mathbf{J}, \mathbf{n}) = 0 \quad \text{on} \quad \partial\Omega\backslash\Gamma_\pm \tag{3}$$

$$U(x_0, y_0, z_0) = 0 \tag{4}$$

$$\mathbf{J} = \mathbf{C}\nabla U \tag{5}$$

where Ω is the computational domain, $\partial\Omega$ is its boundary, $\Gamma_\pm$ are electrode contact surfaces, $\mathbf{n}$ is an external unit normal vector, U is an electric potential, $\mathbf{C}$ is a conductivity tensor, $\mathbf{J}$ is a current density, I_0 is an electric current, $S_\pm$ are areas of the electrode contacts. Equation (1) determines the distribution of electric field in the domain with heterogeneous conductivity $\mathbf{C}$. Equation (2) sets a constant current density on the electrode contact surfaces. Equation (3) defines the no-flow condition on the boundary. Uniqueness of the solution is guaranteed by the equation (4), where (x_0, y_0, z_0) is some point in the domain Ω.

In our study we use the finite element method for solving of 1-5 with P_1 finite elements on unstructured tetrahedral meshes. We assume that each computational element have a constant conductivity coefficient which corresponds to one of the human tissues. For calculations we use Ani3D package [21].

3   Convergence Study

We consider a simple geometrical model of the human torso that was described previously in [16] (Fig. 1) and a series of unstructured tetrahedral meshes with variable element size. Having automatic mesh generation algorithm for this model, we can perform a lot of numerical tests. For each mesh we compute

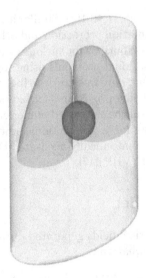

Fig. 1. Simplified geometrical model of the human torso

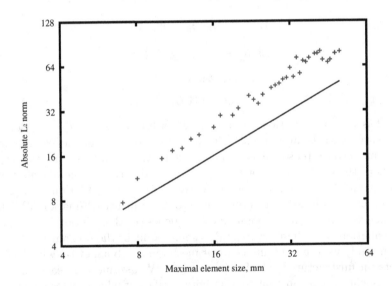

Fig. 2. Convergence study on the series of unmatched meshes

the numerical solution and compare it with the numerical solution obtained on the finest mesh by using L_2-norm to evaluate the difference between numerical solutions. Since different meshes may consist of different vertex sets, we apply a conventional piecewise-linear interpolation from coarse mesh to fine mesh, and compute the discrete L_2-norm on the fine mesh. It should be noted that an extra

Table 1. The results of convergence study on hierarchical meshes

N_V	N_T	Memory, MB	N_{it}	Time, s	L_2-norm
2032	9359	7.16	13	0.02	1.24E-03
14221	74872	37.3	23	0.18	9.31E-04
106509	598976	299.1	58	3.70	5.07E-04
824777	4791808	2437.5	127	68.55	1.53E-04
6492497	38334464	20015.3	353	2634.15	–

interpolation error is added in the case of two unmatched meshes as compared to hierarchical meshes. We consider both series of unmatched unstructured meshes and of hierarchical meshes.

The numerical results of the convergence study with unmatched meshes are presented in Fig. 2. The numerical solution obtained on the finest mesh with maximal element size 5 mm is considered as a control solution. Solutions on other meshes with maximal element size from 7 mm to 50 mm are compared to this control solution. The values in the Fig. 2 are well distributed along the line parallel to the bisector of the coordinate axes of absolute L_2 norm and the maximal element size h, meaning that the proposed method demonstrates first-order convergence on the unmatched meshes.

Now we consider the series of hierarchical meshes. The initial coarse mesh contains 9359 tetrahedrons. Starting from this mesh, we split each tetrahedron into 8 smaller tetrahedra by splitting each face into four triangles by the middle points on the edges [21]. We call this operation a uniform refinement of the mesh. Now we can apply uniform refinement to the new mesh, and so on. At each step the element size of the mesh decreases two times. The vertex set of the finest mesh fully covers the vertex sets of all previous meshes, meaning that the extra interpolation errors are not introduced in L_2-norm computation. The finest mesh in the series of five meshes has more than 38 million tetrahedrons and requires nearly 20 GB of the memory for computation. We used GMRES based iterative linear solver with the second-order ILU preconditioner [11,21].

The results of the convergence study on the series of hierarchical meshes are presented in Table 1. The first two columns show the number of vertices N_V and the number of tetrahedrons N_T. The next three columns show the memory usage, the number of linear solver iterations N_{it} needed for 10^{12}-fold reduction of an initial residual, and the overall time usage respectively. The last column contains the relative L_2-norm that reduces asymptotically with roughly the second order convergence.

In summary, our tests demonstrated first-order convergence of the proposed numerical methods on a series of unmatched meshes and nearly second order convergence on a series of nested meshes.

4   Sensitivity Analysis and Mesh Generation of Model, Based on Real Human Anatomy

Our high resolution human body geometrical model was constructed in two steps. First, the geometrical model of the human torso was created for Visible Human man data. The data were clipped and downscaled to an array of $567 \times 305 \times 843$ colored voxels with the resolution $1 \times 1 \times 1$ mm. The initial segmented model of the VHP [17] human torso was kindly provided by the Voxel-Man group [9]. This model has been produced primarily for visualization purposes, contained a significant amount of unclassified tissue and, thus, was not entirely suited for numerical purposes. Therefore, a further processing of the segmented model was needed. It was performed semi-automatically using ITK-SNAP segmentation software program [20]. At the final stage, we used several post-processing algorithms for filling remaining gaps between tissues and final segmented data smoothing. Our segmented model of the human torso contains 26 labels and describes major organs and tissues.

Several meshing techniques were tested for the mesh generation of segmented data. In our work we opted for the Delaunay triangulation algorithm from the CGAL-Mesh library [15]. This algorithm enables defining a specific mesh size for each model material. In order to preserve geometrical features of the segmented model while keeping a feasible number of vertices, we assigned a smaller mesh size to blood vessels and a larger mesh size to fat and muscle tissues. After initial mesh generation we applied mesh cosmetics from Ani3D package. This essential step reduces discretization errors and the condition number of the resulted systems of linear equations. The segmented model and the generated mesh with 413 508 vertices and 2 315 329 tetrahedra are presented in Fig. 3. This mesh retains most anatomical features of the human torso.

The whole body segmented model is based on the torso model. Missing parts were segmented using ITK-SNAP software. The final model is a $575 \times 333 \times 1878$ voxels array with the resolution $1 \times 1 \times 1$ mm segmented in 30 materials.

We used the proposed techniques to construct the computational mesh for the whole body model based on VHP data. The related segmented model and generated mesh containing 574 128 vertices and 3 300 481 tetrahedrons are shown in Fig. 4.

After mesh generation, we added a skin layer and multilayered electrodes to the surface of the constructed mesh. Boundary triangulation was used to create a prismatic mesh on the surface, and then each prism was split into three tetrahedrons resulting in a conformal mesh.

Along with conventional tetrapolar wrist-to-ankle measurement configuration, two schemes of segmental BIA were considered: an eight-electrode one with the placement of current and potential electrodes 5 cm apart on the back surfaces of the wrists and ankles, and also ten-electrode scheme with an additional electrode pair located on the forehead. Accordingly, five pairs of thin bilayer square objects 23×23 mm in size simulating electrode properties were added on the forehead and distal parts of arms and legs of the segmented model.

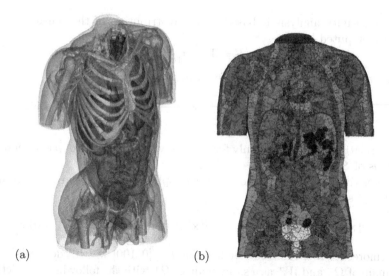

Fig. 3. Geometrical model of the segmented image (a) and unstructured tetrahedral mesh (b)

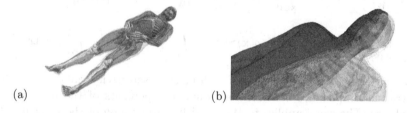

Fig. 4. Segmented whole body model of the Visible Human Man (a) and a part of generated mesh (b)

As described in [7,6] we introduce the reciprocal lead field $\mathbf{J}'_{\text{reci}}$ which is equal to density vector field generated by a unit current excitation using the two PU electrodes. Field $\mathbf{J}'_{\text{reci}}$ is computed from 1-5, with electrode surfaces $\Gamma_{\pm}$ corresponding to PU electrodes and $I_0 = 1$.

The lead field may be used for sensitivity distribution analysis of the PU electrodes for CC electrodes. We will use the following two equations: the general transfer signal equation

$$u = \int_{\Omega} \rho \, \mathbf{J}_{\text{CC}} \cdot \mathbf{J}'_{\text{reci}} \, \mathrm{d}x, \tag{6}$$

and the general transfer impedance equation:

$$Z_{\text{t}} = \int_{\Omega} \rho \, \mathbf{J}'_{\text{cc}} \cdot \mathbf{J}'_{\text{reci}} \, \mathrm{d}x. \tag{7}$$

In these equations u is the measured signal between PU electrodes, ρ is the resistivity, $\mathbf{J}_{\text{CC}}$ is computed from (1)-(5) with electrode surfaces $\Gamma_{\pm}$ corresponding to the current carrying electrodes, Z_{t} is the transfer impedance, and $\mathbf{J}'_{\text{cc}} = \mathbf{J}_{\text{cc}}/I_0$.

The sensitivity analysis is based on the distribution of the sensitivity field, which is computed by

$$S = \mathbf{J}'_{cc} \cdot \mathbf{J}'_{reci}.$$ (8)

Using this notation we have the following relations:

$$Z_t = \int_\Omega \rho S \, dx, \quad \Delta Z_t = \int_\Omega \Delta \rho S \, dx.$$ (9)

The last relation is applicable only for relatively small changes of ρ and moderate variations of S.

For sensitivity analysis purposes we will split Ω in three parts according to the value of sensitivity field:

$$\Omega^- = \{x | S(x) < 0\}, \quad \Omega^+ = \{x | S(x) > 0\}, \quad \Omega^0 = \{x | S(x) = 0\}.$$ (10)

Furthermore, for a specific threshold value $t \in [0, 100]$ we will define W_t^- as a subdomain of Ω^- and W_t^+ as a subdomain of Ω^+ with the following resctrictions:

$$\inf_{x \in \Omega \backslash W_t^-} \rho(x)S(x) \geqslant \sup_{x \in W_t^-} \rho(x)S(x), \quad \int_{W_t^-} \rho S \, dx = \frac{t}{100} \int_{\Omega^-} \rho S \, dx,$$ (11)

$$\sup_{x \in \Omega \backslash W_t^+} \rho(x)S(x) \leqslant \inf_{x \in W_t^+} \rho(x)S(x), \quad \int_{W_t^+} \rho S \, dx = \frac{t}{100} \int_{\Omega^+} \rho S \, dx.$$ (12)

In other words, W_t^+ is the region of high positive sensitivity values, which have the transfer impedance contribution equal to t percents of the total transfer impedance. The same applies to W_t^-, which is the region of the most negative sensitivity values.

We will also define in the same way the following subdomains: V_t^+ and V_t^+.

$$\sup_{x \in \Omega \backslash V_t^\pm} \pm S(x) \leqslant \inf_{x \in V_t^\pm} \pm S(x), \quad \int_{V_t^\pm} S \, dx = \frac{t}{100} \int_{\Omega^\pm} S \, dx.$$ (13)

These regions are the most sensitive regions of small local resistivity changes.

In our sensitivity analysis we investigate the shape of the subdomains W_t^+ and V_t^+. These body regions represent the most sensitive parts of the human body in specific measuring scenario. The shape of W_t^+ describes the part of the body in which one measures the transfer impedance. The shape of V_t^+ represents the part which is the most sensitive to local changes of conductivity. This analysis may be applied for validation of an empirically designed electrode schemes.

5   Adaptation to Position of Extremities

The preparation of the 3D model takes a lot of time. It consists of two stages: image segmentation and mesh generation. While the latter may be automated using tetrahedral mesh generation techniques, the former still requires a lot of manual operations. An accurate 3D model requires the high resolution patient data like CT or MRI for the whole body, which in most cases is not available. However the anthropometrical measurements of the body are easily accessible, and in some cases we may have local CT/MRI images with patient specific features. In [23] we proposed several techniques for adaptation of the once segmented human model to different patients or measurements conditions, including anthropometrical scaling, control points mapping and geometrical modification of body extremities positions. The last one may be crucial in modelling of measurement techniques involving the specific position of the patient, as it may influence the results of the measurements.

An example is adaptation of the model with regard to the geometrical position of the body parts, e.g. position of the arms, legs, or standing / sitting position. In these cases one must perform particular segmented model transformations. Let us consider the modification of arms position. Our proposal is to cut the arms along the virtual interface crossing the center of the shoulder joint. Each arm is rotated around the center of the shoulder joint. The overlapping parts are resolved based on priority of the body parts or labeled tissues. The void sectors, occuring after the rotation, are filled with sweeping of the segmented image trace on the virtual cut surface.

In our previous work [22] we presented the results of sensitivity analysis for segmental bioimpedance measurements. This work was performed with the VHP man segmented model in his original position with his arms placed along the body. In practice these measurements are performed with the angle between the arm and the body nearly equal to $45°$. This angle may have some influence on the result of measurements.

In the present work we adapted the initial model of VHP man with respect to the conventional position of the arms. This adaptation was performed as described above. The constructed mesh has 479 198 vertices and 2 725 980 tetrahedra. We simulated bioimpedance measurements at the electrical current frequency 50 kHz using our FEM model. The electrical conductivity parameters for labeled tissues were taken from [5].

The model has ten electrodes located in pairs on the forehead, both arms and both legs as described in [22]. The sensitivity field for the conventional tetrapolar scheme has a uniform sensitivity distribution near the shoulder as opposed to our previous results [22] obtained for the original model with arms placed along the torso.

As we are interested in comparing our results with our previous model with parallel arms, we computed the sensitivity fields for all six segmental measurement schemes and combined their W_{97}^+ regions, see Fig. 5. The combined region represents the part of the body which may be accessed by at least one of these schemes. As opposed to our previous result, we do not observe the blind zones in lateral parts of shoulders with the conventional position of the arms. These results indicate importance of the empirically proposed arms position for segmental bioimpedance measurements.

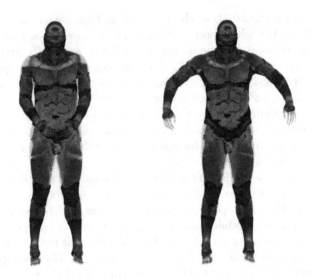

Fig. 5. The combined regions W_{97}^+ of contribution for ten-electrode scheme: arms along torso [22] (left), conventional position of arms (right)

6 Numerical Results

We simulated BIA measurements at the electrical current frequency 50 kHz using FEM.

Current density fields were calculated from the finite-element model, and the corresponding sensitivity field distributions were obtained for various configurations of electrode sites. Fig. 6 shows the high sensitivity body regions for all

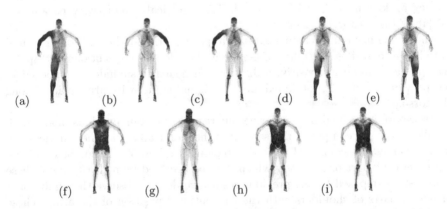

Fig. 6. High sensitivity areas for conventional tetrapolar scheme (a), left (b) and right (c) arms and right (d) and left (e) legs with 10 electrode scheme, head-neck-torso (f) and-head-neck-upper-torso (g) schemes, and crossover (h) and parallel (i) torso schemes

ten-electrode schemes of segmental measurements. For detailed explanation of electrode positions refer to Figure 1 and Table 1 in [22].

7   Conclusion

In this work we proposed the techniques for mathematical modelling of bio-electric impedance analysis. The numerical results on a simplified human torso model demonstrate at least first order convergence of the proposed scheme. We compared our previous results of segmental bioimpedance analysis using VHP man model with modified model with corrected position of the arms. The numerical results demonstrate that the correct position of the arms is crucial for accessing the lateral parts of the shoulders. The modified model also shows uniform sensitivity distribution near the shoulders for conventional tetrapolar scheme.

Acknowledgments. This work has been supported in part by RFBR grant 14-01-00830, and by the Russian President grant MK-3675.2013.1.

References

1. Beckmann, L., van Riesen, D., Leonhardt, S.: Optimal electrode placement and frequency range selection for the detection of lung water using bioimpedance spectroscopy. In: Proc. 29th Annual Int. Conf. of the IEEE, August 22–26, pp. 2685–2688 (2007)
2. Caon, M.: Voxel-based computational models of real human anatomy: a review. Radiat. Environ. Biophys. 42(4), 229–235 (2004)
3. Cherepenin, V., Karpov, A., Korjenevsky, A., et al.: Three-dimensional EIT imaging of breast tissues: system design and clinical testing. IEEE Trans. Med. Imaging 21(6), 662–667 (2002)
4. Cybulski, G.: Ambulatory impedance cardiography. Springer, Heidelberg (2011)
5. Gabriel, C., Peyman, A., Grant, E.: Electrical conductivity of tissues at frequencies below 1 MHz. Phys. Med. Biol. 54(16), 4863–4878 (2009)
6. Geselowitz, D.B.: An application of electrocardiographic lead theory to impedance plethysmography. IEEE Trans. Biomed. Eng. 18(1), 38–41 (1971)
7. Grimnes, S., Martinsen, O.G.: Bioimpedance and bioelectricity basics. Elsevier, Amsterdam (2008)
8. Hoffer, E.C., Meador, C.K., Simpson, D.C.: Correlation of whole-body impedance with total body water volume. J. Appl. Physiol. 27(4), 531–534 (1969)
9. Höhne, K.H., Pflesser, B., Pommert, A., et al.: A realistic model of human structure from the Visible Human data. Meth. Inform. Med. 40(2), 83–89 (2001)
10. Holder, D.S.: Electrical impedance tomography. Institute of Physics Publishers, Bristol (2005)
11. Kaporin, I.E.: High quality preconditioning of a general symmetric positive definite matrix based on its $u^t u + u^t r + r^t u$-decomposition. Numer. Linear Algebra Appl. 5(6), 483–509 (1998)

12. Kauppinen, P.K., Hyttinen, J.A., Malmivuo, J.A.: Sensitivity distributions of impedance cardiography using band and spot electrodes analyzed by a three-dimensional computer model. Ann. Biomed. Eng. 26(4), 694–702 (1998)
13. Kushner, R.F., Schoeller, D.A.: Estimation of total body water by bioelectrical impedance analysis. Am. J. Clin. Nutr. 44(3), 417–424 (1986)
14. Lukaski, H.C., Johnson, P.E., Bolonchuk, W.W., Lykken, G.I.: Assessment of fat-free mass using bioelectrical impedance measurements of the human body. Am. J. Clin. Nutr. 41(4), 810–817 (1985)
15. Rineau, L., Yvinec, M.: A generic software design for Delaunay refinement meshing. Comp. Geom. Theory Appl. 38(1-2), 100–110 (2007)
16. Vassilevski Yu, V., Danilov, A.A., Nikolaev, D.V., et al.: Finite-element analysis of bioimpedance measurements. Zh. Vych. Mat. Matem. Fiz. 52(4), 733–745 (2012) (in Russian)
17. The Visible Human Project, http://www.nlm.nih.gov/research/visible/
18. Xu, X.G., Eckerman, K.F.: Handbook of anatomical models for radiation dosimetry. CRC Press, Boca Raton (2009)
19. Yang, F., Patterson, R.P.: A simulation study on the effect of thoracic conductivity inhomogeneities on sensitivity distributions. Ann. Biomed. Eng. 36(5), 762–768 (2008)
20. Yushkevich, P.A., Piven, J., Hazlett, H.C., et al.: User-guided 3D active contour segmentation of anatomical structures: Significantly improved efficiency and reliability. Neuroimage 31(3), 1116–1128 (2006)
21. 3D generator of anisotropic meshes, http://sourceforge.net/projects/ani3d
22. Danilov, A.A., Kramarenko, V.K., Nikolaev, D.V., Rudnev, S.G., Salamatova, V.Yu., Smirnov, A.V., Vassilevski, Yu.V.: Sensitivity field distributions for segmental bioelectrical impedance analysis based on real human anatomy. J. Phys.: Conf. Ser. 434, 012001 (2013), doi:10.1088/1742-6596/434/1/012001
23. Danilov, A.A., Kramarenko, V.K., Nikolaev, D.V., Yurova, A.S.: Personalized model adaptation for bioimpedance measurements optimization // Russ. J. Numer. Anal. Math. Modelling 28(5), 459–470 (2013)
24. Danilov, A.A., Nikolaev, D.V., Rudnev, S.G., Salamatova, V.Yu., Vassilevski, Yu.V.: Modelling of bioimpedance measurements: unstructured mesh application to real human anatomy. Russ. J. Numer. Anal. Math. Modelling 27(5), 431–440 (2012)

Flow Simulations on 3D Segmented Images Using Reinitialization and Anisotropic Mesh Adaptation

Luisa Silva[1], Jia-Xin Zhao[1], Hugues Digonnet[1], and Thierry Coupez[2]

[1] MINES ParisTech, CEMEF - CNRS UMR 7635, Sophia Antipolis, France
[2] Ecole Centrale de Nantes, ICI, Nantes, France
luisa.silva@mines-paristech.fr

Abstract. In this paper, we introduce a new method to perform image segmentation by reinitializating an implicit function coupled to an anisotropic mesh adaptation technique. One of the advantages of such methodology is that the mesh produced can be directly used for scientific computations. In fact, finite element flow computations on images composed of multiphase structures will illustrate and validate our approach.

1 Introduction

In recent years, imaging techniques, like X-ray tomography, have been used to obtain accurate geometrical and topological information, which made extraordinary contributions in different fields. For scientific computation, accuracy of numerical representations may play a key role. The passage from the image to a finite element mesh allows on one hand, the construction of a numerical representation but, on the other hand, may also reduce the size of the stored data. The first step (before building a mesh) is usually to perform the image segmentation, that is, to partition the image into its multiple objects, so that it becomes easier to analyze it. The result of this segmentation can be regions of the image where the pixels are similar with respect to a characteristic or property (like, for example, the color), or extracted contours. Secondly, a mesh is built from the segmented image until the optimal mesh is obtained, by using different techniques [1]. One class of segmentation techniques is based on on an implicit description of the phases, using level set functions [2], employed also for binary and multi-phase image segmentation [3].

In this paper, we propose to simultaneously segment the image and produce an adapted mesh adequate to perform numerical simulations using the image data. These simulations concern mainly multiphase flows and, in particular, flows through solid fibrous media. For that, we begin by building the Immersed Image Method, which is the interpolation of the image's pixel/voxel values (a sort of topographic distance function) on the nodes of an initial mesh. The obtained field can approximately represent the original image, depending on the discretization and on the overall number of nodes. Optimization of the number of necessary nodes can be performed through anisotropic mesh adaptation using

Y.J. Zhang and J.M.R.S. Tavares (Eds.): CompIMAGE 2014, LNCS 8641, pp. 339–350, 2014.

an appropriate error estimator [4], so that the obtained field accurately represents the original image (but is also enoughly enriched to perform the necessary computation, as we will see later). To further progress towards segmentation, we choose to adapt the mesh not on the interpolated topographic distance function (the pixel/voxel value), but on its regularized Heaviside. To build this Heaviside, which is a smooth hyperbolic tangent varying on a certain thickness ϵ around a predetermined value of the topographic distance, we have implemented a reinitialization method. This procedure, coupled to mesh adaptation, allows segmentation but allows also to build up a mesh with a smooth representation of a phase function distribution, usable in the aimed type of application. Flow is then computed in an Eulerian framework, by solving the Navier-Stokes equations with heterogeneous material properties, whose discontinuity representation throughout the phases will be well represented only if the thickness ϵ is small enough, and if it contains enough elements to represent correctly the chosen Heaviside function. Numerical resolution of these equations is performed using a stabilized finite element method [5]. The proposed approach is applied on images obtained by 3D X-Ray tomography.

2   The Immersed Image Method

In this method, an image voxel (in 3D) or pixel (in 2D) value (grey-scale or RGB) is mapped in an initial mesh, building a function within it, that we name here as topographic distance. Classically, from this function, we recognize N phases by building $N-1$ phase functions and, in the literature, $N-1$ surface meshes are then extracted, most often using the Marching Cubes method [6]. We propose here an alternative, by skipping this step and building directly the mesh from the voxel data. Moreover, an unique mesh is automatically performed containing all the phases and allowing direct multiphase computation.

2.1   Interpolation of the Image Pixel/Voxel Values on the Mesh

Nowadays, images may be two (picture), three (scan) our four (movie) dimensional. In digital imaging, a pixel is the smallest controllable element of a picture represented in two-dimensions. A voxel is a volume element, representing a value on a regular grid in three dimensions. After reading the image (under different possible formats), the pixel/voxel values from the image $\tilde{u}$ are interpolated in the mesh, providing a distributed field, that we choose to designate as the topographic distance function u. In 2D, one may define the image, $\tilde{u}$, as:

$$\tilde{u} = \{\text{pixel}^k(\tilde{x}^k) \in \tilde{u}, k = 1, ..., L \times H\} \tag{1}$$

where $\tilde{x}^k$ are the vector coordinates of pixel^k, in the image space. Pixel values are between 0 and 255, extreme values representing, respectively, the black and white colors. For a sake of simplicity, we note $\tilde{u}^k$ the value of pixel k.

Let us now consider an initial 2D mesh with N nodes, where each node i has a coordinate x^i, for $i = 1, ..., N$, set of nodes of the mesh. The values of $\tilde{u}$ on each mesh node i are interpolated from the pixel values as follows:

$$u^i = u(x^i) = \frac{\tilde{u}^k}{255}, x^i = \frac{\tilde{x}^k}{255} \tag{2}$$

and k is the pixel for which $255 \cdot x^i$ belongs (or is projected). The same reasoning can be extended to 3D, for a $L \times H \times W$-sized image, and is what we call 'image immersion'. In fact, the solution $u \in \mathcal{V}_h$, which is a simple P^1 finite element approximation space, such that $u_h|_K \in P^1(K), K \in \mathcal{K}$ where $\Omega = \bigcup_{K \in \mathcal{K}} K$ is the computational domain, K is a simplex (segment, triangle, tetrahedron) and $\mathcal{K}$ is the set of elements of the mesh.

As an example, let us consider the 2D greyscale image given by Figure 1(a), which is a well known image used for compression algorithms [7]. The original image is a binary greyscale image (BMP, 512x512) containing 262144 pixels ($L \times H = 512 \times 512$), $\tilde{u}$. Firstly, we immerge this image in an isotropic mesh (given in Figure 1(b)), containing 140 nodes ($N = 140$), providing a rather coarse mesh size. Figure 1(c) presents the values of the computed topographic distance function u_h, obtained from the pixel with the same projected coordinate on the image space. We observe that, even if we recognize the global pattern, coarseness of the mesh results in a poor representation of the original image. Increasing the number of nodes overcomes this loss of definition, as expected (Figure 2).

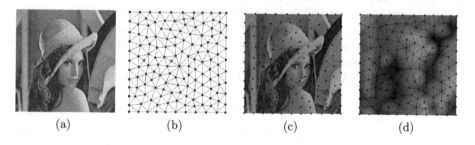

(a)   (b)   (c)   (d)

Fig. 1. Illustration of the interpolation of a 2D grey-scale image in a mesh with 140 nodes: (a) original image; (b) initial mesh; (c) image and node; (d) interpolated image on the mesh

2.2 Compressing Information by Building an Anisotropic Mesh

Mesh Adaptation Based on a Metrics Field. To be able to deal with large-size images (over 1 billion of voxels), mesh adaptation is performed in parallel. For that purpose, we have chosen not to parallelize the mesher, but to use it in a parallel context [8]. In that case, the global domain to which meshing is applied is partitioned and each partition is handled by a dedicated processor that will perform an anisotropic adaptation, based on a metrics field and constructed from

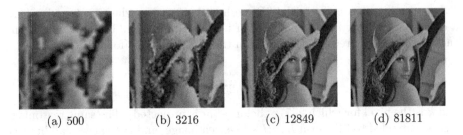

| (a) 500 | (b) 3216 | (c) 12849 | (d) 81811 |

Fig. 2. Application of the interpolation of the image in a mesh in 2D, for meshes with different number of nodes N

an edge based error estimator [4]. The mesh generator used has been developed in previous works [9]. It is based on the iterative improvement (adaptation) of an initial unsatisfactory mesh by performing local operations. In the adaptation process, two principles are enforced: the minimal volume, which assures the conformity of the mesh, with no element overlaps; the geometrical quality, which is evaluated for each element.

The anisotropic adaptation involves building a mesh conforme to a computed metric map. In fact, if we consider an element K of the mesh, its metrics M_K can be built using the affine transformation to a reference element which has to be equilateral of edge length equal to unity. Such a construction leads to a piecewise constant tensor field and thus discontinuous from element to element. However, a continuous metric field will be here constructed, which presents several advantages [4]. In this case, we will designate M^i as the metrics at node i. To compute the mesh metric map, let us recall that $x^i \in \mathcal{R}^d$, $i = 1, \cdots, N$ is the set of nodes of the mesh and the vector connecting nodes i and j, can be noted $x^{ij} = x^j - x^i$. The set of nodes connected to node i is $\Gamma(i) = \{j, \exists K \in \mathcal{K}, x^i, x^j$ are nodes of $K\}$. We introduce in [4] $X^i = \frac{d}{|\Gamma(i)|} \sum_{j \in \Gamma(i)} x^{ij} \otimes x^{ij}$ as the length distribution tensor at node x^i, and we use this tensor to construct the metrics by

$$M^i = (X^i)^{-1} \tag{3}$$

Edge Based Error Estimation and New Metrics Field. The basic idea of adaptive mesh is to balance the error, to be equal everywhere through the mesh. The basic idea of edge based techniques is to compute a length of edge such that the error is equally distributed over the edges, meaning it must be the same everywhere. Because this error is linked to the length of the edge, then the way to get this is to compute a new length for each edge, by applying a stretching factor s^{ij} to the edge, so that

$$x\text{new}^{ij} = s^{ij} x^{ij} \tag{4}$$

This stretch factor will be obtained from the *a posteriori* error analysis of the solution (in our case, u). Let us denote by u^i the nodal value of u at x^i. We note Π_h the Lagrange interpolation operator from $\mathcal{V}$ to $\mathcal{V}_h$ so that $\Pi_h u(x^i) = u(x^i) = u^i$, $\forall i = 1, \cdots, N$. Even if the gradient of u_h is a piecewise constant vector field, $\nabla u \in \mathcal{C}^1(\Omega)$, its projection along the edges is continuous

$$\nabla u_h \cdot x^{ij} = u^{ij} \tag{5}$$

being $u^{ij} = u^j - u^i$. Using the analysis carried out in [4], we can set that the norm of the difference between the projection of the gradient along the edges and the interpolated value of the gradient can be upper bounded by:

$$\|\nabla u_h \cdot x^{ij} - \nabla u(x^i) \cdot x^{ij}\| \leq \max_{y \in [x^i, x^j]} |H(u)(y) x^{ij} \cdot x^{ij}| \tag{6}$$

where $H(u) = \nabla^2 u$ is the associated Hessian of u. For that, the second derivative of u is necessary and its projected value can be established using equation 5 and the interpolation operator, to write

$$\left[\nabla(\Pi_h \nabla u) x^{ij}\right] \cdot x^{ij} = \nabla u(x^{ij}) \cdot x^{ij} \tag{7}$$

Using a mean value argument, one may establish that

$$|H(u)(y) x^{ij} \cdot x^{ij}| = \left| \left[\nabla u(x^j) - \nabla u(x^i)\right] \cdot x^{ij} \right| \tag{8}$$

and use this result to approximate the error along the edge, as

$$e^{ij} = \left[\nabla u(x^j) - \nabla u(x^i)\right] \cdot x^{ij} \tag{9}$$

Nevertheless, this value cannot be evaluated exactly as it requires knowing the gradient of u at the nodes of the mesh, and also its continuity. For that reason, a gradient recovery procedure [4] is used, by building the nodal gradient as

$$\nabla^i u(x^i) = (X^i)^{-1} \sum_{j \in \Gamma(i)} u^{ij} x^{ij} \tag{10}$$

where X^i is, as defined previously, the length distribution tensor at node x^i. The error of approximation is thus re-evaluated as

$$e^{ij} = \left[\nabla^j u(x^j) - \nabla^i u(x^i)\right] \cdot x^{ij} \tag{11}$$

One may then fix a target error to the edge, $\bar{e}^{ij}$, and compute the stretching factor to apply to the edge ij as

$$(s^{ij})^2 = \frac{\bar{e}^{ij}}{e^{ij}} \tag{12}$$

to simply define the new metric as

$$M_{\text{new}}{}^i = \frac{|\Gamma(i)|}{d}(\tilde{X}^i)^{-1} = \frac{1}{d} \sum_{j \in \Gamma(i)} (s^{ij})^2 x^{ij} \otimes x^{ij} \tag{13}$$

Controlling the Number of Nodes. In the overall adaptation procedure, one needs to control the generated number of nodes of the mesh to avoid reaching too fine meshes and be optimal in terms of computational cost, since when scaling a edge by a factor s^{ij}, the error changes quadratically. The procedure to obtain the total number of created nodes is detailed in[5] and only the main points are summarized here. In fact, assuming that an uniform totally balanced error is imposed along the edge $\bar{e}^{ij} = e = $ constant, a direct relation between the total number of nodes in the mesh, N, and e can be established:

$$e(N) = \left(\frac{N}{\sum_i n^i(1)} \right)^{-\frac{2}{d}} \tag{14}$$

being d the dimension and n^i the total number of created nodes per node i. Therefore, the stretching factors to be computed in order to obtain the new metric field, under the the constraint of a fixed number of nodes N are given by

$$s^{ij} = \left(\frac{e}{e(N)} \right)^{-\frac{1}{2}} \tag{15}$$

An example of application is illustrated in Figure 3, where a comparison of the evolution on the interpolated value of the image on the mesh is given for different anisotropic adapted meshes. One observes that the result qualitatively improves with the number of nodes. Furthermore, when comparing Figures 2(g) and 3(c), that have approximately the same number of nodes but that are adapted, respectively, isotropically and anisotropically, one notices that a better quality is obtained in the later.

3 Segmentation through Reinitialization Coupled to Adaptation

In the previous example, we have focused on a binary grey-scale image, the value of pixel or voxel is between 0 and 255, 0 being the black and 255 the white. Let us suppose now that we have an image in which we want to identify a region (to segment) that can be either in a grey-scale format (Figure 5(a)) or even already segmented using a thresholding value (Figure 5(b)). The main purpose behind this is that images that are being treated are slightly different from the ones that illustrated our purpose before, and will be mainly devoted to perform scientific computations on it. Furthermore, these computations require: a single mesh containing all the existing objects of the image; each object should be represented by an implicit function within the mesh. Even if the image immersion in the mesh has provided a function of this type, it does not directly provides an object (or *phase*) function, corresponding to the presence (or not) of the object in a given point in the mesh. For that, the first immediate idea is to perform a thresholding to the image $\tilde{u}$ to obtain $\tilde{u}_{seg}$: over a certain value, the new pixel value is $\tilde{u}_{seg}^k = 255$, under it $\tilde{u}_{seg}^k = 0$; and $\tilde{u}_{seg}$ is nothing else than an Heaviside

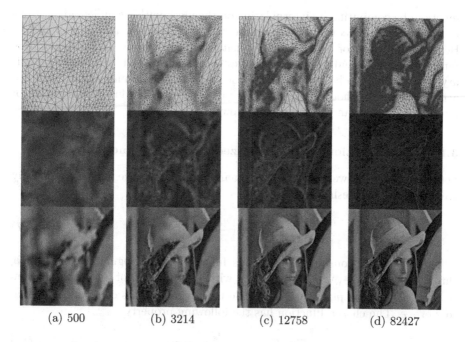

(a) 500   (b) 3214   (c) 12758   (d) 82427

Fig. 3. Obtained anistropic mesh, computed error and resulting interpolation of the image in the new mesh, for four different number of imposed nodes N

function of $\tilde{u}$. However, using our mesh adaptation algorithm on $\tilde{u}_{seg}$ results in a mesh with a poor quality, even not adapted at all, since $\tilde{u}_{seg}$ is not regular enough and the global mesh iteration procedure will oscillate due to the fact that the interpolated gradient may change sign throughout the different steps.

Hence, different authors have developed techniques like the active contour method to build, from a threshold segmented (or not) image, an implicit function representing the boundary of an object (or several functions for several objects) existing in an image. The most commonly used is the *level set* function, $\tilde{u}_d$, which is a signed distance function from pixel k to the boundary of the object Ω. Nevertheless, adapting the mesh on this function will not also provide the expected result. In fact, interpolation or direct resolution on the mesh to obtain $\tilde{u}_d$ (or its interpolated value u_d) implies that

$$||\nabla u_d||_2 = 1 \tag{16}$$

Thus, equidistribution of the error will necessarily provide a mesh that is anisotropically adapted, but with constant mesh sizes $h_{//}$ along each level set contour and $h_\perp$ in the normal direction. To overcome with this difficulty, we have decided to build, from $\tilde{u}$, not u_d, but directly its regularized Heaviside function, by computing its interpolation on the mesh with a coupled adaptation-reinitialization procedure. Hence: segmentation is performed since we build an Heaviside function of an object's implicit function defining its boundary; this function is regular and provides well adapted meshes around the object's boundary. For that, we solve an Hamilton-Jacobi equation, inspired from both the active contour method [10] and the reinitialization procedure in advection of interfaces in, for example, multiphase flows [11].

3.1   Reinitialization of a Regularized Heaviside Function

Let us suppose that we wish to obtain a narrow band distance function, smoothly truncated, in the mesh, u_ε, as

$$u_\varepsilon = \varepsilon \tanh(\frac{u_d(x, \partial\Omega)}{\varepsilon}) \tag{17}$$

There is a relationship between this function and a regularized Heaviside, through $H_\varepsilon = 1 + \frac{u_\varepsilon}{\varepsilon}$, where ε is related with the thickness of the regularization, so that $|u_\varepsilon| < \varepsilon$ for $|u_d| < \sqrt{2}\varepsilon$. Outside these values, u_ε is constant and equal to ε or $-\varepsilon$. The chosen function has the following property:

$$||\nabla u_\varepsilon||_2 = 1 - (\frac{u_\varepsilon}{\varepsilon})^2 = g(u_\varepsilon) \tag{18}$$

To reconstruct this function, one may solve a Hamilton-Jacobi type equation

$$\frac{\partial u_\varepsilon}{\partial \tau} + S(\tilde{u}) \left[||\nabla u_\varepsilon||_2 - g(u_\varepsilon)\right] = 0 \tag{19}$$

where $\Delta\tau$ is an increment step that can be computed from stability conditions for the resolution of this equation, and $S(\tilde{u})$ is the sign function. Equation 19 can be rewritten as a pure convection equation, like performed in [11]. Let us define the reinitialization velocity, v_r, as

$$v_r = S(\tilde{u})\frac{\nabla u_\varepsilon}{||\nabla u_\varepsilon||_2} \tag{20}$$

such that $||\nabla u_\varepsilon||_2 = v_r \cdot \nabla u_\varepsilon$. Then, equation 19 becomes

$$\frac{\partial u_\varepsilon}{\partial \tau} + v_r \cdot \nabla u_\varepsilon = S(\tilde{u})g(u_\varepsilon) \tag{21}$$

The choice of the increment step, $\Delta\tau$, is thus related with the Courant-Friedenriechs-Lewy (CFL) condition. Since $||v_r||_2 \leq 1$, then

$$\Delta\tau < \frac{h}{||v_r||_2} = h \tag{22}$$

being h the mesh size in the reinitialization direction, necessarily in the normal direction of u_ε, such that $h = h(u_\varepsilon)$. Equation 21 resolution is based, as assumed previously for u, that the solution is also $u_\varepsilon \in \mathcal{V}_h$, which is a simple P^1 finite element approximation space. An Euler implicit scheme is applied for time discretization, and an SUPG method to stabilize the convective term. In our case, $S(\tilde{u})$ can be directly obtained from the image: at each point of the mesh, x, the corresponding pixel value is seek and, from the defined thresholding value, one may see if whether the point is inside, on or outside the object to be segmented. In fact, obtaining the sign from the original image is the key point to perform an efficient and non-oscillating reinitialization. Furthermore, at each increment step, if the solution of equation 21 implies, on one node, that u_ε is not of the same sign of the image, a corrector is applied, to avoid oscillating the solution and a more difficult convergence. Figure 4 illustrates the construction of u_ε from an image, on which we wish to segment a particular zone, corresponding to a black circle.

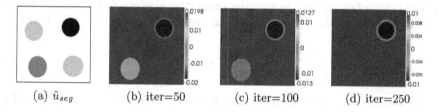

(a) $\tilde{u}_{seg}$ (b) iter=50   (c) iter=100   (d) iter=250

Fig. 4. Illustration of the reinitialization procedure: (a) original image, on which we wish to segment the black circle; (b) u_ε after 50 reinitialization iterations; (c) after 100 iterations; (d) after 250 iterations; the thickness is $\varepsilon = 0.01$

3.2 Application to Images and Adaptation Coupling

The iterative procedure to pass from the image to a representation of its regularized Heaviside in the adapted mesh includes, at each increment step $\Delta\tau$, the resolution of equation 21, followed by the generation of the new mesh with the metrics field given by equation 13, but where the variable on which we adapt (or on which the interpolation error is minimized) is u_ε.

Figure 5 shows the application of the described technique in an image of $200 \times 200 \times 220$ voxels, already segmented (Figure 5a), with a voxel size of $10\mu m$. One may compute the signed distance function by setting $\varepsilon = \infty$ (Figure 5b) or the regularized Heaviside function (Figure 5c). In this case, $\varepsilon = 0.01$, $\Delta\tau = 1e^{-5}$ and $N = 125000$ nodes, being the number of performed increments to convergence 40. The final adapted mesh is illustrated in Figure 5d.

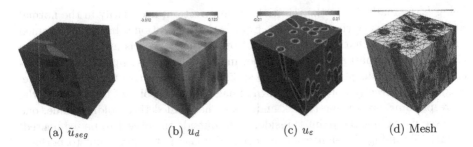

(a) $\tilde{u}_{seg}$ (b) u_d (c) u_ε (d) Mesh

Fig. 5. Original image, computed signed distance function, computed regularized Heaviside function, final adapted mesh

4   Flow Modelling on Images

Flow will be computed in an Eulerian framework, by solving the Navier-Stokes equations with heterogeneous material properties, corresponding to each phase. General form of these equations, for an incompressible Newtonian fluid, are:

$$\begin{cases} \rho\dfrac{dv}{dt} - \eta\Delta v + \nabla p = \rho g \ , \ x \in \Omega \times [0,T] \\ \nabla \cdot v = 0 \end{cases} \qquad (23)$$

The natural boundary conditions are $v = v_D$ on Ω_D and $n \cdot \sigma = F_N$ on Ω_N, being Ω_D and Ω_N complementary subsets of Ω, n is the unit normal vector and v_D and F_N are given functions. Also, the initial condition is $v(x,0) = v_0(x)$ assumed to be consistent with the boundary conditions. To compute velocity v and pressure p, these are approximated in finite dimensional spaces of continuous piecewise polynomials, such that $v_h|_K \in P^1(K)^d$ and $p_h|_K \in P^1(K)$, $\forall K \in \mathcal{K}$. Convergence of the mixed finite element problem will be ensured by enriching the velocity space with a space of bubbles (a finer scale), to satisfy the inf-sup condition, using a polynomial function of order one, with a value equal to unity at the center of the element and vanishing at its boundary. This mixed finite element is named MINI-element (P1+/P1). The problem is also non-linear because of the the non-linear nature of the convective term, which is linearised using a Newton algorithm and a stabilisation technique of the SUPG type is implemented to upwind the derivative and avoid oscillations.

The regularized Heaviside function, u_ε, will be useful when solving these equations in a multiphase context. Let us consider that our image represents a two-phase system (fluid and solid) and that η and ρ are scalar fields, defined by the material parameters (η_s and η_l, ρ_s and ρ_l) and sharing an interface defined in the mesh by an implicit function, such as u_d or u_ε. In fact, these properties are discontinuous from one phase to the other, but dealing with such discontinuity is not affordable by any standard numerical method. We propose to use a smooth transition, for instance using u_ε. Several types of mixture laws are possible, under the condition that $\lim_{\varepsilon \to \infty} \eta_\varepsilon \to \eta$. In the case of viscosity, we have (same reasoning may be applied to density):

$$\eta = \eta_\varepsilon = \frac{\eta_l}{2}(1 - \frac{u_\varepsilon}{\varepsilon}) + \frac{\eta_s}{2}(1 + \frac{u_\varepsilon}{\varepsilon}) \tag{24}$$

To assess the feasibility and capability of our overall procedure, a 3D test case is presented (Figure 6). An image ($900 \times 900 \times 220$ voxels) issuing from 3D X-Ray tomography [12] concerning a mat-reinforced sample is treated and a phase function equal to inside the fibres (solid) and - in the resin (fluid) phases is built. Finite element resolution of these equations is done using the above described mixed stabilized finite element method, with a generated mesh of 5 millions of nodes, from the image. In terms of computational time, mesh generation, with the overall adaptation procedure, was performed in 3 hours, whereas the Navier-Stokes resolution took only 10 min, on 96 CPUs. Results detailed in Figure 6, were obtained by imposing a pressure gradient through the sample on one direction, and imposing no-velocity in the fibers, showing that: the mesh is well adapted at the fluid-solid interface; the definition of this interface is very accurate, as illustrated by the isocontour 0 of u_ε; the computed velocity field enhances the acceleration in the interstitial spaces.

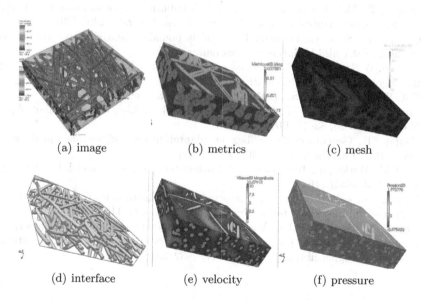

(a) image   (b) metrics   (c) mesh

(d) interface   (e) velocity   (f) pressure

Fig. 6. Original image with 178.2 millions of voxels, von Mises equivalent of the computed metrics field, final mesh of about 5 millions of nodes, isocontour 0 of the regularized Heaviside, final adapted mesh, computed velocity and pressure fields

5   Conclusions and Perspectives

We have proposed a new methodology to simultaneously segment an image and produce an adapted mesh adequate to perform numerical simulations of multiphase flows using the image data. It is based on the Immersed Image Method, which is the interpolation of the image's pixel/voxel values on the nodes of an initial mesh and optimization of the number of necessary nodes is performed through anisotropic mesh adaptation on a regularized Heaviside function. Flow is computed by solving the Navier-Stokes equations with heterogeneous material properties. Examples throughout this paper have shown the application of this technique on real images, in particular issuing from 3D X-Ray tomography. Immediate perspectives of this work concern application of the methodology to other 3D images (biomedical, for example), but also its extension to point cloud data (3D surface data), instead of voxel representations.

References

1. Shapiro, L., Stockman, G.: Computer Vision. Prentice Hall (2001)
2. Munford, D., Shah, J.: Optimal approximation by piece-smooth functions and associated variational problems. Comm. Pure App. Math. 42, 577–685 (1989)
3. Vese, L., Chan, T.: A multiphase level set framework for image segmentation using the Mumford and Shah model. Int. J. Comp. Vis. 50, 271–293 (2002)
4. Coupez, T.: Metric construction by length distribution tensor and edge based error for anisotropic adaptive meshing. J. Comp. Phys. 230, 2391–2405 (2011)
5. Coupez, T., Silva, L., Hachem, E.: Implicit boundary and adaptive anisotropic meshing. EMA SIMAI Springer Series (submitted)
6. Loresen, W.E., Cline, H.E.: Marching cubes: a high resolution 3D surface construction algorithm. Comp. Graph. 21, 163–169 (1987)
7. USC-SIPI Image Database (2010), http://sipi.usc.edu/database
8. Coupez, T., Digonnet, H., Ducloux, R.: Parallel meshing and remeshing. Appl. Math. Model. 25, 83–98 (2000)
9. Coupez, T.: Generation de maillage et adaptation de maillage par optimisation locale. Rev. Eur. Elem. Fin. 9, 403–423 (1999)
10. Kass, M., Witkin, A., Terzopoulos, D.: Snakes: active contours model. Int. J. Comp. Vision 1, 321–331 (1988)
11. Ville, L., Silva, L., Coupez, T.: Convected level set method for the numerical simulation of fluid buckling. Int. J. Num. Meth. Fl. 66, 324–344 (2010)
12. Orgeas, L., Dumont, P.J.J., Vassal, J.P., Guiraud, O., Michaud, V., Favier, D.: In-plane conduction of polymer composites plates reinforced with architectured networks of copper fibres. J. Mat. Sci. 47, 2932–2942 (2012)

UAVision: A Modular Time-Constrained Vision Library for Color-Coded Object Detection

António J.R. Neves, Alina Trifan, and Bernardo Cunha

IRIS Group, DETI / IEETA
University of Aveiro, 3810–193 Aveiro, Portugal
{an,alina.trifan}@ua.pt, mbc@det.ua.pt

Abstract. The ultimate goal of Computer Vision has been, for more than half of century, to create an artificial vision system that could imitate the human vision. The artificial vision system should have all the capabilities of the human vision system but must not carry the same flaws. Robotics and Automation are just two examples of research areas that use artificial vision systems as the main sensorial element. In these areas, the use of color-coded objects is very common since it relieves the burden of information processing while being an unobtrusive restraint of the environment. We present a novel computer vision library called UAVision that provides support for different video sensors technologies and all the necessary software for implementing an artificial vision system for the detection of color-coded objects. The experimental results that we present, both for the scenario of robotic soccer games and for traffic sign detection, show that our library can work at more than 50fps with images of 1 megapixel.

1 Introduction

Color segmentation has been one of the most popular approaches in time-constrained machine vision processing. This is due to the fact that segmenting a region based on colors is still easier and less heavy from the point of view of the computational resources involved than the detection of objects based on geometric features. In areas such as Robotics and Automation, the environment is often reduced to a set of objects of interest that are color-coded or color-labeled. The precise detection of these objects almost always stands at the basis of the correct functioning of the system. However, there is little work done in a structural manner in what concerns color-coded object detection.

In this paper we present a library for color-coded object detection, named UAVision. We call the design of the library as being modular as the library can be stripped down into several independent modules that will be presented in the following sections. Moreover, the architecture of our software is of the type "plug and play", meaning that it offers support for different vision sensors technologies. The software created using the library is easily exportable and can be shared between different types of vision sensors. Another important aspect of our library is that it takes into consideration time constraints. All the algorithms behind this

Y.J. Zhang and J.M.R.S. Tavares (Eds.): CompIMAGE 2014, LNCS 8641, pp. 351–362, 2014.
© Springer International Publishing Switzerland 2014

library have been implemented focusing on maintaining the processing time as low as possible. In Robotics, the notion of "realtime" is an extremely important issue and even though there is not a strict definition of realtime, almost always it refers to the amount of time elapsed between the acquisition of two consecutive frames. Realtime processing means processing the information captured by the vision sensors within the limits of the frame rate. The vision system for color-coded object detection that we have implemented using the UAVision library can work with frame rates up to 50fps and the processing time obtained will be presented in the Experimental Results Section.

The research area of robotic vision is greatly evolving by means of international competitions such as the RoboCup Federation [1]. The RoboCup initiative, through competitions like RoboCup Robot Soccer, RoboCup Rescue, RoboCup@Home and RoboCupJunior is designed to meet the need of handling real world complexities, while maintaining an affordable problem size and research cost. The games of robotic soccer have been used as the test environment for the modular vision library that is being presented. Within the RoboCup soccer competitions, autonomous mobile robots have to play soccer obeying to the FIFA rules. In the RoboCup soccer games, the objects of interest are color-coded, which makes these competitions suitable for employing the proposed library.

The library that we are proposing is an important contribution for the Computer Vision community since so far, there are no machine vision libraries that take into consideration time constraints. CMVision [2], a machine vision library developed at the Carnegie Mellon University was one of the first approaches of building such a library but it remained quite incomplete and has been discontinued in 2004. Several other machine vision libraries, such as Adaptive Vision [3], CCV [4] or RoboRealm [5] provide machine vision software to be used in industrial and robotic application but they are not free. UAVision aims at being an open-source, free library that can be used for robotic vision applications that have to deal with time constraints.

This paper is structured into four sections, first of them being this introduction. Section 2 describes the modules of the vision library. Section 3 presents two practical scenario in which the library has been used and the results that have been achieved. Section 4 concludes the paper and future lines of research are highlighted. Finally, in Section 4 the institutions supporting this work are acknowledged.

2   Library Description

The library that we propose contains software for image acquisition from video cameras supporting different technologies, for camera calibration and for blob formation, which stands at the basis of the object detection. The library can be divided into three main modules, that can be combined for implementing a time-constrained vision system or that can be used individually. These modules will be presented in the following subsections.

2.1 Image Acquisition

UAVision provides the necessary software for accessing and capturing images from three different camera interfaces: USB cameras, Firewire cameras and Ethernet cameras. For this purpose, the Factory Design Pattern [6] has been used and a factory called "Camera" has been implemented. The user can choose from these three different types of cameras in the moment of the instantiation. An important aspect to be mentioned is that UAVision uses some of the basic structures from the core functionality of OpenCV library [7]: the *Mat* structure as a container of the frames that are grabbed and the *Point* structure for the manipulation of points in 2D coordinates.

The module of Image Acquisition also provides methods from converting images between the most used color spaces: RGB to HSV, HSV to RGB, RGB to YUV and YUV to RGB.

2.2 Camera Calibration

The correct calibration is very important in every vision system of all the parameters related to the system. The module of camera calibration includes algorithms for calibration of the intrinsic and extrinsic camera parameters, the computation of the inverse distance map, the calibration of the colormetric camera parameters and in some vision systems, namely in catadioptric vision systems, the detection of the mirror, robot center and the definition of the regions of the image that have to be processed.

The result of the vision system calibration can be stored in a configuration file which contains four main blocks of information: camera settings, mask, map and color ranges.

The camera settings contain the basic information about the resolution of the image acquired, the Region of Interest regarding the CCD or CMOS of the camera and colormetric parameters among others.

The mask is a binary image containing the information about the pixels to be processed by the vision system. For example, in a catadioptric vision system it is not worthy to process the robot's body. Ignoring the pixels that belong to the body of the robot is significant for reducing both the noise in the image, as well as the processing time.

The map is a matrix containing the correspondence between a pixel position in the image and the corresponding position in the real world, considering a specific work plane, for example the ground. This can be used in a specific application as a Look Up Table to translate the position of the objects from pixels to real coordinates.

The color ranges contain the color regions for each color of interest (at most 8 different colors as we will explain later) in a specific color space (ex. RGB, YUV, HSV, etc.). In practice, it contains the lower and upper bounds of each one of the three color components for a specific color of interest.

The UAVision library contains algorithms for the self-calibration of most of the parameters described above, including some algorithms developed previously within our research group, namely the algorithm described in [8] for the automatic calibration of the colormetric parameters and the algorithms presented in [9] for calibration of the intrinsic and extrinsic parameters of catadioptric vision systems used to generate the map. For the calibration of the intrinsic and extrinsic parameters of a perspective camera, we have used and implemented the algorithm for the "chessboard" calibration, presented in [10].

2.3   Color-Coded Object Detection

The color-coded object detection is composed by four sub-modules that are presented next.

• Look-Up Table

For fast color classification, color classes are defined with the use of a look-up table (LUT). A LUT represents a data structure, in this case an array, used for replacing a runtime computation with a basic array indexing operation.

This approach has been chosen in order to save significant processing time. The images can be acquired in the RGB, YUV or Bayer format and they are converted to an index image (image of labels) using an appropriate LUT for each one of the three possibilities.

The table consists of 16,777,216 entries (2^{24}, 8 bits for R, 8 bits for G and 8 bits for B) with one byte each. The table size is the same for the other two possibilities (YUV or Bayer), but the meaning of each of the components changes. Each bit in the table entries expresses if one of the colors of interest (white, green, blue, yellow, orange, red, blue sky, gray - no color) is within the corresponding class or not. A given color can be assigned to multiple classes at the same time. For classifying a pixel, first the value of the color of the pixel is read and then used as an index into the table. The 8-bit value then read from the table is called the "color mask" of the pixel. It is possible to perform image subsampling in this stage in systems with limited processing capabilities in order to reduce even more the processing time. The color classification is only applied in the valid pixels if a mask exists.

• Scanlines

To extract color information from the image we have created three types of search lines, which we also call scanlines: radial, linear (horizontal or vertical) and circular. The radial search lines are constructed based on the Bresenham line algorithm [11]. They are constructed once, when the application starts, and saved in a structure in order to improve the access to these pixels in the color extraction module. This approach is extremely important for the reduction of processing time. In Fig. 1 the three different types of scanlines are illustrated.

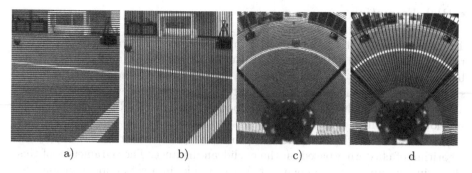

a)   b)   c)   d

Fig. 1. Examples of different types of scanlines: a) horizontal scanlines; b) vertical scanlines; c) circular scanlines; d)radial scanlines

• Run Length Encoding (RLE)

For each scanline, an algorithm of Run Length Encoding is applied in order to obtain information about the existence of a specific color of interest in that scanline. In more detail, we iterate through its pixels and we calculate the number of runs of a specific color and the position where they occur. Moreover, we extended this idea and it is optional to search, in a window before and after the occurrence of the desired color, for the occurrence of other colors. This allows the user to determine both color transitions and color occurrences using this approach.

When searching for run lengths, the user can specify the color of interest, the color before, the color after, the search window for these last two colors and three thresholds that can be used to filter what can be the valid information.

As a result of this module, we obtain a list of positions in each scanline, and if needed for all the scanlines, where a specific color occurs and also the amount of pixels in each occurrence (Fig. 2).

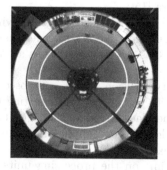
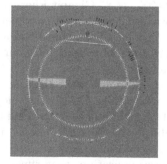

Fig. 2. On the left, an image captured using the Camera Acquisition module of the UAVision library. On the right, the run length information annotated.

- **Blob Formation**

To detect objects with a specific color in a scene, we have to be able to detect regions in the image with that color, usually named blobs, and validate those blobs according to some characteristics, namely area, bounding box, solidity, skeleton, among others. In order to construct these regions, we use information about the position where a specific color occurs based on the Run Length module previously described (Fig. 2).

We iterate through all the run lengths of a specific color and we apply an algorithm of clustering based on the euclidean distance. The parameters of this clustering are application dependent. For example, in a catadioptric vision system, the distance in pixels to form blobs changes radially regarding the center of the image.

While the blob is being built, its descriptor is being updated. The description of the blobs currently calculated are, to name a few, center, area, width/height relation, solidity, etc.

3   Experimental Results

We have chosen as a first testbed of the UAVision library the game of robotic soccer, promoted by the RoboCup initiative. We have used the Middle-Size League [12] team of robots CAMBADA [13] from the University of Aveiro (Fig. 3(a)). These robots are completely autonomous, able to perform holonomic motion and are equipped, in terms of hardware, with a catadioptric vision system that allows them to have omnidirectional vision [14]. In order to play, a robot has to detect, in useful time, the ball, the limits of the field and the field lines, the goal posts and the other robots that are on the field. These robots can move with a speed of up to 4m/s and the ball can be kicked with a velocity of up to 10m/s, which leads to the need of having fast object detection algorithms. In the RoboCup MSL soccer games, the objects of interest are color coded making thus the soccer games a suitable application for the use of the UAVision library. The camera used by the CAMBADA robots is an *IDS UI-5240CP-C-HQ-50i Color CMOS 1/1.8"* Gigabit Ehernet camera [15].

We provide along with this paper three video sequences exemplifying the scenarios that have been tested and a configuration file [17], in order that other researchers are able to reproduce our results, as well as, to serve as a reference for future work.

Using the modules of the UAVision library, a vision system composed of two different applications has been developed with the purpose of detecting the orange ball, the white lines of the field and the black robots or obstacles that are present during the soccer games on the field. The two applications are of the type client-server and they are described next.

The core application, that runs in realtime on the processing units of the robots, was implemented as a server that accepts the connection of a calibration tool client. This client is used for configuring the vision system (color ranges,

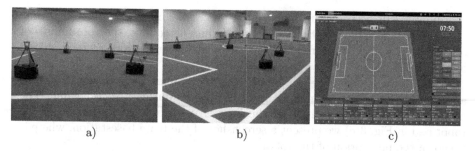

Fig. 3. On the left and center images, an example of a robot setup during a soccer game. On the right, the world as the robot understands it displayed on the team basestation.

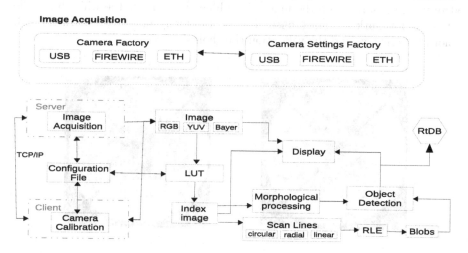

Fig. 4. Software architecture of the vision system developed based on the UAVision library

camera parameters, etc.) and for debug purposes. The main task of the server application is to perform realtime color-coded object detection. The pipeline of the object detection procedure, presented in Fig. 4, is the following: after having an image acquired, using a LUT previously built, the original image is transformed into an image of labels. This image of color labels, also denominated in our software by index image, will be the basis of all the processing that follows. The index image is scanned using one of the three types of scanlines previously described (circular, radial or linear) and the information about transitions between the colors of interest is run length encoded. Transitions between green and other colors of interest (white, ball color, black) are searched in order to garantee that the objects detected are inside the field area. Blobs are formed by merging adjacent RLEs of the ball color. The blob is then labeled as ball if the blob area/distance from the robot respects a certain function that has been experimentally determined. Moreover, the width/height relation and solidity are also used for ball validation. If a given blob passes the validation criteria, its center coordinates will be passed to higher-level processes and shared on a Real-time Database(RtDB) [18]. For the obstacles and line detections, the coordinates of the detected points of interest are passed to higher-level processes and shared on the RtDB.

In Fig. 3 we present an example of the soccer games environment. Fig. 3(a) and Fig. 3(b) show a common setup of the robots during a soccer game. The information about the position of the lines is used for the localization of the robot and in Fig. 3(c) we present a screenshot of the team basestation, where it is shown the perception of the robot.

Figure 5(a) shows an image captured by the omnidirectional vision system of the CAMBADA robots and in Fig. 5(b) we have the results of the color detection algorithms, annotated on the image. The blue circles mark the white lines, the white circles mark the black obstacles and the mangenta circles mark the ball color blobs that passed the validation thresholds.

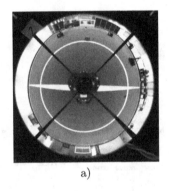 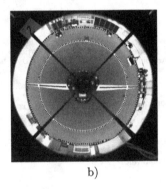

a)   b)

Fig. 5. On the left, an image acquired by the omnidirectional vision system. On the right, the result of the color-coded object detection. The blue circles mark the white lines, the white circles mark the black obstacles and the mangenta circles mark the orange blobs that passed the validation thresholds.

The intermediate steps of the vision pipeline are presented in Fig. 6. In Fig. 6(a) we present the index image, in which all the colors of interest have been assigned a label. Fig. 6(b) presents the color classified image and in Fig. 6(c) we present the "reality" of the robot.

To prove the use of the proposed library in other applications, we installed a digital camera as perspective vision system in a regular vehicle and we made some experiments. Similar results to the ones obtained in soccer robots are presented in Fig. 7. In this case we detect the position of the traffic signs and lines on the road. This could be seen as pre-processing step of a vision system for an autonomous vehicle. The camera used was a Firewire *Point Grey Flea 2, 1 FL2-08S2C with a 1/3" CCD Sony ICX204* [16]. We present results achieved by using the UAVision library for two different cameras, but the architecture of the vision system is the same and it is presented in Fig. 4.

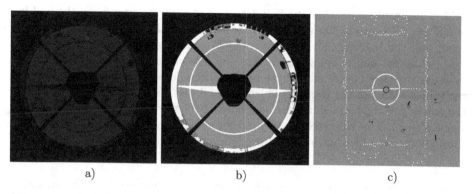

Fig. 6. On the left, the index image in which all of the colors of interest are labeled. In the middle, the color classified image (a colored version of a)) and on the right, the surrounding world from the perspective of the robot.

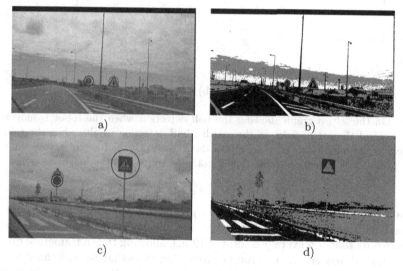

a)   b)

c)   d)

Fig. 7. Results obtained using a perspective camera on a vehicle. (a) and (b) where obtained on a highway and (c) and (d) on a national road. In (a) and (c) - the acquired image where the position of traffic signs and lines on the road are marked; (b) and (d) - color classified image.

Several game scenarios have been tested using the autonomous mobile robots CAMBADA. In Fig. 8(a) we present a graphic with the result of the ball detection when the ball is stopped in a given position, in this case, the central point of the field and the robot is moving. The graphic shows a consistent ball detection while the robot is moving in a tour around the field. The field lines are also properly detected, as it is proved by the correct localization of the robot in all the experiments. The second scenario that has been tested is illustrated in Fig. 8(b). The robot is stopped on the middle line and the ball is sent across the field. This graph shows that the ball detection is accurate even when the ball is found at a distance of 9m away from the robot. Finally, in Fig. 8(c) both the robot and the ball are moving. The robot is making a tour around the soccer field, while the ball is being sent across the field. In all these experiments, no false positives were detected and the ball has been detected in more than 90% of the frames. Most of the times in which the ball was not detected, it was due to the position of the ball behind the bars holding the mirrorof the omnidirectional vision system. The video sequences used for generating these results, as well as the configuration file that has been used are available at [17].

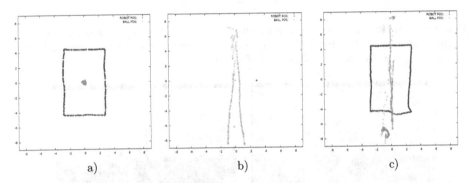

a)   b)   c)

Fig. 8. On the left, a graph showing the ball detection when the robot is moving in a tour around the soccer field. In the middle, ball detection results when the robot is stopped on the middle line on the right of the ball and the ball is sent across the field. On the right, ball detection results when both the robot and the ball are moving.

The processing time shown in Table. 1 proves that the vision system built using the UAVision library is extremely fast, the full execution of the vision pipeline software only takes on average a total of 12 ms, allowing thus a framerate greater than 80fps. Moreover, the maximum processing time that we measured was 13 ms, which is a very important detail since it shows that the processing time is almost independent of the scene complexity. The time results have been obtained in a computer with a Intel Core i5-3340M CPU @ 2.70GHz 4 processor. In the implementation of this vision system we didn't use multi-threading, however both image classification and the next steps can be parallelized if needed.

The cameras that we have used can provide 50fps at full resolution when acquiring images in the Bayer format. As described before, the LUT in the vision library can work with the Bayer format and the experimental results show that the detection performance is not affected.

There are two initialization processes that are part of the vision pipeline and that take place only once during the execution of the vision system. The execution times of these processes are presented in Table 2.

The LUT is created once, when the vision process runs for the first time and it is saved in the cache file. If the information from the configuration file has not

Table 1. Average processing times measured using the video sequences that we provide along with this paper

Operation	Time (ms)
Image acquisition	1
Run length coding of scanlines	4
Blob creation	2
Bob validation and RtDB filling	3
Total	**10**

Table 2. Processing times for the initialization of the LUT and scanlines

Operation	Time (ms)
LUT creation	5864
LUT loading from a cache file	25
Scanlines initialization	28

been altered, during the following runs of the vision software, the LUT will be loaded from the cache file, reducing thus the processing time of this operation by approximately 25 times. Only when the information in the configuration file changes, the LUT has to be recreated.

For the video sequences that we provide, the following number of scanlines have been built during the performance of the vision software:

- 720 radial scanlines for the ball detection.
- 98 circular scanlines for the ball detection.
- 170 radial scanlines for the lines and obstacle detection.
- 66 circular scanlines for the lines detection.

4 Conclusions and Future Work

In this paper we have presented a novel computer vision library that supports the development of artificial vision systems for the detection of color coded objects. The proposed library, UAVision, encompasses algorithms for camera calibration, image acquisition and color coded object detection. These algorithms take into consideration time constraints, making the library suitable for applications that have to run in a specific, limited, interval of time. As future work, we aim at providing software support for image acquisition from more types of cameras and complement the library with algorithms for generic object detection.

Acknowledgements. This work was developed in the Institute of Electronic and Telematic Engineering of University of Aveiro and was partially supported by FEDER through the Operational Program Competitiveness Factors - COMPETE and by National Funds through FCT - Foundation for Science and Technology in a context of a PhD Grant (FCT reference SFRH/BD/85855/2012) and the project FCOMP-01-0124-FEDER-022682 (FCT reference PEst-C/EEI/UI0127/2011).

References

1. http://www.robocup.org (last visited March, 2014)
2. http://www.cs.cmu.edu/~jbruce/cmvision/ (last visited March, 2014)
3. https://www.adaptive-vision.com/en/home/ (last visited March, 2014)
4. http://libccv.org/ (last visited March, 2014)
5. http://www.roborealm.com/index.php (last visited March, 2014)
6. Gamma, E., Helm, R., Johnson, R., Vlissides, J.: Design Patterns: Elements of Reusable Object-oriented Software. Addison-Wesley Longman Publishing Co., Inc., Boston (1995)
7. http://docs.opencv.org (last visited March, 2014)
8. Alina Trifan, A.J.R.: Neves and Bernardo Cunha. Self-calibration of colormetric parameters in vision systems for autonomous soccer robots. In: Proc. of RoboCup 2014 Symposium (2014)
9. Neves, A.J.R., Pinho, A.J., Martins, D.A., Cunha, B.: An efficient omnidirectional vision system for soccer robots: from calibration to object detection. Mechatronics 21(2), 399–410 (2011)
10. Zhang, Z.: Flexible camera calibration by viewing a plane from unknown orientations. In: ICCV, pp. 666–673 (1999)
11. Jack, E.: Bresenham. Algorithm for computer control of a digital plotter. IBM Systems Journal 4(1), 25–30 (1965)
12. http://wiki.robocup.org/wiki/Middle_Size_League (last visited March, 2014)
13. http://robotica.ua.pt/CAMBADA (last visited March 2014)
14. Neves, A.J.R., Corrente, G., Pinho, A.J.: An omnidirectional vision system for soccer robots. In: Neves, J., Santos, M.F., Machado, J.M. (eds.) EPIA 2007. LNCS (LNAI), vol. 4874, pp. 499–507. Springer, Heidelberg (2007)
15. https://en.ids-imaging.com (last visited March, 2014)
16. http://www.ptgrey.com/products/flea2/flea2_firewire_camera.asp (last visited March, 2014)
17. http://sweet.ua.pt/an/uavision/ (last visited March, 2014)
18. Neves, A., et al.: CAMBADA soccer team: from robot architecture to multiagent coordination. In: Papic, V. (ed.) Robot Soccer, ch. 2. I-Tech Education and Publishing, Vienna (2010)

Time-of-Flight Camera Based Virtual Reality Interaction for Balance Rehabilitation Purposes

Danilo Avola[1], Luigi Cinque[2], Stefano Levialdi[2], Andrea Petracca[1],
Giuseppe Placidi[1], and Matteo Spezialetti[1]

[1] Department of Life, Health and Environmental Sciences, University of L'Aquila
Via Vetoio Coppito 2, 67100, L'Aquila, Italy
{danilo.avola,andrea.petracca,giuseppe.placidi,
matteo.spezzialetti}@univaq.it
[2] Department of Computer Science, Sapienza University
Via Salaria 113, 00198, Rome, Italy
{cinque,levialdi}@di.uniroma1.it

Abstract. The 3D Human Body Models (3D HBMs) and the 3D Virtual Reality Environments (3D VREs) enable users to interact with simulated scenarios in an engaging and natural way. The Computer Vision (CV) based Motion Capture (MoCap) systems allow us to obtain user models (i.e., self-avatars) without using cumbersome and uncomfortable physical tools (e.g., sensor suites) which could adversely affect user experience. This last point is of great importance in developing interactive applications for balance rehabilitation purposes where the recovery of lost skills is related to different factors (e.g., patient motivation) including spontaneity of the interaction during the virtual rehabilitative exercises. This paper presents an overview of the Customized Rehabilitation Framework (CRF), a single range imaging sensor based system oriented to patients who experienced with brain strokes, head traumas or neurodegenerative disorders. In particular, the paper is focused on the implementation of two new ad-hoc virtual exercises (i.e., Surfboard and Swing) supporting patients in recovering physical and functional balance. Observations on accuracy of user body models and their real-time interaction ability within rehabilitative simulated environments are presented. In addition, basic experiments concerning usefulness of the proposed exercises to support balance rehabilitation purposes are also reported.

Keywords: 3D human body models, 3D virtual reality environments, motion capture, Time-of-Flight camera, self-avatars.

1 Introduction

The modeling and the movement analysis of the human body have numerous applications in different research fields including rehabilitation. The early CV based MoCap systems equipped with one or more synchronized RGB cameras [1] promoted the modeling and the motion capture of the body by means of visual expedients (e.g., visual markers, coloured bodysuits) which encouraged to leave

Y.J. Zhang and J.M.R.S. Tavares (Eds.): CompIMAGE 2014, LNCS 8641, pp. 363–374, 2014.

physical tools (e.g., haptic devices, sensor suites), but caused a substantial increasing of algorithmic complexity and related computational overhead due to the difficulty of extracting coherent foreground information from single or multi-view RGB images. The depth maps provided by the current range imaging sensors [2] (e.g., Time of Flight (ToF) cameras, Structured Light (SL) scanners) have allowed us to redesign crucial operations of the RGB image based motion capture processes (e.g., segmentation, tracking, background subtraction) obtaining a new generation of reliable and fast CV based MoCap markerless systems able to accurately model and track the human body [3]. The naturalness and the free body interaction are key issues of many application contexts, in rehabilitation area they can have even greater importance allowing the recovering of lost skills without using physical measurement interfaces of performance which could adversely affect re-education and progress results of the patients [4, 5]. In particular, recent studies have shown that in balance rehabilitation tasks the free body interaction to model and control self-avatars in real-time, while acting within immersive VREs, provides patients opportunities to engage rehabilitative exercises in enjoyable and purposeful way [6, 7]. These last points positively influence personal motivation, frequency, and duration of the exercises producing a further improving of the effectiveness of the rehabilitation.

The movement analysis as well as the rehabilitation experience can be advantageously supported by using self-avatars fitted as much as possible with the main physical features of the patients (e.g., shape, height, volume). This allows us both to obtain more realistic measurements of the patient movements and to support a more genuine interactive experience [8–10]. In this context takes on importance the algorithmic design of the HBM whose data structure has to facilitate diversified types of movement analysis of the whole body (or parts of it), maintaining a light format to computationally support synchronization and real-time interaction aspects. A single range imaging sensor arranged to capture poses of a user body provides a set of depth images (depending on the fixed frames per second (fps)) in which each foreground can be seen as a partial surface of a whole shaped volume (i.e., the body) according to the camera viewpoint. The adopted body modeling approach uses a fixed set of homogeneous and overlapping geometrical spheres which suitably sized and arranged are used to fill (on each frame) the assessed user body volume [11]. The spheres have some attractive properties that make them particularly suitable to represent a human body [12]. First of all, they appear the same shape from any viewing position, besides their geometrical attributes (e.g., boundaries, spatial coordinates, radius) are easy to compute and handle. Finally, the curved surface of the spheres tends to naturally approximate the different parts of the human body maintaining all its physical features, in addition the regular form of the spheres sustains a harmonized visual rendering and provides a realistic synthesis of the human body. For all these reasons, the obtained self-avatars can be considered a suitable compromise, between manageability and accuracy, able to support a truthful feedback to the patients and, at the same time, to assist interactive computational aspects. A final consideration on the use of 3D HBMs and 3D

VREs in rehabilitation field is that rehabilitative virtual exercises can be easily and inexpensively customized according to patient requirements. Moreover, these techniques allow us to have historical visualization and monitoring of the patient progresses which can be evaluated over time from different therapists. In addition, the digital information related to patient model and movement analysis can facilitate (where possible) a fully supervised system to remotely monitor the maintenance of the rehabilitation that patients do at home.

This paper introduces an architectural upgrade of the CRF, a our previously presented single ToF camera based system for fast prototyping and implementing of general exercises for rehabilitation purposes [13]. The system was designed to define a versatile architecture for hosting our previous experiences in markerless movement analysis of the full body, including hands, for rehabilitation purposes [14, 15] and [16]. The upgrade has regarded the introduction of two modules to equip the system with a plug-in based feature. The first module, Self-Avatar Generator (SAG), allows us to introduce into the framework new algorithms to process the depth maps and return different kinds of self-avatar. The aim of the module is to enable system in having available a family of methods to model the human body in different shapes. In this way, the framework has been equipped with a mechanism by which to generate different self-avatars of the same patient to satisfy different requirements, such as: accuracy of the model, types of movement analysis, interactive features. In this context, we do not have completely designed a new modeling algorithm, but we have integrated and customized a robust Natural User Interface (NUI) (iisu^{TM} Middleware, [17]) and a well-known high performance real-time 3D engine (IrrLicht, [18]) to reconstruct a sphere based self-avatar compliant with the mentioned requirements. The second module, Rehabilitative Exercise Generator (REG), supports an eXtensible Markup Language (XML) parsing approach to permit us the insertion into the framework of new rehabilitative exercises. This module has been designed to allow us a fast implementation of VREs (i.e., exercises) where self-avatars of patients are loaded. The focus of the paper is the description of the Surfboard and Swing exercises (i.e., the two new plug-ins) which were studied to support the equilibrium recovery of patients suffering of postural instability. The proposed approach has been designed with the intent to be an alternative cheaper and practical system with respect to more advanced and expensive ones, such as: Vicon [19], PTI 3D MoCap System [20], and RV Grabber [21].

The rest of the paper is organized as follows. Sections 2 discusses some main works representing the state-of-the-art of the rehabilitation systems based on HBMs and VREs. Section 3 presents an overview of the current version of the CRF architecture, including SAG and REG modules. Afterwards, it describes the two introduced plug-ins, that is the balance rehabilitation exercises: Surfboard and Swing. Section 4 presents observations regarding the user body models including notes on the real-time interaction and synchronization matters. In addition, extensive experiments regarding both evaluation of the system and patient convenience in using exercises are also reported. Finally, Section 5 concludes the paper and introduces future research directions.

2   Related Work

This section discusses works focused on the recovery of skills using self-avatars interacting with virtualized serious exercises. We have considered only those works that more than other are compliant with our intents and architecture.

2.1   MOCAPs and VREs in Rehabilitation Systems

The work in [22] presents a MoCap and analysis system based on a single Microsoft Kinect[TM] [23] in combination with the Microsoft SDK [24] to assess anatomical landmark position and angular displacement data during clinical tests of postural control. The authors conclude that such a system can be used to support a wide variety of fields with important postural control strategy information that are not currently obtainable in the clinical setting. On the same device is based the system shown in [25], where the authors propose a tool for static body posture analysis and dynamic range of movement estimation of the skeleton joints based on 3D anthropometric information from multi-modal data. The system takes a set of key-points to align RGB and depth data, reconstruct the depth surface, match the key-points, and compute accurate measurements about posture and spinal curvature. Although the joined use of the RGB and depth information is encouraged to improve the modeling of the foreground [26, 27], our aims allow us to adopt only the depth maps obtaining remarkable results. The authors in [28] describe a non-invasive technique and validation results for posture classification which can be suitably used in several in-home scenarios. Their single ToF based framework uses two complementary descriptors which work on the volumetric and topological representations of the human body, respectively. A different work is introduced in [29], where a system which enables chronic pain patients to train their motor skills in a serious game is implemented. This work integrates within the framework two different CV based MoCap systems: iotracker device [30] (a passive marker based infrared motion tracking), and the Microsoft Kinect[TM]. The authors conducted technical evaluations of both MoCap systems deduced that an iotracker setup would be too expensive for home use and also too difficult to handle by therapists and/or patients. They observed that Microsoft Kinect[TM] worked very well as an alternative MoCap system. These last points on this as in other original works (e.g., [31–33]) have confirmed the high accuracy achieved by the current range imaging sensor based MoCap systems. The work presented in [34] describes the main role of the VREs within the rehabilitation field. It highlights as the virtual reality supports applications in neuroscience research including rehabilitation and study of the brain activity. On the same direction is the work illustrated in [35], where the authors develop a virtual reality proprioceptive rehabilitation system that can manipulate the visual feedback during upper-limb training and ask the patient to rely only on proprioception feedback. A final work is introduced in [36], where a fast 3D modeling algorithm is proposed. Their system allows them to accurately model each object within any environment. This technology can provide new scenarios in rehabilitation fields as well as other application contexts.

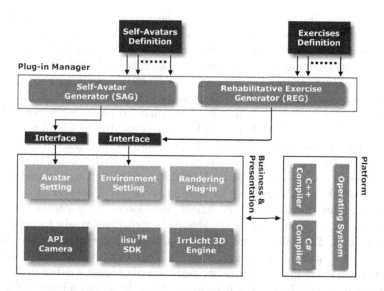

Fig. 1. The plug-in based Customized Rehabilitation Framework (CRF) architecture. It is composed of three tiers: Platform, Business & Presentation, and Plug-in Manager

3   The Framework Architecture and Plug-Ins

This section starts introducing the plug-in based architectural upgrade of the previously presented CRF (for details see: [13]). In particular, an overview of the first release of the CRF and the integration of the new SAG and REG modules is presented. The section continues showing some details about the implementation of the self-avatar by the iisu^{TM} Middleware and the 3D IrrLicht engine, and ends proposing the two new developed plug-ins: Surfboard and Swing.

3.1   The Plug-in Based CRF Architecture

As shown in Fig. 1, the current framework architecture is composed of three tiers. The first two (*Platform*, and *Business & Presentation*) are inherited from the previous release of the framework, while the third (*Plug-in Manager*) represents the new tier by which to import new self-avatars and rehabilitative exercises.

The Platform represents the lower tier of the framework which requires the C++ and C# compilers to support both the framework functionalities and the iisu^{TM} Middleware as well as IrrLicht features.

The Business & Presentation is composed of three components: *API Camera*, *Library Module* (iisu^{TM} SDK, and IrrLicht 3D Engine), and *Development Module* (Avatar Setting, Environment Setting, and Rendering Plug-in). The *API*

Camera interfaces the framework with the range imaging sensor using the related API management package provided with the device. Although our framework has been designed to deal with different kinds of camera, currently we are using the OptriCam™ 311 [37], an USB ToF camera. The *Library Module* is composed of two reliable products adapted to our needs: iisu™ SDK, and IrrLicht 3D Engine. The first has been chosen as a complementary component of the ToF camera, the latter has been selected as a suitable element to easily represent 3D virtual scenarios. The iisu™ SDK is a middleware compatible with all major ToF cameras currently available, moreover it supports different gesture recognition functions. The ToF camera produces depth maps and RGB images of the scene including: people, walls and objects. Raw data are passed to the middleware which analyses them and performs background removal. Moreover, it calculates information about the subject (e.g., height, location of body parts), thus providing them to our framework in suitable data structures ready to be used in building avatars. To achieve such an integration level, we included the iisu™ data model ([17]) within our data structures. The Irrlicht 3D Engine is an open source cross-platform high performance real-time 3D engine written in C++. A careful evaluation has shown that it includes all the basic and advanced features we need to reach our fixed aims. In particular, it uses D3D [38] and OpenGL [39], the two reference graphical libraries to perform 2D and 3D real-time rendering. Finally, it integrates a fast XML parser [40] to achieve three important technical purposes: loading of features of avatars and environments by manageable property files; dumping and storing of information of exercises within versatile report files; exchange of information by suitable transfer files. The *Development Module* extends the library module (inheriting all data structures and functions of the lower layers) to integrate the current VRE with the HBM. This module is composed of three sub-environments: Avatar Setting, Environment Setting, and Rendering Plug-in. The first is implemented to collect the RGB and 3D spatial information of the user interaction. The second is designed to create and manage both the avatar and the virtual environments. The last is developed to join and render the avatar and virtual environment:

- *Avatar Setting*: it deals with two tasks, Camera Dynamic Calibration (CDC), and Avatar Feature Setting (AFS). The first is accomplished by a GUI through which the basic camera calibration parameters (e.g., centre of the scene, brightness, contrast) are defined. The second is carried out by another GUI through which the avatar parameters are specified;
- *Environment Setting*: it deals with three tasks, Virtual Space Definition (VSD), Environment Feature Setting (EFS), and Rules Setting (RS). The first defines the geometrical space (e.g., cube) in which the whole virtual environments and avatars are considered. The second supports the design of each scenic element belonging to the virtual environment. The third defines the interaction rules between elements and avatars;
- *Rendering Plug-in*: it finalizes the acquisition of both self-avatar data and virtual environment, moreover it supports the running process synchronizing, rendering and animating the whole scenario.

The Plug-in Manager is composed of two components: *Self-Avatar Generator (SAG)*, and *Rehabilitation Exercise Generator (REG)*:

- *SAG*: this component has been designed to support the implementation of different kinds of self-avatars. As just mentioned, in this context we do not have developed a new modeling algorithm, but we have adopted the native features of the iisu™ SDK and IrrLicht 3D Engine to build a suitable human model. Our main contribution on this task has been (over the technical and methodological efforts to align the previous architecture with the new plug-in mechanism) to define an XML communication protocol to transmit (on-the-fly) sphere features (e.g., number, radius, colour) to the framework. Moreover, we are just working in implementing different self-avatar plug-ins conceived to support different kinds of exercises and ability games;
- *REG*: this component has been designed to parse a well structured XML file to derive all the useful information to implement a specific exercise. The REG knows that the framework will start from a pre-defined environment (e.g., a homogeneous coloured background: black or white). Each extracted element from the XML file will enrich this environment. A simple classification of the available elements is the following: scenic elements (e.g., walls, doors, windows) and those that the patient manages, touches or grasps (e.g., tools, objects, equipments); interaction rules, that is the role of each SE and the rules describing how the patient can interact with the scenic elements, typically forces and constraints (e.g., gravity, motion rules, movement limits); GUI elements, that is the addition of functions (e.g., buttons) or control elements (e.g., check box) on the basic GUI to manage the exercise.

3.2 The Self-Avatar Implementation

Once that the configuration file has been produced by the SAG, a sphere based self-avater can be obtained. In fact, the middleware is able to detect (on each frame and in real-time) a set of centroids, related the user foreground, by which to synthesize each part of the human body. These centroids are in turn supplied to the 3D engine which uses them (according to the configuration file specifications) to draw a centred spheres.

3.3 The Surfboard and Swing Plug-ins

This sub-section presents the Surfboard and Swing plug-ins. These two exercises have been developed to support patients having postural instability due to residual cognitive impairments. Our previous experiences in evaluating the cortical activation during balance tasks ensure the effectiveness of the proposed exercises [41, 42]:

The Surfboard exercise, shown in Fig. 2, is a balance recovering task where the patient, interacting with its avatar, has to maintain the equilibrium over a virtual surfboard placed over a pivot around which the board can rotate. The target

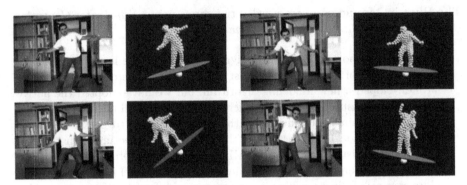

Fig. 2. Screenshots of the Surfboard exercise

of the exercise is to maintain as much as possible the Surfboard in horizontal equilibrium according to a fixed angle of tolerance. The weight of the patient above the board is simulated by considering the distribution and position of the spheres composing the avatar, with respect to the vertical axis passing through the patient centre of mass. In this context, we can assume that the spheres have the same weight, this fact does not influence the rehabilitative aim. The patient controls his balance over the surfboard by bringing his centre of gravity on the right or on the left. As the subject oscillates with respect to his centre of gravity, his 3D representation is distributed on his feet proportionally. The patient, while watching his avatar on the screen, has to keep his body balanced enough to avoid that the tilt angle of the surfboard exceeds a threshold. The board colour changes when the equilibrium is lost (i.e., the board inclination is above a given angle). The first two couples of screenshots (up-left and up-right) show an acceptable inclination of the board, the third couple (down-left) highlights a wrong inclination, while the last couple (down-right) shows again a balanced situation. We also have introduced two parameters. The first allows to manage friction between the pivot and the surfboard to change the reaction of the patient accordingly. The second consists on a random perturbation of the surfboard inclination to force the patient to restore the equilibrium state. The exercise ends when expires a fixed time interval.

The Swing exercise, shown in Fig. 3, has been designed by considering that the patient has to maintain the equilibrium standing on a virtual long arms Swing. The board of the Swing is subjected to external impulsive perturbations, occurring randomly in time, intensity and direction (back or forth). The patient is forced to recover the equilibrium by tilting back and forth his body, taking the arms along his body and remaining fixed on the feet. The exercise has been implemented in the following way. An invisible node, a pivot, is placed at an height of 2.5 meters from the floor. At each frame, the centre of gravity, Cg, of the user model and the centre of gravity of the part of the user model above Cg, Cu, are calculated. A sphere is visualized on the floor of the scene corresponding to the perpendicular of Cu with respect to the floor (to avoid this point is

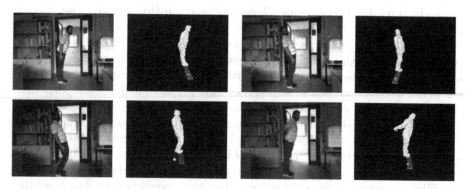

Fig. 3. Screenshot of the Swing exercise

obscured by the user body model, it is represented on the user side as a yellow ball), called COM. The board of the swing receives external perturbations, the user is required to follow the board thrusts by maintaining his COM inside the board: if not, the board colour becomes red and a fault is annotated. After the perturbation, the board returns, autonomously and slowly, to its original equilibrium condition. Also in this case the therapists can manage different parameters, such as: user weight, static and dynamic friction, duration, and so on. A yellow sphere indicating the subject centre of mass was mathematically calculated by the mass of the spheres and projected onto a virtual blue board. During the balance task, the subject was required to maintain his projected centre of mass onto the virtual board keeping his feet apart at shoulder distance width and the hands at his sides.

4   Experimental Results

The experimental phase has been divided in two parts. During the first, we have performed some empirical observations regarding both the real-time interaction and the self-avatar representation. In both cases, we believe we have achieved remarkable results. A first set of qualitative observations measuring the similarity (i.e., shape volume) from the real human body and the related self-avatar, have shown a difference of less than 14%. The measurements have been performed on a sample of 22 persons (10 images/frames for person in different common poses) on which the difference from the RGB and related self-avatar has been computed. The second and significant part of the experimental session has regarded the test of the developed exercises in terms of qualitative results of the balance rehabilitation tasks. To formalize this second parts we have conduct a basic case study.

4.1   Case Study

The case study has been performed on 15 patients (10 males, and 5 females) suffering of light and medium balance disorders. We have classified their disorder degree in three levels (i.e., 1:low, 2:average, and 3:high). We have tested each patient for a month, three times for week. Each individual session taken 1 hour: 25 minutes for each one of the two exercises, and 10 minutes of rest between the two exercises. To evaluate the effectiveness of the proposed exercises we have involved 5 therapists. They have followed each patient for each session. At the end of the whole experimental session they have prepared individual reports that can be summarized as reported in Table 1. We have divided the 15 patients in 3 groups according to their level of disorder. The first group was composed by 8 patients (6 males, and 2 females), the second by 4 patients (1 male, and 3 females), the last group by 3 patients (3 males). Each therapist judged three aspects of the framework (effectiveness, neutralness, and usability, respectively) providing a numerical value (from 1:very bad to 6: excellent). As shown, all the therapists have considered the developed framework and the related exercises a useful tool to support and improve the degree of disability in patient suffering of balance disorders. Table 1 also shows that the level of disability is tied to the usability criteria feeling by patients during the interaction processes.

Table 1. Case Study

Therapists/Groups	$Group_1$	$Group_2$	$Group_3$
1 Therapist	[6, 5, 5]	[6, 5, 6]	[5, 5, 6]
2 Therapist	[5, 5, 6]	[5, 5, 4]	[5, 5, 4]
3 Therapist	[6, 6, 5]	[6, 5, 5]	[6, 5, 4]
4 Therapist	[6, 5, 6]	[5, 5, 6]	[6, 5, 6]
5 Therapist	[4, 5, 6]	[5, 4, 5]	[4, 4, 3]

5   Conclusions

The upgraded version of the CRF allows us to define rehabilitative VREs in easy way adopting a simple plug-and-play architecture. The CRF is also ready to support the insertion of HBMs (this feature will be formalized in a next work). The used software platforms and required hardware configuration based on a single ToF camera allow us to obtain a low-cost and open system that can be used in different application contexts. We have tested the new version of the CRF by implementing two new plug-ins oriented to the recovery of the postural instability: Surfboard, and Swing. Experimental observations performed by a set of therapists have confirmed the usefulness of the proposed exercises. Moreover, the upgraded version of the CRF is easy to use, practical, and robust. Currently, we are working in implementing two different self-avatar algorithms designed to provide a more realistic human body representation.

References

1. Moeslund, T.B., Hilton, A., Krüger, V.: A survey of advances in vision-based human motion capture and analysis. Computer Vision and Image Understanding 104(2), 90–126 (2006)

2. Berman, S., Stern, H.: Sensors for gesture recognition systems. IEEE Transactions on Systems, Man, and Cybernetics, Part C 42(3), 277–290 (2012)
3. Chen, L., Wei, H., Ferryman, J.: A survey of human motion analysis using depth imagery. Pattern Recognition Letters 34(15), 1995–2006 (2013)
4. Zannatha, J.M.I., Tamayo, A.J.M., Sanchez, A.D.G., Delgado, J.E.L., Cheu, L.E.R., Arevalo, W.A.S.: Development of a system based on 3d vision, interactive virtual environments, ergonometric signals and a humanoid for stroke rehabilitation. Computer Methods and Programs in Biomedicine 112(2), 239–249 (2013)
5. Chang, Y.J., Han, W.Y., Tsai, Y.C.: A kinect-based upper limb rehabilitation system to assist people with cerebral palsy. Research in Developmental Disabilities 34(11), 3654–3659 (2013)
6. Bohil, C.J., Alicea, B., Biocca, F.A.: Virtual reality in neuroscience research and therapy. Nature Reviews Neuroscience 12, 752–762 (2011)
7. Chang, Y.J., Chen, S.F., Huang, J.D.: A kinect-based system for physical rehabilitation: A pilot study for young adults with motor disabilities. Research in Developmental Disabilities 32(6), 2566–2570 (2011)
8. Suau, X., Ruiz-Hidalgo, J., Casas, J.R.: Detecting end-effectors on 2. 5d data using geometric deformable models: Application to human pose estimation. Computer Vision and Image Understanding 117(3), 281–288 (2013)
9. Shen, J., Yang, W., Liao, Q.: Part template: 3d representation for multiview human pose estimation. Pattern Recognition 46(7), 1920–1932 (2013)
10. Westfeld, P., Maas, H.G., Bringmann, O., Grollich, D., Schmauder, M.: Automatic techniques for 3d reconstruction of critical workplace body postures from range imaging data. Journal of Photogrammetry and Remote Sensing 85, 56–65 (2013)
11. Mohr, R., Bajcsy, R.: Packing volumes by spheres. IEEE Transactions on Pattern Analysis and Machine Intelligence 5(1), 111–116 (1983)
12. Badler, N., O'Rourke, J., Toltzis, H.: A spherical representation of a human body for visualizing movement. Proceedings of the IEEE 67(10), 1397–1403 (1979)
13. Avola, D., Spezialetti, M., Placidi, G.: Design of an efficient framework for fast prototyping of customized human-computer interfaces and virtual environments for rehabilitation. Computer Methods and Programs in Biomedicine 110(3), 490–502 (2013)
14. Spezialetti, M., Avola, D., Placidi, G., De Gasperis, G.: Movement analysis based on virtual reality and 3d depth sensing camera for whole body rehabilitation. In: Computational Modelling of Objects Represented in Images. Fundamentals, Methods and Applications, pp. 367–372. CRC Press, Taylor & Francis Group (2012)
15. Placidi, G.: A smart virtual glove for the hand telerehabilitation. Computers in Biology and Medicine 37(8), 1100–1107 (2007)
16. Placidi, G., Avola, D., Iacoviello, D., Cinque, L.: Overall design and implementation of the virtual glove. Computers in Biology and Medicine 43(11), 1927–1940 (2013)
17. IISU^{TM} (2014), http://www.softkinetic.com/products/iisumiddleware.aspx
18. IrrLicht (2014), http://irrlicht.sourceforge.net
19. Vicon (2014), http://www.vicon.com/
20. PTI^{TM} (2014), http://www.ptiphoenix.com
21. STT (2014), http://www.stt-systems.com/en/
22. Clark, R.A., Pua, Y.H., Fortin, K., Ritchie, C., Webster, K.E., Denehy, L., Bryant, A.L.: Validity of the microsoft kinect for assessment of postural control. Gait & Posture 36(3), 372–377 (2012)

23. MicrosoftKinect^{TM} (2014),
    http://www.microsoft.com/en-us/ kinectforwindows
24. MicrosoftSDK (2014),
    http://www.microsoft.com/en-us/ kinectforwindowsdev/start.aspx
25. Reyes, M., Clapés, A., Ramírez, J., Revilla, J.R., Escalera, S.: Automatic digital biometry analysis based on depth maps. Computers in Industry 64(9), 1316–1325 (2013)
26. Hernández-López, J.J., Quintanilla-Olvera, A.L., López-Ramírez, J.L., Rangel-Butanda, F.J., Ibarra-Manzano, M.A., Almanza-Ojeda, D.L.: Detecting objects using color and depth segmentation with kinect sensor. Procedia Technology 3, 196–204 (2012)
27. Camplani, M., Salgado, L.: Background foreground segmentation with rgb-d kinect data: An efficient combination of classifiers. Journal of Visual Communication and Image Representation 25(1), 122–136 (2014)
28. Diraco, G., Leone, A., Siciliano, P.: In-home hierarchical posture classification with a time-of-flight 3d sensor. Gait & Posture 39(1), 182–187 (2014)
29. Schonauer, C., Pintaric, T., Kaufmann, H., Jansen Kosterink, S., Vollenbroek-Hutten, M.: Chronic pain rehabilitation with a serious game using multimodal input. In: International Conference on Virtual Rehabilitation (ICVR), pp. 1–8 (2011)
30. IOTracker (2014), http://www.iotracker.com/
31. Zhu, Y., Dariush, B., Fujimura, K.: Kinematic self retargeting: A framework for human pose estimation. Computer Vision and Image Understanding 114(12), 1362–1375 (2010)
32. Shum, H.P.H., Ho, E.S.L., Jiang, Y., Takagi, S.: Real-time posture reconstruction for microsoft kinect. IEEE Transaction on Cybernetics 43(5), 1357–1369 (2013)
33. Metcalf, C., Robinson, R., Malpass, A., Bogle, T., Dell, T., Harris, C., Demain, S.: Markerless motion capture and measurement of hand kinematics: Validation and application to home-based upper limb rehabilitation. IEEE Transactions on Biomedical Engineering 60(8), 2184–2192 (2013)
34. Rose, F.D., Brooks, B.M., Virtual, A.R.: reality in brain damage rehabilitation: Review. CyberPsychology & Behavior 8(3), 241–262 (2005)
35. Cho, S., Ku, J., Cho, Y.K., Kim, I.Y., Kang, Y.J., Jang, D.P., Kim, S.I.: Development of virtual reality proprioceptive rehabilitation system for stroke patients. Computer Methods and Programs in Biomedicine 113(1), 258–265 (2014)
36. Yue, H., Chen, W., Wu, X., Liu, J.: Fast 3d modeling in complex environments using a single kinect sensor. Optics and Lasers in Engineering 53, 104–111 (2014)
37. OptriCam^{TM}311 (2014), http://www.softkinetic.com/solutions
38. Direct3D (2014), http://msdn.microsoft.com/en-us/directx/aa937781.aspx
39. OpenGL (2014), http://www.opengl.org/
40. XML (2014), http://www.ambiera.com/irrxml
41. Moro, S.B., Bisconti, S., Muthalib, M., Spezialetti, M., Cutini, S., Ferrari, M., Placidi, G., Quaresima, V.: A semi-immersive virtual reality incremental swing balance task activates prefrontal cortex: A functional near-infrared spectroscopy study. NeuroImage 85(pt. 1), 451–460 (2014)
42. Ferrari, M., Bisconti, S., Spezialetti, M., Basso Moro, S., Palo, C., Placidi, G., Quaresima, V.: Prefrontal cortex activated bilaterally by a tilt board balance task: A functional near-infrared spectroscopy study in a semi-immersive virtual reality environment. Brain Topography, 1–13 (2013)

A Random Decision Forests Approach to Face Detection

M. Hassaballah and Mourad Ahmed

Department of Mathematics, Faculty of Science, South Valley University, Qena 83523, Egypt
m.hassaballah@svu.edu.eg; mourad.ahmed@sci.svu.edu.eg

Abstract. Face detection has been considered one of the most important areas of research in computer vision due to its wide range of use in human face-related applications. This paper addresses the problem of face detection using Hough transform employed within the random forests framework. The proposed Hough forests-based method is a task-adapted codebooks of local facial appearance with a randomized selection of features at each split that allow fast supervised training and fast matching at test time, where the codebooks are built upon a pool of heterogeneous local appearance features and the codebook is learned for the face appearance features that models the spatial distribution and appearance of facial parts of the human face. Experimental results are included to verify the effectiveness and feasibility of the proposed method.

1 Introduction

Because of its various uses in several applications, face detection has received a considerable attention in the last decade. The human face is the main source of information during human interaction and in vision-based Human Computer Interaction (HCI) systems. Thus, any system integrating vision-based HCI requires fast and reliable face detection [1]. The first step of any face processing system is detecting locations in images where faces are present. Face detection is also a required preliminary step to automated face recognition whose performance greatly impacts recognition rates.

According to [2] the face detection problem can be described as: given an arbitrary image, determine whether there are any human faces in the images, and if there are, return the location of each face in the image. Generally, face detectors return the image location of a rectangular bounding box containing the face. This bounding box serves as the starting point for the above mentioned applications. Automatic detection of the human face is one of the most difficult problems in pattern recognition and computer vision because the face is a non-rigid object that has a high degree of variability with respect to head poses (off-plane rotations), illumination, facial expression, occlusion, aging, image quality, and cluttered backgrounds may cause great difficulties [3].

On the other hand, random decision forests [4,5] have become popular in many applications of computer vision such as Bioinformatics [6], image classification [7], and computational genomics [8] as well as object detection/tracking [9]. Because it provides a unique combination of prediction accuracy and model interpretability among popular machine learning methods. Random Forest (RF) includes an ensemble of decision trees and incorporates a randomized selection of features at each split and interactions naturally in the learning process, which can deal with small sample size, high-dimensional

Y.J. Zhang and J.M.R.S. Tavares (Eds.): CompIMAGE 2014, LNCS 8641, pp. 375–386, 2014.
© Springer International Publishing Switzerland 2014

feature space, and complex data structures. Gall et al. [10] examined using random forests for three tasks: object detection, tracking, and action recognition. They proved the efficacy of forests-based method for these tasks and specifically Hough forests perform well compared to the state of the art for all the three tasks. In [11], a non-maxima suppression method is proposed for detecting multiple object instances in images using Hough transform. To obtain the probabilistic votes, the Hough forest are learned on a training data set from images with the objects of interest (pedestrians) at a fixed scale and from the set of background images. The Hough-based method copes better with multiple occluding instances; and according to the experiments conducted by the authors, a significant increase in accuracy is obtained.

Motivated by these works, in this paper, we investigate the ability of random forests for detecting the human face in digital images by employing the Hough transform within the random decision forests framework. In this respect, a direct mapping between the facial landmarks appearance and its Hough vote in the Hough space can be learned. This Hough forests-based approach can be regarded as task-adapted codebooks of local facial features appearance that allow fast supervised training and fast matching at test time. The set of leaf nodes of each tree in the Hough forest forms a discriminative codebook, where each leaf node makes a probabilistic decision whether a patch corresponds to the facial part or not, and casts a probabilistic vote about the centroid position with respect to the patch center. As far as we know, this is the first time that Hough forest is utilized for the face detection problem. The proposed method-based Hough forests is very efficient at runtime, since matching a sample against a tree is logarithmic in the number of leaves. Therefore, the method is able to sample patches densely, while maintaining acceptable computational performance. In contrast to other methods, the proposed method is less sensitive to geometrical distortion, noise and partial occlusion. Experimental results on the widely used face database (i.e., CMU+MIT database) are presented to demonstrate the efficacy of the proposed method.

The rest of this paper is organized as follows. A brief review on existing face detection methods is presented in Section 2. The principles of Hough forests are discussed in Section 3, while the proposed method for detecting faces is introduced in Section 4. Experimental results are provided in Section 5. Conclusion along with future direction is summarized in Section 6.

2   Literature Review

As mentioned before, detection of the human face in an image is a difficult task in pattern recognition because the face is a non-rigid object that has a high degree of variability as well as variations in occlusions, illumination changes, and background clutter. Though the difficulties, the last years have shown a great deal of research effort put into face detection technology. Numerous methods have been proposed to detect faces in images. Many of these methods are reviewed in two surveys by Yang et al. [2] and by Hjelmas and Low [12]. These methods can be broadly classified into two main categories: appearance-based approaches and feature-based approaches. Appearance-based approaches are known to be better suited for detecting non-frontal faces and more successful in complex scenes, however in simple scenes feature-based approaches are more successful. In contrast to the appearance-based approaches, feature-based approaches make explicit use of face knowledge. They are usually based on the detection of local invariant features of the face such as eyes, eyebrows, nose, mouth, and the structural relationship between these facial features. Based on the detected facial features, a statistical model is built to describe their relationships and to verify the existence of a face. There are other face detection methods that use a combination of both approaches in order to achieve a more robust and better performance [13].

Viola and Jones [14] present a machine learning approach for face detection, which has been integrated into OpenCV library with five Haar-cascade classifiers. Their method is probably the best known face detection method and it has gained a wide spread acceptance due to the availability of an open source implementation. The novelty of this method comes from the integration of a new image representation (integral image), a learning algorithm (based on AdaBoost to build a very rapid cascade classifier based on weak classifiers ("Haar-like basis functions"), and a method for combining the classifiers cascade. The original work on frontal faces has been extended to detect tilted and non-frontal faces by extending the set of basic features and by introducing pose estimators. Variations of the framework that use different basis sets have been presented using Gabor wavelets, local orientations of gradient and Laplacian based filters [15,16]. Li et al. [17] modify the monotonic assumption of the Adaboost algorithm proposed by Viola and Jones [14] to develop the so-called Floatboost algorithm for the training of face and non-face classifiers. By implementing these classifiers using a coarse-to-fine and simple-to-complex pyramidal structure, the authors successfully develop a computationally efficient multi-view face detection system. However, the proposed classifiers used in such boosted cascades operate independently of each other and therefore discard useful information between layers, resulting in convergence problems during the training process. In addition, non-face samples collected by the bootstrap procedure are incorporated within the database during the training process and hence increase the complexity of the classification task. Moreover, during the latter stages of the training process, the pattern distributions of the face and non-face regions may become so complicated that it is virtually impossible to distinguish between them on the basis of their Haar-like features as reported in [18].

Chen and Lien [18] develop a statistical system for automatic multi-view face detection and pose estimation consisting of five modules, Their statistical multi-view face detection system is based on significant local facial features (or subregions) rather than the entire face. The low and high frequency feature information of each subregion of the facial image are extracted and projected onto the eigenspace and residual independent basis space in order to create the corresponding PCA (principal component analysis) projection weight vector and ICA (independent component analysis) coefficient vector, respectively. Therefore, the system has an improved tolerance toward different facial expressions, wide viewing angles, partial occlusions and lighting conditions due to projecting on feature subspaces. Furthermore, either projection weight vectors or coefficient vectors in the PCA or ICA space have divergent distributions and are therefore modeled by using the weighted Gaussian mixture model (GMM) rather than a single Gaussian model. The GMM weights and parameters of the GMM are estimated iteratively using the Expectation Maximization (EM) algorithm. Face detection is then performed by conducting a likelihood evaluation process based on the estimated joint probability of the weight and coefficient vectors and the corresponding geometric positions of the subregions. Regarding the overall performance of this multi-view face detection method, as the authors reported the system can successfully function under various imaging conditions with the accurate detection rate of higher than 91% and can estimate the pan-rotation angles of more than 90% of the input patches to within $\pm 10°$ of their ground-truth values. Though this high detection rate, this method depends basically on different types of thresholds and several parameters should be adapted in advance in different databases. So the method is neither simple nor applicable.

Yang et al. [19] incorporate a genetic algorithm into the AdaBoost training to optimize the detection performance given the number of Haar features for embedded systems. While, in [20], a bank of Gabor filters is utilized to search for ten facial features (eye corners, eye centers, nostrils and mouth corners). Each feature is modeled using a Gaussian Mixture Model (GMM) of feature responses. Any triplet of feature detections with an acceptable spatial orientation produce a face location hypothesis. These face candidates are then normalized using an affine transformation and tested using a SVM region classifier. The highest ranking candidate based on the SVM discriminant function is declared the location of the face. The method detects 91% of faces in the XM2VTS database and 65% of BioID database within 10% of the true inter-ocular distance. The proposed approach in this paper is closely related to this family of facial feature-based methods.

3   The Hough Decision Forests

This section describes the necessary general background of the Hough forests framework and the notation that we will use in the rest of the paper. Hough forests consist of a collection of randomized trees where each tree consists of split nodes and leaves. During training, in each splitting node the algorithm tries to split the given training data $\{z_i; v_i\}_{i=1}^{N}$ where $z_i \in R^D$ is a D-dimensional feature vector, $v_i \in \{1, \ldots, C\}$ is the corresponding class label, and N is the number of training samples. By predefined the number of splitting functions, this recursive algorithm continues to split the data until either the maximum depth of the tree is reached; the subset of the data in a node is pure, or the number of samples is below a threshold. If any of these conditions is met, a leaf node is created and the class probability $p(v|z)$ is estimated.

Hough forests work on small patches extracted at random locations within a given bounding box from positive and negative training images of a face, each patch is described with several features, termed channels. Positive samples additionally store an offset vector pointing to the center of the face. Hough Forests then try to separate positive from negative patches and simultaneously cluster together similar positive patches according to their offset vectors. The splitting functions at each node in the Hough Forests randomly selects a feature channel and two pixels within the patch and calculates the difference of the feature values. This difference is then thresholded to determine which patches are forwarded to the left or the right child node. While, in the test phase, each image patch is passed through all trees in parallel, in each non-leaf node, a simple binary test is performed. The test is applied to each patch that arrives in the node, and its output defines the child that the patch will proceed to. The set of leaf nodes of each tree in the Hough forest can be regarded as a discriminative codebook. Each leaf node makes a probabilistic decision whether a patch corresponds to a part of the face or to the background, and casts a probabilistic vote about the centroid position with respect to the patch center in a probabilistic generalized Hough transform, and the maxima in the Hough voting space (Hough image) correspond to face hypotheses.

4   The Proposed Methodology

Figure 1 shows steps of the proposed method using Hough forests to detect faces in images, which can be summarized as follows: first, the different views of a human face can be handled by a single codebook B with entries $B_1, \ldots, B_b$ for each face pose in the images. The training procedure first extracts a set of patches which are sampled from a set of bounding box annotated positive images of facial landmarks and a set of background images. The set of training patches P_j^{train} are randomly sampled from the examples used to construct each tree T on the Hough forests, where the set of patches is $\{P_j^{train} = (a_j, l_j, o_j)\}$, where a_j are the extracted image feature channels Γ of the patch (facial appearance), l_j is the class label for the patch, and o_j is a offset vector from the patch center to the centroid. The patches sampled from the negative set (background patches) are assigned the class label $l_j = 0$, while the patches sampled from the interior of the face bounding boxes are assigned $l_j = 1$. Each face patch is also assigned a 2D offset vector o_j equal to the offset from the centroid of the bounding box to the center of the patch. Based on such a set of patches, the Hough forests trees are then constructed recursively starting from the root.

Second, the selection of random tests is based on how well they separate the input set of patches, the quality of the separation is measured by one of two uncertainty measures: class label uncertainty μ_1 measuring the impurity of the class labels l_j and offset uncertainty μ_2 measuring the impurity of the offset vectors o_j

$$\mu_1(\mathcal{A}) = |\mathcal{A}| . \ \mathcal{E}(\{l_j\}) \tag{1}$$

$$\mu_2(\mathcal{A}) = \sum_{j : l_j = 1} \| (o_j - \mathcal{O}_m) \|^2 \tag{2}$$

Where $\mathcal{A}$ is the set of patches assigned to a node $\mathcal{A} = \{P_j^{train}\}$, $|\mathcal{A}|$ is the number of patches in the set $\mathcal{A}$, and $\mathcal{O}_m$ is the mean offset of this set. $\mathcal{E}$ is Shannon entropy, used to maximize the classification information gain. The class label entropy is

$$\mathcal{E}(\{l_j\}) = - \sum_{l \in \{0,1\}} \mathcal{P}(l_j | \mathcal{A}) \ log \left(\mathcal{P}(l_j | \mathcal{A}) \right) \tag{3}$$

Where $\mathcal{P}(l_j | \mathcal{A})$ is the proportion of patches with class label l_j in the set $\mathcal{A}$. The first measure μ_1 tries to create two subsets of patches that are as pure as possible in terms of their class labels, while the second measure μ_2 forces the patch offsets to be spatially coherent. When the number of patches is below a certain threshold or the maximum predefined height of the tree is reached, the node is declared a leaf. For each leaf node

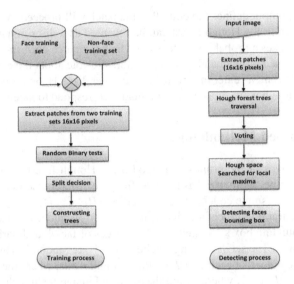

Fig. 1. Flowcharts of the training and detecting processes of the proposed face detection method

L in the constructed tree, the information about the patches that have reached this node at train time is stored. Thus, we store the proportion $\mathcal{F}_L$ of the facial patches (i.e., $\mathcal{F}_L = 1$ means that only facial patches have reached the leaf) and the list $\mathcal{O}_L = o_j$ of the offset vectors corresponding to the facial patches. In this context, the leaves of the tree in the forest form a discriminative codebook with the assigned information about possible locations of the face center. At runtime, this information is used to cast the probabilistic Hough votes about the existence of the face at different positions.

Third, the appearance of the patch a_j for each non leaf node in each tree is assigned a binary test during training. The patches have a fixed size of pixels at both train and test time; the appearance of the patch can be written as $a_j = (\Gamma_j^1, \Gamma_j^2, \ldots, \Gamma_j^c)$, where c is the number of the extracted feature channels. The binary tests on a patch appearance $\mathcal{T}(a) \rightarrow \{0, 1\}$ is defined as simple pixel-based tests. Such a test simply compares the values of a pair of pixels in the same channel with some threshold. The test is defined by a channel $\alpha \in \{1, 2, \ldots, c\}$, two positions p, q in the patch image, and a real threshold value r. The test $\mathcal{T}_{(\alpha,p,q,r)}(a)$ is defined as:

$$\mathcal{T}_{(\alpha,p,q,r)}(a) = \begin{cases} 0, \text{ if } \Gamma^\alpha(p) - \Gamma^\alpha(q) < r \\ 1, \text{ otherwise} \end{cases} \tag{4}$$

Using (1) and (2) for uncertainty measures μ_1 and μ_2, a pool of binary tests $\{\mathcal{T}\}$ can be generated by sampling α, p, and q uniformly given a training set of patches P^{train}. The threshold value r for each test is chosen uniformly from the range of differences observed on the data randomly. Then, the random decision is made whether should minimize the class label uncertainty μ_1 or the offset uncertainty μ_2 at the non-leaf node.

We choose this with equal probability unless the number of negative patches is small than 5%, in the case of the non-leaf node it is chosen to minimize the offset uncertainty μ_2. Finally, the set of patches arriving at the non-leaf node is evaluated with all binary tests in the pool and the binary test satisfying the minimization target Ω, which is sum of the respective uncertainty measures to split the training set, Ω can be defined as:

$$\Omega_k = min\left(\mu_\gamma\left(\{P_j | T^k(a_j) = 0\} \right) + \mu_\gamma\left(\{P_j | T^k(a_j) = 1\} \right) \right) \qquad (5)$$

Where $\mu_\gamma = \mu_1$ or μ_2 depending on the random choice. By choosing the non-leaf nodes that decrease the class label uncertainty μ_1 with the non-leaf nodes that decrease the offset uncertainty μ_2, the tree construction process ensures that the sets that reach the leaf have low variations in both class labels and offsets (leaves represent patches for the facial features only).

In general, the tree construction for generating the codebook follows the common Hough forests framework [9]. During the construction, each node receives a set of training patches. If the depth of the node is equal to the maximal one ($\mathcal{D}_{max} = 15$) or the number of patches is small ($\mathcal{N}_{min} = 20$), the constructed node is declared a leaf and the leaf vote information ($\mathcal{F}_L, \mathcal{O}_L$) is accumulated and stored. Otherwise, a non-leaf node is created and an optimal binary test is chosen from a large pool of randomly generated binary tests. For detecting the face, image patches are sampled from the test image and passed through the trees, every patch of the test image P_i^{test} is matched against the codebook B and its probabilistic votes are cast to the Hough image, the image patches can be densely sampled or subsampled as for training. Consider a patch $P^{test}(y) = (a(y), l(y), o(y))$ centered at the position y in the test image, where, y lies inside the face bounding box $\mathcal{B}(x)$ centered at x. Here, $a(y)$ is the appearance of the patch, $l(y) = 1$ is the hidden class label and $o(y)$ is the hidden offset vector from the center of the face bounding box to y. Furthermore, $E(x)$ denotes the random event corresponding to the existence of the face centered at the location x in the image. The probabilistic evidence $\mathcal{P}(E(x)|a(y))$ that the appearance $a(y)$ of the patch brings about the availability $E(x)$ at different positions x in the image is defined as:

$$\mathcal{P}(E(x)|a(y)) = \mathcal{P}(E(x), l(y) = 1|a(y)) =$$
$$\mathcal{P}(o(y) = y - x|l(y) = 1, a(y)) \cdot \mathcal{P}(l(y) = 1|a(y)) \qquad (6)$$

Assuming that for a tree T the patch appearance ends up in a leaf L, the first factor can then be approximated using the probability density estimation methods [21] based on the offset vectors D_L collected in the leaf at train time, while the second factor can be straightforwardly estimated as the proportion C_L of face patches at train time. For a single tree T, the probability estimate is

$$\mathcal{P}(E(x)|a(y); T) = \left[\frac{1}{|\mathcal{O}_L|} \sum_{o \in \mathcal{O}_L} \frac{1}{2\pi\delta^2} \exp\left(-\frac{\|(y - x) - o\|^2}{2\delta^2} \right) \right] \cdot \mathcal{F}_L \qquad (7)$$

Where $\delta^2 I_{(2\times2)}$ is the covariance of the Gaussian Parzen-Window, for the entire forest $\{T_t\}_{t=1}^{F}$, we simply average the probabilities (7) coming from different trees

$$P(E(x)|a(y); \{T_t\}_{t=1}^{F}) = \frac{1}{F} \sum_{t=1}^{F} P(E(x)|a(y); T_t) \qquad (8)$$

Equations (7) and (8) define the probabilistic vote cast by a single patch about the existence of the face. To integrate the votes coming from different patches, we accumulate them in an additive way into a 2D Hough image $H(x)$ using

$$H(x) = \sum_{y \in \mathcal{B}(x)} P(E(x)|a(y); \{T_t\}_{t=1}^{F}) \qquad (9)$$

The detection procedure simply computes the Hough image H and returns the set of its maxima locations and values $\{\overline{x}, H(\overline{x})\}$ as the face hypotheses. The Hough image $H(x)$ is then obtained by Gaussian filtering the vote counts accumulated in each pixel. An alternative way to find the maxima of the Hough image would be to use the mean-shift procedure as it is done in [11]. To handle scale variations, let us first assume that the size of the detected face bounding boxes is fixed to $w \times h$ during both training and testing. The test image is resized by a set of scale factors $\sigma_1, \sigma_2, \dots, \sigma_z$. The Hough images $H^1, H^2, \dots, H^z$ are then computed independently at each scale. After that, the images are stacked in a 3D scale vector, the Gaussian filtration is performed across the third (scale) dimension, and the maxima of the resulting function are localized in 3D

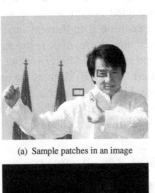

(a) Sample patches in an image

(b) Probability of each patch in (a)

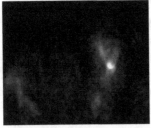

(c) Aggregating all votes

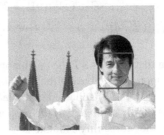

(d) Face location in the image

Fig. 2. Aggregating the votes of patches into the Hough space; the Hough image peak is the face

scale vector. The resulting face hypotheses have the form $(\overline{x}, \overline{\sigma}, H^{\overline{\sigma}}(\overline{x}))$. Finally, the hypothesized bounding box in the original image is then centered at the point $\frac{\overline{x}}{\overline{\sigma}}$, has the size $\frac{w}{\overline{\sigma}} \times \frac{h}{\overline{\sigma}}$, and the face detection confidence $H^{\overline{\sigma}}(\overline{x})$ as illustrated in Fig. 2.

5 Experimental Results

For training, we use a set of 500 face images with a fixed size of 24×24 pixels. While, non-face training set contains 2,750 images cropped manually and collected by random sampling non-face regions of different images downloaded from the Internet. A total of 15000 random binary tests are considered for each node. Furthermore, each tree was trained on 20000 positive and 20000 negative patches. It should be noted that in the proposed approach, the positive patches (facial features) need to collaborate somehow to detect the searched faces. The extracted features of the patches are as follows; the first two channels contain the pixel values and normalized ones to avoid the effect of illumination, the first and second derivatives in x,y directions, and the rest of channels are the HOG descriptors respectively. Other local features descriptors such as SURF and SIFT, or Gabor wavelets may be used, but in this work we examine the HOG descriptor [22]. This is because the definition of split functions (4) is in general based on local image features (i.e., locations and descriptors). Furthermore, for time-efficiency reasons and memory, split functions need to be simple but should also be designed for maximizing the information gain.

The performance of the proposed face detection is evaluated in terms of the receiver operating characteristics (ROC) curve. Where, the two quantities of interest are clearly the number of correct detections, which one wishes to maximize, and the number of false detections, which should be minimize. The ROC curve plots the true positive rate

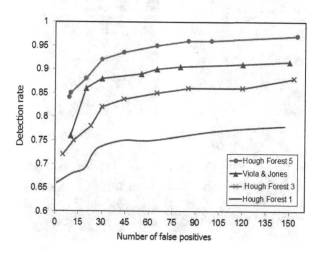

Fig. 3. ROC curves for Hough forests method with different tree number and Viola &Jones [14] method on CMU+MIT database

versus the false positive rate. We investigate the effect of trees number in the forest; thus the detector is trained for three different Hough forests trees number with same setting and training data used in constructing the trees. The first detector is trained for Hough forests of only one tree, the second detector of three trees, while the last detector of five trees. The ROC curves are obtained for each one of the three detector using the CMU+MIT database [23]. From this experiment, we note that there is a significant variation in the performance between the three detectors. The detector of five trees (i.e., Hough Forests 5) performs best compared to the other detectors achieving a high detection rate of 96% at 60 false positives as shown in Fig. 3. The Hough forests detector with five trees in the forest is compared with the baseline face detector of Viola and Jones [14] using CMU+MIT database. Figure 3 shows also the ROC curves for this comparison; the presented results on the curves are extracted from author's publication without any modifications. It is clear that the Hough forests based method with five trees outperforms the compared Viola & Jones' method achieving the highest detection rate of 97.4% at 156 false positives. In particular, the implementation of OpenCV 2.4.2 with the default frontal face classifier configuration (i.e., *haarcascadefrontalface-default.xml*) of Viola & Jones method is used. Some examples that are successfully detected by Hough forests based method but failed in Viola & Jones method are given in Fig. 4.

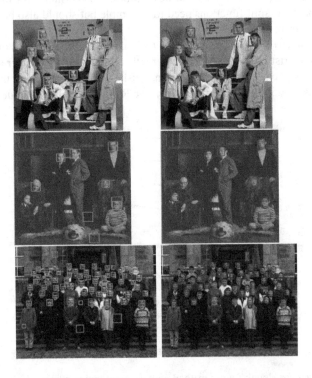

Fig. 4. Comparison detection examples using Viola & Jones' method (green left) and Hough forests method (red right) on test images from the CMU+MIT database

6   Conclusions

This paper introduced a method for face detection based on Hough forests that can learn a mapping from local image or depth patches to a probability over the parameter space. We chose Hough forests approach, because it is capable to handle large training datasets, high generalization power, fast computation, and ease of implementation. A simple experimental evaluation is conducted on the CMU+MIT database for face detection and the obtained results are encouraging. The performance of the proposed method is compared to the baseline face detector of Viola and Jones. There is still a room to further improve the detection performance, so our future work includes using non-maxima suppression that can be combined with Hough forests to improve the detection results. Investigating the aggregating of local descriptors SIFT, SURF, or HOG-LBP into Hough forests is another promising approach for improving the detection accuracy.

References

1. Hassaballah, M., Murakami, K., Ido, S.: Face detection evaluation: A new approach based on the golden ratio Φ. Signal, Image and Video Processing (SIViP) Journal 7(2), 307–316 (2013)
2. Yang, M., Kriegman, D., Ahuja, N.: Detecting faces in images: A survey. IEEE Trans. on Pattern Analysis and Machine Intelligence 24(1), 34–58 (2002)
3. Tsao, W.-K., Lee, A.J.T., Liu, Y.-H., Chang, T.-W., Lin, H.-H.: A data mining approach to face detection. Pattern Recognition 43(3), 1039–1049 (2010)
4. Breiman, L.: Random forests. Machine Learning 45(1), 5–32 (2001)
5. Criminisi, A., Shotton, J., Konukoglu, E.: Decision forests: A unified framework for classification, regression, density estimation, manifold learning and semi-supervised learning. Foundations and Trends in Computer Graphics and Vision 7(2-3), 81–227 (2011)
6. Barrett, J., Cairns, D.: Application of the random forest classification method to peaks detected from mass spectrometric proteomic profiles of cancer patients and controls. Statistical Applications in Genetics and Molecular Biology 7(2), 1544–6115 (2008)
7. Moosmann, F., Nowak, E., Jurie, F.: Randomized clustering forests for image classification. IEEE Trans. on Pattern Analysis and Machine Intelligence 30(9), 1632–1646 (2008)
8. Chen, X., Ishwaran, H.: Random forests for genomic data analysis. Genomics 99(6), 323–329 (2012)
9. Gall, J., Lempitsky, V.: Class-specific Hough forests for object detection. In: Proc. IEEE Conf. on Computer Vision and Pattern Recognition, pp. 1022–1029 (2009)
10. Gall, J., Yao, A., Razavi, N., Gool, L.-V., Lempitsky, V.: Hough forests for object detection, tracking, and action Recognition. IEEE Trans. on Pattern Analysis and Machine Intelligence 33(11), 2188–2202 (2011)
11. Barinova, O., Lempitsky, V., Kohli, P.: On detection of multiple object instances using Hough transforms. IEEE Trans. on Pattern Analysis and Machine Intelligence 34(9), 1773–1784 (2012)
12. Hjelmas, E., Low, B.: Face detection: A survey. Computer Vision and Image Understanding 83(3), 236–274 (2001)
13. Tabatabaie, Z., Rahmat, R., Udzir, N.B., Kheirkhah, E.: A hybrid face detection system using combination of appearance-based and feature-based methods. International Journal of Computer Science and Network Security 9(5), 181–185 (2009)

14. Viola, P., Jones, M.J.: Robust real-time face detection. International Journal of Computer Vision 57(2), 137–154 (2004)

15. Brubaker, S.C., Wu, J., Sun, J., Mullin, M., Rehg, J.: On the design of cascades of boosted ensembles for face detection. International Journal of Computer Vision 77(1-3), 65–86 (2008)

16. Xiaohua, L., Lam, K.-M., Lansun, S., Jiliu, Z.: Face detection using simplified Gabor features and hierarchical regions in a cascade of classifiers. Pattern Recognition Letters 30(8), 717–728 (2009)

17. Li, S., Zhang, Z.: Floatboost learning and statistical face detection. IEEE Trans. on Pattern Analysis and Machine Intelligence 26(9), 1112–1123 (2004)

18. Chen, J.-C., James Lien, J.-J.: A view-based statistical system for multi-view face detection and pose estimation. Image and Vision Computing 27(9), 1252–1271 (2009)

19. Yang, M., Crenshaw, J., Augustine, B., Mareachen, R., Wu, Y.: Adaboost based face detection for embedded systems. Computer Vision and Image Understanding 114(11), 1116–1125 (2010)

20. Hamouz, M., Kittler, J., Kamarainen, J.-K., Paalanen, P., Kälviäinen, H., Matas, J.: Feature-based affine-invariant localization of faces. IEEE Trans. on Pattern Analysis and Machine Intelligence 27(9), 1490–1495 (2005)

21. Parzen, E.: On estimation of a probability density function and mode. Annals of Math. Statistics 33(3), 1065–1076 (1962)

22. Dalal, N., Triggs, B.: Histograms of oriented gradients for human detection. In: IEEE Conf. on Computer Vision and Pattern Recognition, pp. 886–893 (2005)

23. Schneiderman, H., Kanade, T.: A statistical method for 3D object detection applied to faces and cars. In: IEEE Conf. on Computer Vision and Pattern Recognition, pp. 741–751 (2000)

A Data-Driven Investigation and Estimation of Optimal Topologies under Variable Loading Configurations

Erva Ulu, Rusheng Zhang, Mehmet Ersin Yumer, and Levent Burak Kara

Carnegie Mellon University, Pittsburgh, PA, USA
{eulu,rushengz}@andrew.cmu.edu, {meyumer,lkara}@cmu.edu

Abstract. We explore the feasibility and performance of a data-driven approach to topology optimization problems involving structural mechanics. Our approach takes as input a set of images representing optimal 2-D topologies, each resulting from a random loading configuration applied to a common boundary support condition. These images represented in a high dimensional feature space are projected into a lower dimensional space using component analysis. Using the resulting components, a mapping between the loading configurations and the optimal topologies is learned. From this mapping, we estimate the optimal topologies for novel loading configurations. The results indicate that when there is an underlying structure in the set of existing solutions, the proposed method can successfully predict the optimal topologies in novel loading configurations. In addition, the topologies predicted by the proposed method can be used as effective initial conditions for conventional topology optimization routines, resulting in substantial performance gains. We discuss the advantages and limitations of the presented approach and show its performance on a number of examples.

Keywords: Data-driven design, topology optimization, dimensionality reduction.

1 Introduction

Efficient use of material is a key priority for designers in many industries including automotive, aerospace and consumer product industries [1–3]. Optimizing material layout to satisfy a specific performance criteria, i.e. topology optimization is thus a crucial part of engineering design process. With recent advances in manufacturing technologies, topology optimization now attracts even more attention [2]. So far, various optimization algorithms including genetic algorithms, method of moving asymptotes, level sets and topological derivatives have been studied for structural topology optimization [1, 4–8].

Although structural optimization algorithms are becoming computationally more efficient with time, the need for a large number of iterations can rarely be avoided due to the essence optimization theory. Even with very small alterations in the design constraints, a structurally optimum topology can not be predicted

Y.J. Zhang and J.M.R.S. Tavares (Eds.): CompIMAGE 2014, LNCS 8641, pp. 387–399, 2014.

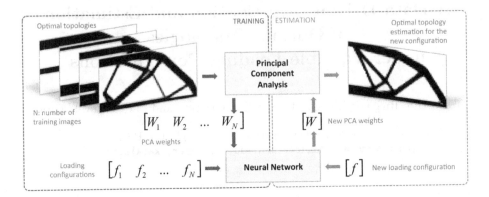

Fig. 1. Overview of our approach for optimal topology estimation

directly by a human from physical principles due to the complex nature of the problem. Based on this observation, we explore how known solutions to topology optimization problems can be exploited to generate a new design for a novel set of loading configurations. Here, the main challenge is to find a mapping between design constraints and the resulting optimal topologies. With this motivation, we present a data-driven approach to topology optimization involving structural mechanics and explore its feasibility and performance.

Our approach takes as input a set of images representing optimal 2D topologies, each resulting from a conventional optimization method, and generates an optimal topology estimation for a novel set of design constraints (Fig. 1). In this study, only the variation in loading configurations is explored under a fixed set of structural boundary conditions. In the proposed method, the set of input images (known optimal topologies) which are represented in a high dimensional image space are projected onto a lower dimensional space using Principal Component Analysis (PCA). Once the dimensionality is reduced, a mapping between the loading configurations and the optimal topologies represented as PCA component weights is computed using a feed-forward neural network. Using the trained mapping, we estimate the PCA component weights for a novel loading configuration, and use the resulting estimation to synthesize a solution in the image space. This image represents our estimation of the optimal topology, given a novel loading configuration.

The primary goal of this study is to explore the feasibility and effectiveness of a data-driven approach to structural topology optimization problems. Our results show that the proposed method can successfully predict the optimal topologies in different problem settings, but the results are sensitive to the complexity and the size of the design space dictated by the loading configurations. However, independent of the problem complexity, a practical advantage of the proposed system is that the resulting topology estimations serve as effective initial conditions that facilitate faster convergence in conventional topology optimization problems.

2   Related Work

In this section, we review the literature on structural topology optimization techniques, use of data analysis and dimensionality reduction approaches as well as mapping methods.

Structural Topology Optimization: Topology optimization is one of the most powerful technologies in structural design [1, 7]. It optimizes the shape and material connectivity of a domain through the use of finite element methods together with various optimization techniques [8].

Density-based topology optimization approaches including homogenization methods [9, 10] and solid isotropic microstructure with penalty (SIMP) methods [11, 12] are one of the most popular methods in the literature. These methods approach topology optimization in a way that defines geometry by optimizing material distribution in the domain. A detailed review on density based topology optimization methods can be found in [13–15]. Another approach for structural topology optimization is based on topological derivatives and level-sets [8, 16, 17]. The optimization process utilizes the implicit description of the boundary to numerically represent the geometry. A recent work [7] discusses the level-set based topology optimization methods more deeply. In [15], topological derivative and level-set based methods in the literature are claimed to be very promising although they are not widely embraced by industries. Aside from the above methods, evolutionary approaches are also used for topology optimization, e.g. [4, 5]. However, the use of genetic algorithms are computationally expensive, thus they are suitable for only small scale problems [15].

Since topology optimization is an iterative and computationally demanding process, an efficient implementation of the above mentioned methods in various programming languages is also important for designers. In [18, 19], authors present two different versions of an efficient MATLAB code for structural topology optimization of classical Messerschmitt-Blkow-Blohm (MBB) beam problem. As an optimization technique, they implemented an available SIMP approach with slight modifications involving filters. In our approach, we utilize the available code in [18] to generate the initial optimized topologies for different loading conditions as a way to generate the pool of training data.

Data Analysis and Dimensionality Reduction: In data-driven methods, a pre-analysis of available data to extract informative characteristics is essential, especially for large multivariate data sets. To the best of our knowledge, there is no use of dimensionality reduction methods for structural topology optimization in the literature. Such methods are commonly used in engineering design and computer science (e.g. [20–25]). Commonly used dimensionality reduction methods include principal component analysis (PCA) [26], multidimensional scaling (MDS) [27], Isomaps [28] and locally linear embedding (LLE) [29].

PCA is an eigenvector based approach that uses an orthogonal transformation to convert the original data into linearly independent components. Dimensionality reduction is accomplished by representing data in terms of the linearly independent components that best explain the variance in the data. In MDS, high

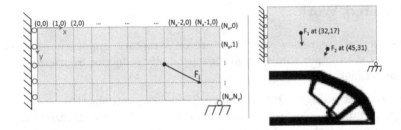

Fig. 2. Left: Design domain for topology optimization problem. Right: Example loading configuration and resulting optimal topology.

dimensional data is embedded into low dimensional space in such a way that pairwise distances between data points are preserved. Isomaps aim to preserve the geodesic distances in the manifold formed by the data. LLE is a neighborhood-preserving dimensionality reduction method. It projects high-dimensional data into lower dimensional global coordinates by utilizing different linear embeddings for each data point locally. In the proposed work, we use PCA to analyze the dominant characteristics of our data set and to reduce the dimensionality accordingly. However, the aforementioned dimensionality reduction methods could be adopted into the workflow of the proposed techniques without loss of generality.

One important aspect of the proposed work is the mapping between an input configuration (in our case the loading configuration) and the resulting optimal topology. Note that a PCA-based learning and topology reconstruction is readily implementable with the available training images. However, the key need is to be able to specify a novel loading configuration, from which the optimal topology can be estimated. In previous work, most methods employ a linear mapping between the input feature vectors and the resulting PCA reconstructions [23, 30]. However, the relationship between the input loading configurations and the resulting topology reconstructions in our domain is highly non-linear as demonstrated in the following sections. To address this challenge, we present a mapping technique that uses feed-forward neural networks. This generative method provides a significant improvement over linear regression models.

3   Problem Formulation

We illustrate our approach using the Messerschmitt-Blkow-Blohm (MBB) beam problem, a classical problem in topology optimization. The rectangular beam is represented by an N_x-by-N_y image as illustrated in Fig.2. The design domain is discretized by square finite elements each of which corresponds to a pixel in the gray-scale images. A number of external forces, F_i $(i = 1, ..., k)$, can be applied to the beam at the nodes represented by (x_i, y_i) coordinates. Applied forces can be in any direction, i.e. they can have both horizontal and vertical components with magnitudes ranging between $[0, 1]$. Boundary support conditions are shown in Fig.2. Note that this model is used to facilitate discussions; the following sections

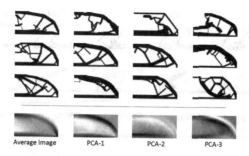

Fig. 3. Top: Example training samples. Bottom: Average image and first three PCA images.

will demonstrate results on variations of the domain, boundary conditions and loading configurations.

Our aim is to estimate the optimal topology for such problems when a novel loading condition is prescribed. For this, we generate a pool of training data where each training sample consists of a known loading configuration, and a corresponding optimal topology. To compute the optimal topologies given the loads, we use a density-based topology optimization algorithm given in [18]. The method assigns a density value between $[0, 1]$ to each pixel in the domain that dictates the Young's modulus for that particular pixel with lighter colors representing weaker portions. The optimization works toward minimizing the compliance resulting from the generated gray-scale structure. Resulting images with a varying Young's modulus field represent the optimal topologies for corresponding loading configurations. Collection of these images establish an input database to our method.

4 Component Analysis

Principal component analysis is useful for analyzing the input data to identify the significant features inherent in the data, as a way to facilitate dimensionality reduction with minimal information loss.

Suppose we have M images each with N_x-by-N_y resolution in our dataset. Then, gray-scale density values for images are stacked into M column vectors $\mathbf{t_j}$ ($j = 1, ..., M$) of length $l = N_x \times N_y$ to form the high-dimensional image space feature vectors. To mean-shift the data, the average image $\bar{\mathbf{t}}$ is calculated and subtracted from each sample in the training dataset, i.e. $\mathbf{t_j} - \bar{\mathbf{t}}$. In Fig.3, a randomly selected subset of the example training dataset (with 1000 samples), the resulting mean image, and the first three PCA component images are shown.

Let the mean centered image be $\mathbf{u_j} = \mathbf{t_j} - \bar{\mathbf{t}}$, we can store our entire data set into lxM matrix $\mathbf{U}$ to perform principal component analysis. Each column of $\mathbf{U}$ represents one mean centered image. In order to obtain the eigenvectors (i.e. principal components), the covariance matrix can then be constructed as $\mathbf{C} = \mathbf{U}\mathbf{U}^\mathrm{T}$. However, size of the matrix $\mathbf{C}$ is l-by-l and calculating l eigenvectors

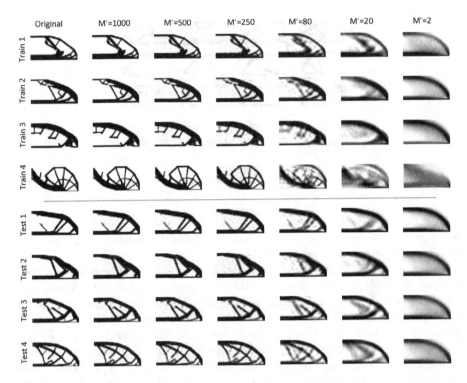

Fig. 4. Reconstruction of example samples relative to the different number of eigencomponents used. Each row corresponds to a different example. The upper half illustrates reconstructions for sample training images. The lower half shows the same for test images (i.e., images not involved in the construction of PCA).

may not be practical. As mentioned in [22], if the number of features is larger than the number of training images ($l >> M$), there can be at most $(M-1)$ useful eigenvectors (corresponding to non-zero eigenvalues) instead of l. These eigenvectors of l-by-l $\mathbf{U}\mathbf{U}^{\mathbf{T}}$ matrix can be determined from the eigenvectors of M-by-M matrix $\mathbf{U}^{\mathbf{T}}\mathbf{U}$ as $\mathbf{c_j} = \mathbf{U}\mathbf{v_j}$ where $\mathbf{v_j}$ is eigenvectors of $\mathbf{U}^{\mathbf{T}}\mathbf{U}$. In this paper, $\mathbf{c_j}$'s will be referred to as eigen-images. Each input topology optimization image can then be represented as a linear combination of these M eigen-images, resulting in a PCA weight vector of $\mathbf{W_i} = [w_1, w_2, ..., w_M]^T$. Even using only a few number of eigen-images, M', associated with the largest eigenvalues, a good approximation of an image can be obtained. In Fig.4, reconstruction of sample topology optimization images with different number of eigen-images are illustrated. In this example images are 80-by-40 pixels. There are 1000 training images generated by random assignments to the loading configurations and solving for the corresponding optimal topologies. Since PCA is limited by the number of training samples (1000 < 3200), the number of non-zero eigen-images is 1000. Here, it can be observed that a remarkably small number of eigen-images

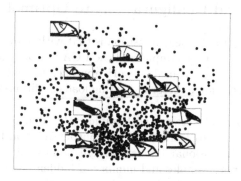

Fig. 5. Training images projected into the 2D space created by the first two PCA components

are sufficient for a high-fidelity reconstruction of the original images. Note that Fig.4 shows example reconstructions of samples that were used during training (train), as well as for novel samples that were not part of the training (test). In remainder of the paper, we will use the first 80 eigen-images in our examples.

Fig.5 shows the dataset of 1000 training images when projected to the space created by the first two eigen-vectors.

To quantify the mismatch between an original image and its reconstruction, we use the L_1 distance between the two images:

$$d(t_1, t_2) = \frac{\|t_1 - t_2\|_{L1}}{length(t)} \tag{1}$$

Fig.6 illustrates this difference. This metric provides a value between $[0, 1]$ where 0 represents identical images.

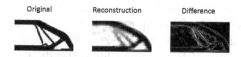

Fig. 6. Difference between an example topology and its reconstruction using first 80 eigen-images

When properly weighted, eigen-images can be linearly combined to create an approximation to a new image representing a new optimized topology. For this purpose, a set of PCA weights associated with the corresponding loading configuration should be estimated. We deal with this problem by introducing a mapping function between the loading configurations, $\mathbf{F}$ and the PCA weights, $\mathbf{W}$ of the training samples. Details of this process will be described in the next section.

5   Mapping Load Configurations to Optimal Topologies

A useful application of PCA decomposition is that with a low dimensional data, a mapping between the original input and the PCA vector space can be created. In this section, we present a neural network approach to generate this mapping, specifically between the force vector indicating load conditions ($\mathbf{F_i}$) and the PCA weights ($\mathbf{W_i}$).

Theoretically, a neural network with sufficiently complicated structure and training samples is able to learn any input-output relationship for regression. However, with high dimensional data, such regression would require considerably high number of training samples and number of hidden layer nodes resulting in impractical convergence time in the training stage [31]. We present results that indicate with limited amount of data and empirically determined number of hidden layer nodes, the neural network can learn the structure of the topology optimization gracefully.

In our experiments, we utilize a fully-connected feed-forward single hidden layer neural network [31] as the learner with the following input and output configurations:

1. The input vector of the neural network is composed of four real numbers (x and y positions and magnitudes) for each force in the problem.
2. The output vector of the neural network is composed of 80 real numbers corresponding to the PCA weights.

We train the resulting neural network with scaled conjugate gradient algorithm [31], we use 80 nodes in the hidden layer for all examples presented in the results section.

6   Results and Discussions

With a sufficient number of training samples, the neural network can generate a precise mapping between the loading configurations and the corresponding PCA weights. However, the resulting estimation can be affected by the number of eigen-images used to express that image. Fig.7 illustrates the performance of our approach on several test samples for a specific design domain (middle configuration in Fig.9. In this configuration, PCA and neural network are trained with 400 samples and tested with randomly generated loading configurations. As previously mentioned , only the first 80 eigen-vectors with highest variances are used for reconstruction and estimation. Fig.7 shows the original samples and their corresponding estimations using our method. Note that estimation involves using the neural network to map the loading configuration into the PCA weight vector, followed by a PCA based reconstruction using 80 samples.

As a convenient method, linear regression is one of the most favored approaches for learning the mapping between a set of feature vectors [23]. However, the relationship between the loading configurations and the PCA weights in such a high dimensional space may not be accurately predicted by this approach. In

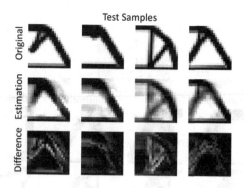

Fig. 7. Difference between example topologies and their neural network estimations using the first 80 eigen-images

Fig.8, we compare the performance of neural network versus linear regression on a sample test image. Both mapping methods are trained with 400 samples. Note that linear regression fails to reproduce some of the details in the optimal topology.

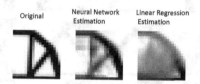

Fig. 8. Comparison of neural network estimation with linear regression estimation of an example topology

Fig.9 illustrates the performance of our algorithm on several test configurations. In the top row, basic representations of the design problems are illustrated. Here, boundary conditions and loading configurations are shown. Red areas represent spaces where forces can be placed. In the following row, reconstructions of several test samples using eigen-images are presented. Since only the first 80 eigen-images are used to construct an image, there are slight differences from the original optimal topologies. We compare our estimation results with the optimal topologies in the third row. As the design problem becomes more complex, the accuracy of resulting estimations reduces since the number of training samples for neural network may fail to be sufficient. Better estimations can be made using a higher number of training samples for more complex problems. In the last row of Fig.9, a histogram showing the distribution of error between the optimal topology and the estimation result of our approach among 100 test samples is given for each design configuration. Although we use a limited number of

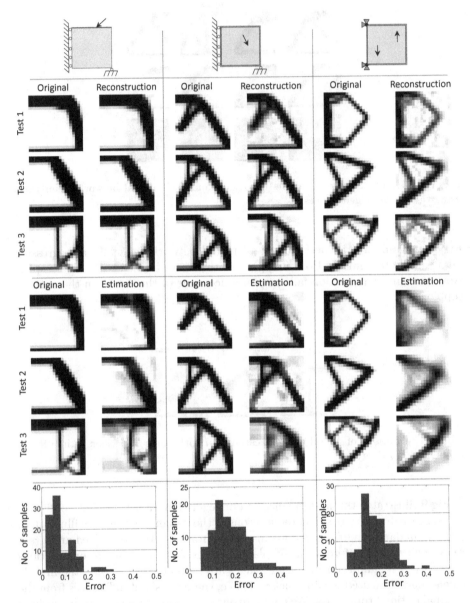

Fig. 9. Performance of our method for different design configurations. Left: single force anywhere on the top surface in any direction and magnitude. Middle: single force anywhere in the domain in any direction and magnitude. Right: two vertical forces anywhere in the domain in any magnitude. Reconstruction refers to the PCA reconstruction of the sample using the eigen-images. Estimation uses the proposed neural network, followed by PCA reconstruction.

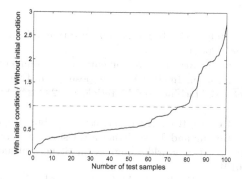

Fig. 10. Convergence time ratio of 100 samples with and without using the neural network result as an initial condition to subsequent optimization. Configuration used: Fig.9(left)

training samples and PCA components, the main structure for optimal topologies can be estimated.

In design problems involving complex loading configurations, the reconstruction accuracy may decrease visually (e.g., estimations in the last column of Fig.9). However, even in those cases, our optimal topology estimates can be used as an initial condition for a conventional topology optimization algorithm, e.g. [18, 19], to reduce the convergence time. Fig.10 shows the effect of using our estimation as an initial condition. For around 70% of 100 test samples, reduction in convergence time is observed for the posed problems. This gain can be even more significant for larger and more complex design domains.

7 Conclusions

We explore the feasibility and performance of a data-driven approach to topology optimization problems involving structural mechanics. We take a set of optimal topology examples for a given configuration, and project them into a lower dimensional space with PCA analysis. We then learn a mapping from loading configurations to optimal topologies using neural networks. Using the trained network, we studied the performance of estimating optimal topologies for novel loading configurations. Our results show that the proposed method can successfully predict the optimal topologies in different problem settings. Moreover, we also prove that the topologies predicted by the proposed method are effective initial conditions for faster convergence in subsequent topology optimization. We believe such time and computational power savings will be greater as the problem size and complexity increase. Thus, a valuable future direction is the application of the proposed method for 3D topology optimization.

References

1. Bendsoe, M.P., Sigmund, O.: Topology Optimization: Theory, Methods and Applications. Springer (2004)
2. Schramm, U., Zhou, M.: Recent Developments in the Commercial Implementation of Topology Optimization. In: IUTAM Symposium on Topological Design Optimization of Structures, Machines and Materials, pp. 239–248. Springer Netherlands (2006)
3. Richardson, J.N., Coelho, R.F., Adriaenssens, S.: Robust Topology Optimization of 2D and 3D Continuum and Truss Structures Using a Spectral Stochastic Finite Element Method. In: 10th World Congress on Structural and Multidisciplinary Optimization (2010)
4. Chapman, C.D., Saitou, K., Jakiela, M.J.: Genetic Algorithms as an Approach to Configuration and Topology Design. Journal of Mechanical Design 116, 1005–1012 (1994)
5. Jakiela, M.J., Chapman, C.D., Duda, J., Adewuya, A., Saitou, K.: Continuum Structural Topology Design with Genetic Algorithms. Computer Methods in Applied Mechanics and Engineering 186, 339–356 (2000)
6. Aage, N., Lazarov, B.S.: Parallel Framework for Topology Optimization Using the Method of Moving Asymptotes. Structural and Multidisciplinary Optimization 47, 493–505 (2013)
7. Dijk, N.P., Maute, K., Langelaar, M., Keulen, F.: Level-Set Methods for Structural Topology Optimization: A Review. Structural and Multidisciplinary Optimization 48, 437–472 (2013)
8. Norato, J.A., Bendsoe, M.P., Haber, R.B., Tortorelli, D.A.: A Topological Derivative Method for Topology Optimization. Structural and Multidisciplinary Optimization 33, 375–386 (2007)
9. Bendsoe, M.P., Kikuchi, N.: Generating Optimal Topologies in Structural Design Using a Homogenization Method. Computer Methods in Applied Mechanics and Engineering 71, 197–224 (1988)
10. Suzuki, K., Kikuchi, N.: A Homogenization Method for Shape and Topology Optimization. Computer Methods in Applied Mechanics and Engineering 93, 291–318 (1991)
11. Bendsoe, M.P.: Optimal Shape Design as a Material Distribution Problem. Structural Optimization 1, 193–202 (1989)
12. Rozvany, G.I.N., Zhou, M., Birker, T.: Generalized Shape Optimization without Homogenization. Structural Optimization 4, 250–252 (1992)
13. Hassani, B., Hinton, E.: A Review of Homogenization and Topology Optimization I–Homogenization Theory for Media with Periodic Structure. Computers and Structures 69, 707–717 (1998)
14. Rozvany, G.I.N.: Aims, Scope, Methods, History and Unified Terminology of Computer-Aided Topology Optimization in Structural Mechanics. Structural and Multidisciplinary Optimization 21, 90–108 (2001)
15. Rozvany, G.I.N.: A Critical Review of Established Methods of Structural Topology Optimization. Structural and Multidisciplinary Optimization 37, 217–237 (2009)
16. Sethian, J.A., Wiegmann, A.: Structural Boundary Design via Level Set and Immersed Interface Methods. Journal of Computational Physics 163, 489–528 (2000)
17. Wang, M.Y., Wang, X., Guo, D.: A Level Set Method for Structural Topology Optimization. Computer Methods in Applied Mechanics and Engineering 192, 227–246 (2003)

18. Andreassen, E., Clausen, A., Schevenels, M., Lazarov, B.S., Sigmund, O.: Efficient Topology Optimization in MATLAB Using 88 Lines of Code. Structural and Multidisciplinary Optimization 43, 1–16 (2011)
19. Sigmund, O.: A 99 Line Topology Optimization Code Written in MATLAB. Structural and Multidisciplinary Optimization 21, 120–127 (2001)
20. Sirovich, L., Kirby, M.: Low-Dimensional Procedure for the Characterization of Human Faces. Journal of Optical Society of America 4, 519–524 (1987)
21. Kirby, M., Sirovich, L.: Application of the Karhunen-Loeve Procedure for the Characterization of Human Faces. IEEE Transactions on Pattern Analysis and Machine Intelligence 12, 103–108 (1990)
22. Turk, M., Pentland, A.: Eigenfaces for Recognition. Journal of Cognitive Neuroscience 3, 71–86 (1991)
23. Allen, B., Curless, B., Popovic, Z.: The Space of Human Body Shapes: Reconstruction and Parameterization from Range Scans. ACM Transactions on Graphics 22, 587–594 (2003)
24. Yumer, M.E., Kara, L.B.: Conceptual Design of Freeform Surfaces From Unstructured Point Sets Using Neural Network Regression. In: ASME International Design Engineering Technical Conferences/DAC (2011)
25. Yumer, M.E., Kara, L.B.: Surface Creation on Unstructured Point Sets Using Neural Networks. Computer-Aided Design 44, 644–656 (2012)
26. Jolliffe, I.: Principal Component Analysis. Wiley Online Library (2005)
27. Cox, T., Cox, M.: Multidimensional Scaling. Chapman and Hall, London (1994)
28. Tenenbaum, J.: Advances in Neural Information Processing 10, vol. 10, pp. 682–688. MIT Press, Cambridge (1998)
29. Roweis, S.T., Saul, L.K.: Nonlinear Dimensionality Reduction by Locally Linear Embedding. Science 290, 2323–2326 (2000)
30. Blanz, V., Vetter, T.: A Morphable Model for the Synthesis of 3D Faces. In: Proceedings of the 26th Annual Conference on Computer Graphics and Interactive Techniques, pp. 187–194. ACM Press/Addison-Wesley (1999)
31. Bishop, C.M., Nasrabadi, N.M.: Pattern Recognition and Machine Learning. Springer, New York (2006)

Innovative On-line Handwriting Identification Algorithm Based on Stroke Features

Danilo Avola[1], Luigi Cinque[2], Stefano Levialdi[2], Andrea Petracca[1],
Giuseppe Placidi[1], and Matteo Spezialetti[1]

[1] Department of Life, Health and Environmental Sciences, University of L'Aquila
Via Vetoio Coppito 2, 67100, L'Aquila, Italy
{danilo.avola,andrea.petracca,giuseppe.placidi,
matteo.spezzialetti}@univaq.it
[2] Department of Computer Science, Sapienza University
Via Salaria 113, 00198, Rome, Italy
{cinque,levialdi}@di.uniroma1.it

Abstract. The handwriting analysis is a field of great interest since supports the study of different personal characteristics of the human beings, including identity, character, and neurological disabilities. In particular, the handwriting identification area, which also includes the handwritten signature verification, is a topic continuously investigated since the freehand writing of a manuscript, as well as the appending of a personal signature on a paper document, are still the most widespread ways to certify documents in legal, financial and administrative fields. The rapid diffusion of devices that enable user interaction by means of freehand or capacity pen based writing, and the growing successes obtained in processing the digital handwriting, are allowing us to extend more and more the boundaries of this fascinating area. The automatic handwriting identification is an engaging matter that supports several application contexts including the personal identification. In this paper we present a novel on-line handwriting identification algorithm based on the computation of the static and dynamic features of the strokes composing an handwritten text. Extensive experiments have demonstrated the usefulness and the accuracy of the proposed method.

Keywords: handwriting analysis, handwriting identification, handwritten signature verification, feature extraction, freehand drawing.

1 Introduction

The handwriting identification is focused in capturing the individuality and uniqueness of the freehand writing. The handwritten signature verification can be considered a specific case in which the handwritten text contains only the signature of the writer [1, 2]. Text and signature authentication still represents the most accredited and legal way to validate paper documents in forensic as in other fields. For these reasons, the last few decades have seen a wide proliferation of applications to support the authentication of manuscripts and handwritten

Y.J. Zhang and J.M.R.S. Tavares (Eds.): CompIMAGE 2014, LNCS 8641, pp. 400–411, 2014.

signatures [3–5]. These applications are designed to acquire a paper document in off-line mode (e.g., scanner), followed by a pre-elaboration phase (e.g., noise reduction, segmentation) to facilitate the acquisition of the handwritten text. Finally, digitalization and post-processing are performed to obtain a suitable data structure representing as accurately as possible the handwritten text. The off-line automatic handwriting identification (off-line AHI) systems, as well as the off-line automatic signature verification (off-line ASV) systems, can only work on the static features (e.g., geometrical) of the handwritten tract since the informative content of the interaction between writer and paper sheet has been lost. Despite this, these systems are still of primary importance since the authentication of manuscripts and signatures on paper documents represents the broader application context. The wide availability of devices that enable user interaction by means of freehand or capacity pen based writing have allowed to diversify and extend the application contexts in which to adopt these techniques. Moreover, these devices have a double advantage; they directly acquire the digitalized handwritten text avoiding noises and heavy pre-processing steps (e.g., segmentation); they can directly acquire dynamic features (e.g., velocity, acceleration) of the handwritten tract to enrich the handwriting identification and signature verification processes. These last points allowed us to develop versatile on-line AHI and ASV systems, which also have a high level of reliability [6–8]. As well known, it is generally accepted that handwriting, including making a signature, can be considered as a combination of features that are unique and identifiable for each writer [9–11]. More specifically, this principle affirms that no other user writes handwritten text whose features are all similar to those of another user. This implies that the handwritten text can be seen as a unique graphical representation whose features can be interrelated to create a complex handwriting formula for each individual. The only technical difference in acquiring a handwritten text in on-line or off-line mode lies in the possibility to have more features with which to characterize the mentioned formula. This last point is of huge importance since, while the theoretical approach to design an effective formula is achievable, its implementation is influenced by different factors (e.g., acquisition tool, application context). Moreover, several particular cases (e.g., short handwriting text) can be better supported with a formula composed by more features. Finally, phenomena as the forgery of manuscripts and signatures require to have a robust set of features. In addition to the mentioned principle, and in agreement with what asserted in different studies, [12–15], it is also our belief that handwritten text (and related features) can be also considered as a personal pattern connected to the physiological process of the brain that occur during the activity of writing. This means that handwritten text can be seen as a graphical abstraction without considering what the user has traced, but only knowing how the handwriting has been made by investigating on the shape of the strokes that compose the text.

In this paper we present a novel on-line handwriting identification algorithm based on stroke features. Our idea, encouraged by an extensive experimental session, is that a handwriting text can be treated as a freehand drawing whose key features can be captured by analysing its spatial and temporal properties. More specifically, we consider a handwriting text as a complex graphical symbol composed by a set of strokes which are (individually, i.e. local, and jointly with others, i.e. global) analysed to derive a feature vector representing the mentioned formula that uniquely characterizes each writer. The whole set of features has been inspired by studying different works in literature regarding the on-line separation between graphical and textual domain, [16, 17], the on-line freehand drawing recognition of graphical multi-domains, [18, 19], and the on-line style identification of drawn graphical shapes, [20]. Note that the proposed system has been designed to work in on-line and off-line mode; in off-line mode (e.g., analysing scanned manuscripts) the formula will not contain dynamic features.

The rest of the paper is organized as follows. Section 2 introduces basic related work supporting our approach from domain separation, freehand drawing recognition, and style identification viewpoints. Section 3 presents an overview of the system architecture, and describes the main global and local feature extractors. Section 4 reports and discusses the experimental results. Finally, Section 5 concludes the paper and shows future developments.

2   Related Work

The freehand drawing processing is a wide topic of interest supporting the human-computer interaction (HCI) field. It faces different issues including domain separation, recognition, and style identification. Although the section is not exhaustive of the many remarkable results achieved in this area, it is aimed in providing an overview of the works that more than others have addressed our conceptual and technical choices. In particular, the global feature extractors have been encouraged by works regarding the domain separation and the style identification, while local feature extractors have been inspired by works concerning the freehand drawing recognition. All the treated works regard the on-line mode, being the off-line a particular case. Note that in this paper we do not discuss about segmentation processes (off-line mode) since they are out the focus of the paper. Moreover, here we are not interested in comparing our work with others since the use of freehand drawing based approaches is a novelty within the handwriting identification field. Finally, an extension of the obtained results is already argument of a new work where the present paper is compared with the current state-of-the-art in handwriting identification.

2.1   Freehand Drawing Processing

We have investigated different approaches regarding the freehand drawing field. The set of basic global features has been derived by the works shown in [16, 17, 20]. The first paper describes an approach to distinguish the freehand drawing from the handwritten text. Their method is only based on the mathematical features of the strokes drawn by the users. Moreover it results effective and robust since it overcomes several critical issues, such as: user actions (e.g., deletion, restyling), and spatial relationship detection (e.g., inclusion, overlapping). The second paper represents an extension of the previous work, where the authors detail SketchSPORE, a framework designed both to distinguish graphical from textual elements within the same sketch, and to recognize freehand drawing as well as handwriting. The system is composed by three main algorithms. The first algorithm detects how many objects have been sketched by users and their related domain. As in our context, it considers an object as set of drawn strokes. The second and the third algorithms recognize the freehand drawing and the handwriting, respectively. Note that, their freehand drawing process has been designed to support the multi-domain and the ambiguity solving issues. These last points highlight the versatile characteristics of the proposed feature extractors. The third paper proposes an approach to formalize the recognition of the different drawing styles (i.e., solid, bold, and dashed). The algorithm computes the direction changes of a stroke depending on a fixed axis; the points identified by these changes jointly with those representing the start and the end of the stroke are used to detect the set of sub-strokes whose areas are used to measure the stroke style. Differently, the set of basic local features has been derived by other works [18, 19]. These two works are designed to define and recognize each set of graphical symbols. Their behaviour is quite similar, but the works detail different viewpoints of the approach. Initially the systems detect all the elements (i.e., closed regions and poly-lines) composing the sketch; subsequently each element is analysed to identify the set of primitives (i.e., lines and ovals) that compose it. These primitives, and a set of spatial constraints, support an exhaustive and unique description of the symbol. Actually, these last works have also led some choices in approaching our overall architecture. Other studies have substantially contributed to our method; works shown in [21, 22] define a set of measures used in our approach to compute some main local features. Their system is based on the computation of a set of complex mathematical and geometrical characteristics by which to recognize a fixed library of shapes. These latter are recognized independently from their size, rotation, arbitrary angle or drawing style (solid or bold). Another interesting work is presented in [23], where the authors describe a framework to auto-complete and recognize sketched symbols. In [24] a multi-domain sketch recognition engine is described. The system can be applied to a variety of domains by providing structural descriptions of the shapes in that domain; no training data or programming is necessary. According to our target, we have taken into account some observations related to the recognition of different domains. We conclude by mentioning two last works [25, 26]. The first illustrates LADDER, the first language to describe how sketched diagrams in a domain are drawn, displayed, and edited. The language consists of predefined shapes, constraints, editing behaviours, and display methods, as well as syntax for specifying a domain description sketch grammar and extending the language. The second proposes concepts and architecture for a generic geometry-based recognizer. Both works have supported some reasoning in implementing a strategy to dynamically build the formula for each individual writer.

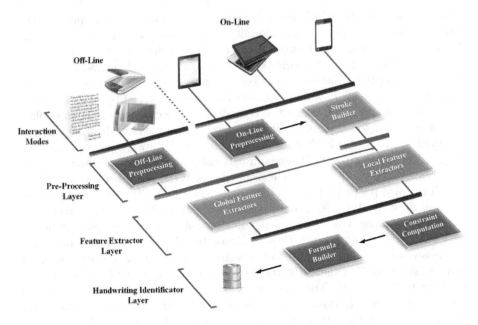

Fig. 1. The architecture of the system is composed of three layers: Pre-Processing Layer (PPL), Feature Extractor Layer (FEL), Handwriting Identificator Layer (HIL)

3 System Design

As shown in Figure 1, the proposed system has been designed to work in on-line and off-line mode. As previously mentioned, the difference between the two modes is that the off-line mode does not have dynamic information to support the implementation of the handwriting formula. Moreover, the second mode requires of a more complex pre-processing activity than the first. According to what stated in the purposes of the paper, we will only treat on-line interaction mode. The architecture of the system is structured into three layers which process the handwriting of a user, up to producing a univocal formula characterizing his/her personal pattern of writing. The first layer, Pre-Processing Layer (PPL), generates a suitable data structure including spatial and temporal information for each stroke drawn by the user. The second layer, Feature Extractor Layer (FEL), takes as input these strokes and computes on them a set of local and global mathematical (and geometrical) measurements. Note that, starting from two specular copies of the data structure regarding the strokes, the local and global measurements can be parallel processed since they are independent computations. Finally, the last layer, Handwriting Identificator Layer (HIL), summarizes the obtained features, computes the additional spatial and temporal constraints (i.e., relationships between strokes), and build the personal formula. The proposed system has been conceived to support two linked tasks; it should identify (after a training phase) the writer provided that he composes

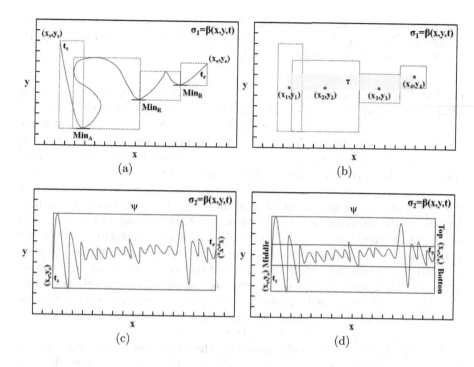

Fig. 2. Global Feature Extractors: Alignment Extractor - (a) building of the bounding boxes, (b) construction of the centres of gravity. Density Extractor - (c) building of the bounding box, (d) building of the bounds

a text with sufficient length; it has to recognize the similarity of two (or more) texts written from the same author which is unknown. Although these issues are very similar they open up different scenarios. In this section we do not provide additional information about the PPL since pre-processing phases are out the focus of the paper; only a basic formalization of the stroke is given to facilitate the understanding of the next two sub-sections. In our context, a stroke σ can be described as a function β of spatial (x, y) and temporal (t) coordinates:

$$\sigma = \beta(x, y, t) \tag{1}$$

3.1 Feature Extractor Layer

The FEL is composed by two main modules. The Global Feature Extractors (GFEs), and the Local Feature Extractors (LFEs). The first module extracts a set of mathematical measures from each "word" of the text. In this context, the term "word" is referred to a set of strokes linked by some spatial (and/or temporal) constraint. The second module first transforms the whole handwriting in a set of shapes (i.e., closed regions and poly-lines), and then, computes on each of them a set of geometrical measures. Note that it is not possible to provide in a single paper an exhaustive explication of the FEL due to its vastness and complexity. The aim of the present subsection is to explore the basic ideas on which the whole feature vector is based.

Global Feature Extractors: The first task of the GFEs is to analyse the whole text to split it into a set of "words". As mentioned, a "word" does not represent an element of a phrase (although they are often coincident), but it can be considered a continuous physiological process of a writer. For this reason, the GFEs try to recompose these "words" by using adaptive spatial and temporal constraints. In particular, two or more strokes belong to the same "word" if a closeness and/or interception relationship occurs among them (see details in [16, 17]). Unlike older implementations of these constraints, in this paper we have introduced the temporal factor to better support the re-composition process. In other words, when the bounding boxes of two (or more) strokes are close, but not enough to be considered as belonging to the same "word", then a temporal comparison is performed. More specifically, if the strokes are temporally consecutive, and their start and/or end points are aligned on compatible directions, then they could be merged within the same "word". However, once GFEs has derived the whole set of "words", for each of them three mathematical features are extracted: Alignment, Density, and Overlapping.

As shown in Figure 2(a) and Figure 2(b), the Alignment feature measures the linearity of a stroke style according to a fixed axis. This feature has been designed to capture the ability of the user in controlling trace amplitude during handwriting movements. To achieve this result, on each stroke (e.g., $\sigma_1 = \beta(x, y, t)$) the feature extractor considers its projection (e.g., $\sigma_{1y} = \beta(y, t)$) on the y axis. Subsequently, on each projection function, all the points of minimum (absolutes/relatives) are computed (e.g., Min_A, Min_R); these points are used to build a set of bounding boxes (e.g., the four bounding boxes in Figure 2(a)) each of which contains a disjointed part of the original stroke. In a further step, the feature extractor computes the centre of gravity of each bounding box (e.g., (x_1, y_1), (x_2, y_2), (x_3, y_3), and (x_4, y_4), Figure 2(b)). These centres are used to build a numerical band (τ) within which to assess the degree of the personal alignment of the writer. Actually, this last measure is composed by several numerical evaluations (e.g., distribution of the centres within τ, density, pattern of the clusters within τ); here we could only describe the basic measure. The Density feature measures the density of a stroke style. This feature has been conceived to capture the ability of the writer in distributing the tracing during a handwriting. To achieve this result, on each stroke (e.g., $\sigma_2 = \beta(x, y, t)$) the feature extractor computes a global bounding box (Ψ, Figure 2(c)). Within the bounding box three bounds are computed (e.g., *Top*, *Middle*, and *Botton*, Figure 2(d)), these bounds represent the statistical distribution of the stroke, the middle band is designed to maximize the quantity of pixels within the related area. Also in this case, we could only show the basic measure and not all the derived evaluations.

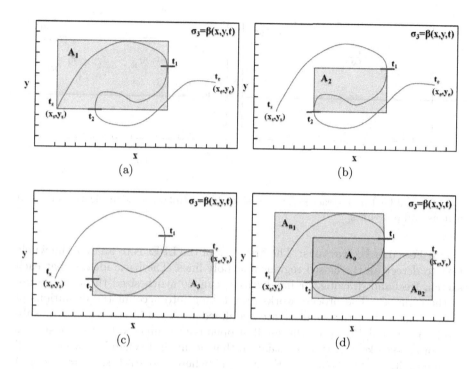

Fig. 3. Global Feature Extractors: Overlapping Extractor - (a)(b)(c) building of the bounding boxes, (d) overlapping of the bounding boxes

The Overlapping feature measures the compactness of a stroke style. Originally, this measure was implemented to distinguish the bold style from the solid style within a sketch-based interface (see details in [20]). In this context, we have adapted this measure to quantify the ability of the user in control tracing extension during a handwriting. To achieve this result, on each stroke (e.g., $\sigma_3 = \beta(x, y, t)$, Figure 3(a)) the feature extractor considers its projection (e.g., $\sigma_{1x} = \beta(x, t)$) on the x axis. This time, the feature extractor is focused in detecting the direction changes of the stroke according to the tracing direction (i.e., x axis). As shown in Figure 3(a), the stroke has two direction changes, the first at time t_1, and the second at time t_2. These direction changes can be used to build a set of bounding boxes. In Figure 3(a), Figure 3(b), and Figure 3(c) the three sub-strokes with their bounding boxes are represented. Note that each bounding box is characterized by the measure of an area (A_1, A_2, A_3). In Figure 3(d) the overlapping of the three bounding boxes is shown. In particular, the resulting areas A_{n1} and A_{n2} are zones that have been covered by no more than one bounding box, while the area A_o is a zone that has been covered by at least two bounding boxes. This means that a greater overlapping highlights a high degree of the compactness of a stroke style. Also in this last case, we have shown only a basic measure from which we have derived different levels of compactness.

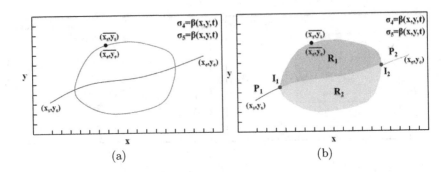

Fig. 4. Local Feature Extractors: (a) crossing of two strokes, (b) identification of closed regions and poly-lines

Local Feature Extractors: The first task of the LFEs is to analyse the whole text to detect all the closed regions and poly-lines. The basic idea is that each sketch, freehand drawing, or handwriting can be synthesized through the use of these shapes. The process works only taking into account the definitions of closed region (i.e., the smallest area confined by a set of strokes and/or sub-strokes), and poly-line (i.e., the smallest open path composed by a set of strokes and/or sub-strokes). A typical situation that occurs in freehand drawing as well as handwriting is presented in Figure 4(a), where two strokes, $\sigma_4 = \beta(x, y, t)$ and $\sigma_5 = \beta(x, y, t)$, are crossed. The resolution process, as shown in Figure 4(b), starts from the intersection points (I_1, I_2). Exhaustively, each path is analysed to search the shapes respecting the given definitions; when the process ends all strokes have been analysed, and each of them belongs to a closed region and/or to a poly-line (e.g., two closed regions: R_1, R_2; and two poly-lines: P_1, P_2). In a further step, the feature extractor replaces each poly-line with a geometrical multi-path line, and each closed region with a suitable composition of geometrical ellipses and arcs (see details in [18]). In this way, the whole handwritten text has been represented by a collection of known geometrical shapes which properties and characteristics (including constraints) can be studied. The result of this study is an individual pattern of how a user draws an ellipse, an arc, or a multi-path line considering also the dynamic features, in particular: velocity and acceleration. As in the previous cases, the understanding of how to characterize the user sketch are only basic measures of the LFEs.

3.2 Handwriting Identificator Layer

All the features computed within the FEL are adopted to define the formula representing the personal pattern handwriting of a user. In particular, we have been inspired by the method described in [27]. Our customization has consisted in dynamically refining the numerical values composing the formula according to the user interaction (i.e., writing) without considering the matching process since here we do not have a specific reference library.

4 Experimental Results

This section presents the protocol that has been implemented to test the developed system. On this first version of the software, we have privileged the checking of the basic ideas of the approach. In particular, we have carefully analysed the building of the formula for each test user, and we have verified that there were no two users able to generate two similar formulas.

Table 1. Matching Rank

	Groups of Users				
Rank (R)	Group 1	Group 2	Group 3	Group 4	Group 5
$0\% \leq R \leq 25\%$	—	—	—	—	✓
$26\% \leq R \leq 50\%$	—	✓	—	—	✓
$51\% \leq R \leq 70\%$	—	✓	—	✓	✓
$71\% \leq R \leq 90\%$	✓	✓	—	✓	✓
$91\% \leq R \leq 100\%$	✓	✓	✓	✓	✓

We have recruited 18 persons between 25 and 35 years old, 14 males and 4 females. Each person had to face both a training and an experimental phase. During the first phase each person was equipped with a graphic tablet (WACOM Intuos Pro L) connected to a PC (Toschiba Satellite, Intel(R) Core(TM) i5-2430M CPU@2.40GHz, 4,00GB) to acquire his/her handwriting style (system developed in Java SE 7, supported by MySQL Cluster 7.3). To achieve this result, each person had to handwrite, by the tablet, a text dictated by a synthetic voice. The training text was the same for each person, and it was composed by 3000 characters (Latin alphabet in cursive). At the end of the first phase the system had automatically generated an individual formula for each writer. Each formula can be seen as a set of numerical intervals where some of them depend on others (i.e., constraints). These formulas were stored within the database in XML format [28] which allowed system a fast parsing and a manageable matching process. During the experimental phase a different dictation was proposed to each person (always composed by 3000 characters). This time the system dynamically compared the newest formula with those stored within the database. The matching process occurred while the persons were writing the text, in this way it was possible to check how much text of the new dictation they had to write to reach the success in the matching process. Table 1 summarizes the obtained results. We have divided the persons in groups that have obtained similar results, in particular: $Group$ 1 (3 $persons$), $Group$ 2 (3 $persons$), $Group$ 3 (7 $persons$), $Group$ 4 (4 $persons$), and $Group$ 5 (1 $persons$). The unique person of the $Group$ 5 obtained the success with just the 25% in handwriting the new dictation, while only seven persons belonging to the $Group$ 3 required at least the 91% of the dictation to obtain a success. However, the system responded appropriately on each person, and the generated formulas always differed one from the others.

5 Conclusions

The paper presents a novel on-line handwriting identification algorithm based on stroke features. The proposed approach can be also used without considering the dynamic features captured during the on-line interaction mode thus making the method suitable for off-line handwriting identification. In this paper, we were interested in testing our idea to check its feasibility, effectiveness, and efficiency. Although the experimental session has been held in a controlled environment, without forgeries, and avoiding other influencing external factors, it has proven that the conceived measures can be used to achieve the stated targets. The proposed system has the advantage to treat the handwriting like a freehand drawing enabling users in writing both text and drawings. This last is an interesting opportunity that should be investigated in signature verification. However, the approach requires much more experiments. Moreover extensive work has to be done on robustness.

References

1. Seki, Y.: What kind of strategies does a document examiner take in handwriting identification? In: Sako, H., Franke, K.Y., Saitoh, S. (eds.) IWCF 2010. LNCS, vol. 6540, pp. 193–199. Springer, Heidelberg (2011)
2. Sukor, N., Muda, A., Muda, N., Huoy, C.: A comparative study of tree-based structure methods for handwriting identification. In: Herawan, T., Deris, M.M., Abawajy, J. (eds.) Proceedings of the First International Conference on Advanced Data and Information Engineering (DaEng-2013). LNEE, vol. 285, pp. 269–276. Springer, Singapore (2014)
3. Plamondon, R., Srihari, S.N.: On-line and off-line handwriting recognition: A comprehensive survey. IEEE Trans. Patt. Anal. Mach. Intell. 22(1), 63–84 (2000)
4. Kalera, M.K., Srihari, S., Xu, A.: Off-line signature verification and identification using distance statistics. International Journal of Pattern Recognition and Artificial Intelligence, 228–232 (2003)
5. Schlapbach, A., Bunke, H.: Off-line handwriting identification using hmm based recognizers. In: Proceedings of the 17th International Conference on Pattern Recognition, ICPR 2004, vol. 2, pp. 654–658 (August 2004)
6. Jain, A.K., Griess, F.D., Connell, S.D.: On-line signature verification. Pattern Recognition 35 (2002)
7. Quan, Z.H., Huang, D.S., Liu, K.H., Chau, K.W.: A hybrid hmm/ann based approach for online signature verification. In: International Joint Conference on Neural Networks, IJCNN 2007, pp. 402–405 (August 2007)
8. O'Reilly, C., Plamondon, R.: Development of a sigma-lognormal representation for on-line signatures. Pattern Recognition 42(12), 3324–3337 (2009)
9. Bulacu, M., Schomaker, L.: Text-independent writer identification and verification using textural and allographic features. IEEE Transactions on Pattern Analysis and Machine Intelligence 29(4), 701–717 (2007)
10. Tan, G.X., Viard-Gaudin, C., Kot, A.C.: Automatic writer identification framework for online handwritten documents using character prototypes
11. Harralson, H., Miller, L.: Developments in Handwriting and Signature Identification in the Digital Age. Forensic studies for criminal justice (2013)

12. Plamondon, R.: A kinematic theory of rapid human movements. Biological Cybernetics 72(4), 295–307 (1995)
13. O'Reilly, C., Plamondon, R.: Looking for the brain stroke signature. In: 2012 21st International Conference on Pattern Recognition (ICPR), pp. 1811–1814 (November 2012)
14. Impedovo, D., Pirlo, G., Plamondon, R.: Handwritten signature verification: New advancements and open issues. In: ICFHR, pp. 367–372 (2012)
15. Plamondon, R., O'Reilly, C., Galbally, J., Almaksour, A., Anquetil, É.: Recent developments in the study of rapid human movements with the kinematic theory: Applications to handwriting and signature synthesis. Pattern Recognition Letters 35, 225–235 (2014)
16. Avola, D., Del Buono, A., Del Nostro, P., Wang, R.: A novel online textual/Graphical domain separation approach for sketch-based interfaces. In: Damiani, E., Jeong, J., Howlett, R.J., Jain, L.C. (eds.) New Directions in Intelligent Interactive Multimedia Systems and Services - 2. SCI, vol. 226, pp. 167–176. Springer, Heidelberg (2009)
17. Avola, D., Cinque, L., Placidi, G.: Sketchspore: A sketch based domain separation and recognition system for interactive interfaces. In: Petrosino, A. (ed.) ICIAP 2013, Part II. LNCS, vol. 8157, pp. 181–190. Springer, Heidelberg (2013)
18. Avola, D., Del Buono, A., Gianforme, G., Paolozzi, S., Wang, R.: Sketchml a representation language for novel sketch recognition approach. In: Proceedings of the 2nd International Conference on PErvasive Technologies Related to Assistive Environments, PETRA 2009, pp. 31:1–31:8. ACM, New York (2009)
19. Avola, D., Del Buono, A., Gianforme, G., Paolozzi, S.: A novel recognition approach for sketch-based interfaces. In: Foggia, P., Sansone, C., Vento, M. (eds.) ICIAP 2009. LNCS, vol. 5716, pp. 1015–1024. Springer, Heidelberg (2009)
20. Avola, D., Ferri, F., Grifoni, P.: Formalizing recognition of sketching styles in human centered systems. In: Apolloni, B., Howlett, R.J., Jain, L. (eds.) KES 2007, Part II. LNCS (LNAI), vol. 4693, pp. 369–376. Springer, Heidelberg (2007)
21. Fonseca, M.J., Jorge, J.A.: Experimental evaluation of an on-line scribble recognizer. Pattern Recognition Letters 22(12), 1311–1319 (2001)
22. Fonseca, M.J., Ferreira, A., Jorge, J.A.: Content-based retrieval of technical drawings. IJCAT 23(2-4), 86–100 (2005)
23. Tirkaz, C., Yanikoglu, B.A., Sezgin, T.M.: Sketched symbol recognition with autocompletion. Pattern Recognition 45(11), 3926–3937 (2012)
24. Alvarado, C., Davis, R.: Sketchread: A multi-domain sketch recognition engine. In: Proceedings of the 17th Annual ACM Symposium on User Interface Software and Technology, UIST 2004, pp. 23–32. ACM, New York (2004)
25. Hammond, T., Davis, R.: Ladder: A language to describe drawing, display, and editing in sketch recognition. In: Gottlob, G., Walsh, T. (eds.) IJCAI, pp. 461–467. Morgan Kaufmann (2003)
26. Brieler, F., Minas, M.: A model-based recognition engine for sketched diagrams. J. Vis. Lang. Comput. 21(2), 81–97 (2010)
27. Avola, D., Bottoni, P., Dafinei, A., Labella, A.: Fcbd: An agent-based architecture to support sketch recognition interfaces. In: DMS, Know. Sys. Ins., pp. 295–300 (2011)
28. XML (2014), http://www.w3.org/xml/

Author Index